Gastrointestinal, Hepatobiliary and Pancreatic Surgery and Hernias

LEXPLICIT
Lecture Notes

for Surgery Residents and Superspecialty Aspirants

Gastrointestinal, Hepatobiliary and Pancreatic Surgery and Hernias

L EXPLICIT Lecture Notes

for Surgery Residents and Superspecialty Aspirants

TV Haridas MS, DNB, FRCS

Associate Professor
Department of Surgery
Government Medical College
Thrissur, Kerala

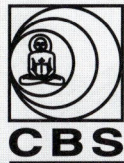

CBS Publishers & Distributors Pvt Ltd

New Delhi • Bengaluru • Chennai • Kochi • Kolkata • Mumbai
Hyderabad • Jharkhand • Nagpur • Patna • Pune • Uttarakhand

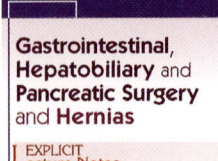

Gastrointestinal, Hepatobiliary and Pancreatic Surgery and Hernias
EXPLICIT Lecture Notes

ISBN: 978-93-90709-16-8

Published by Satish Kumar Jain and produced by Varun Jain for

CBS Publishers & Distributors Pvt Ltd

4819/XI Prahlad Street, 24 Ansari Road, Daryaganj, New Delhi 110 002, India
Ph: 011-23289259, 23266861, 23266867   Website: www.cbspd.com
Fax: 011-23243014   e-mail: delhi@cbspd.com; cbspubs@airtelmail.in
Corporate Office: 204 FIE, Industrial Area, Patparganj, Delhi 110 092
Ph: 011-4934 4934   Fax: 011-4934 4935   e-mail: publishing@cbspd.com;
                                          publicity@cbspd.com

Branches

• **Bengaluru:** Seema House 2975, 17th Cross, K.R. Road, Banasankari 2nd Stage, Bengaluru 560 070, Karnataka
Ph: +91-80-26771678/79   Fax: +91-80-26771680   e-mail: bangalore@cbspd.com
• **Chennai:** 7, Subbaraya Street, Shenoy Nagar, Chennai 600 030, Tamil Nadu
Ph: +91-44-26680620, 26681266   Fax: +91-44-42032115   e-mail: chennai@cbspd.com
• **Kochi:** 42/1325, 1326, Power House Road, Opp. KSEB, Power House, Ernakulam 682018, Kochi, Kerala
Ph: +91-484-4059061-65   Fax: +91-484-4059065   e-mail: kochi@cbspd.com
• **Kolkata:** 6/B, Ground Floor, Rameswar Shaw Road, Kolkata 700014 (West Bengal), India
Ph: +91-33-2289-1126, 2289-1127, 2289-1128   e-mail: kolkata@cbspd.com
• **Mumbai:** PWD Shed, Gala No. 25/26, Ramchandra Bhatt Marg, Next to JJ Hospital, Gate No. 2 Opp. Union Bank of India, Noorbaug, Mumbai 400009, Maharashtra, India
Ph: +91-22-66661880/89   e-mail: mumbai@cbspd.com

Representatives

• **Hyderabad** 0-9885175004 • **Jharkhand** 0-9811541605 • **Nagpur**   0-9421945513
• **Patna**   0-9334159340 • **Pune**   0-9623451994 • **Uttarakhand** 0-9716462459

Printed at Magic International Pvt. Ltd., Greater Noida, UP, India

to
_____

my late parents Mr TK Nair and Mrs Leelavathy
my wife Dr Shalini Nair
my son Akash and daughter Smriti
all my teachers, students and well wishers

Foreword

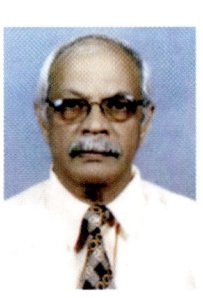

Learning is an ongoing process. It is like searching for horizon. When you feel you have reached it, the horizon moves further away.

In this era of exponential increase in medical literature and the ease of its accessibility, every contribution seems so vital.

Dr Haridas was my postgraduate student in general surgery. His unquenchable thirst for knowledge was evident in the formative years.

I must consider myself lucky to be in company with such brilliant disciples.

Dr Haridas has taken great pains to bring out a wonderful book mostly covering the difficult aspects of gastro sciences and other topics.

This book surely will be a great support for students preparing for surgery examination and for entrance exam preparation for superspecialty (MCh) courses.

He had training in UK which refined him as a precious gem. He is a faculty in gastrosurgery MCh entrance classes in Kerala, which have helped him in filtering important topics from the vast literature and explaining them in a simple language for the students to understand.

I have great pleasure and take pride in writing the Foreword to the extremely useful book my dear student has brought forth.

My heartfelt blessings.

Prof P Rajan MS, FRCS (Glasgow)
Emeritus Professor
Former Head, Department of Surgery
Government Medical College, Calicut, Kerala

Preface

This book is a compilation of my postgraduate notes and is prepared for the benefit of postgraduate students who are doing MS or DNB in surgery and for those who are preparing for MCh entrance examinations after completing MS/DNB for various specialities.

This book will also be useful to a select group of undergraduate students who are enthusiastic about surgery. This book is prepared in the form of notes, as the title indicates. This will enable students to have a quick read during their training period and allow easy revision during examinations.

The references used in preparation of this book are the standard textbooks in general surgery, gastrointestinal surgery, hepatobiliary and pancreatic surgery and the information given in this book is highly reliable. Due to the conflict in data given in various books, I have tried to convey it by putting the different sources in brackets. The charts and tables in this book are very crisp and to the point.

The last chapter includes the TNM staging for various cancers. Each organ system is described as a chapter and various topics under it are described under subtitles.

I sincerely hope this humble effort will be useful to each one of the readers.

TV Haridas

Acknowledgements

I am grateful to my senior residents Dr Anu N. Kumar, Dr Tinu Sasi, Dr Lakshmi Radhakrishnan and Dr Jasira PM for their timely help during various stages. I also thank the junior residents Dr Rajiv Sajan Thomas and Dr Agil Babu for their time and efforts. Special thanks to Dr Agil Babu, who helped me in designing the pages and was a constant source of encouragement. I also thank Dr Vishnu, my house surgeon, for helping me in drawing all the illustrations in digital format.

I am grateful to our Head of Department, Prof PJ Babu, and all my colleagues for their encouragement.

I express my gratitude to our Principal, Prof MA Andrews, for his support.

I also express my sincere gratitude towards CBS Publishers and Distributors for publishing this book.

TV Haridas

Contents

Esophagus

1.1 ANATOMY

- Muscular tube approximately 25 cm long
- It mainly occupies posterior mediastinum
- Extends from UES (cricopharyngeus muscle) to cardia
- Upper esophagus and UES have striated muscle
- Followed by transitional zone

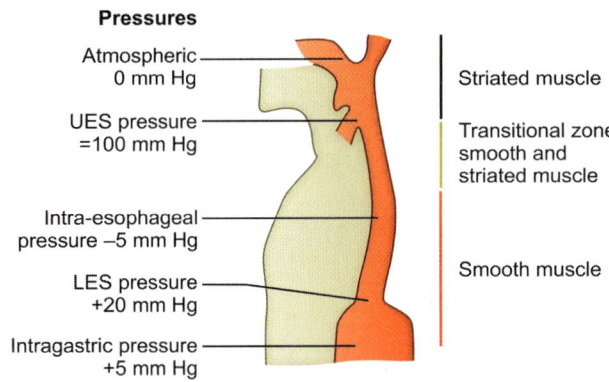

- Lower half consists of smooth muscle
- There are 3 minor deviations
  - At the base of neck—towards left—in cervical approach of esophagus through left side will be easier
  - At T7 level—towards right
  - GE junction towards left
- Cervical esophagus—from EUS to sternal notch (15–20)
- Upper thoracic esophagus—(sternal notch to azygos 20–25 cm)
- Mid-thoracic esophagus—azygos vein to inferior pulmonary vein (25–30 cm)
- Lower thoracic esophagus—IPV to EGJ (30–40 cm)
- Abdominal esophagus—EGJ to 3–4 cm below.

Arterial supply esophagus has 'shared vasculature' with no esophageal artery

Arterial Supply of Esophagus

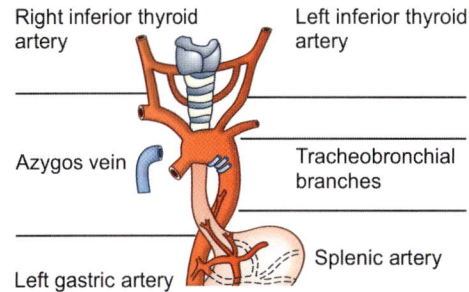

Anchoring Structures of Esophagus

- Cricopharyngeal muscles
- Cricopharyngeal tendon
- Bronchoesophageal fibers
- Pleuroesophageal fibers
- Gastrosplenic ligament
- Lesser omentum
- Phrenoesophageal membrane
- Phrenoesophageal membrane, also known as *Laimer ligament or Allison membrane*

Layers of Esophagus

- Adventitia
- Muscle
  - Outer longitudinal
  - Inner circular
- Submucosa
- Mucosa
  - Muscularis mucosa
  - Lamina propria
  - Nonkeratinizing squamous epithelium
- Esophageal veins have no valves

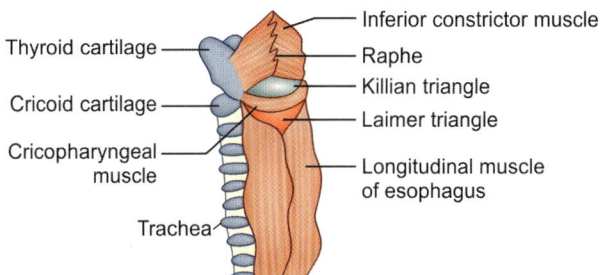

Lymphatics

- Watershed line is at carina, above this lymph drains to neck, below drains towards abdomen.

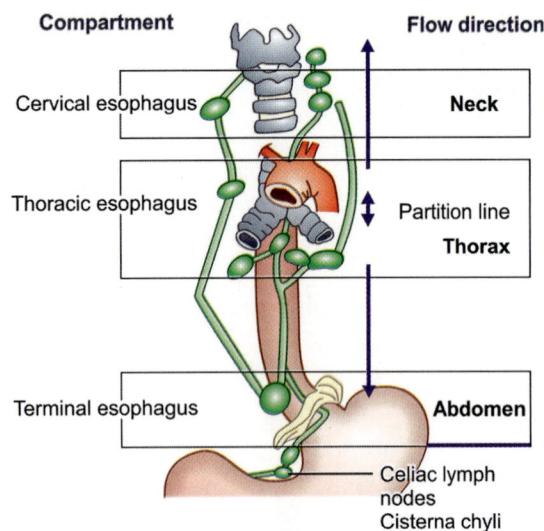

Concept of lymphatic drainage

Thoracic Duct

- Starts at cisterna chyli at L1-L2
- Passes through aortic foramen: T12
- Ascends through posterior mediastinum
- Continues on left of dorsal of esophagus
- At T5 level just cranial to azygos vein—inclines to left
- Joins at junction of left subclavian and IJV

Nerve Supply

- Parasympathetic from vagus—synaptic connections to myenteric plexus
- Submucosal Meissner's plexus is sparse in esophagus
- UES has powerful striated muscles.
- LES has a subtle—asymmetrical arrangement of muscle fibers just above EG junction

Physiology of Swallowing

- Oral is voluntary phase
- Pharyngeal and esophageal phases—involuntary
- Propulsion of food with air happens in primary peristalsis—vagal mediated
- UES is normally closed, a protective factor
- LES 3–4 cm long
- Normal humans swallow 500 times/day
- Food from pharynx takes 8–10 seconds to reach distal esophagus

- Secondary peristalsis—follows primary
- Tertiary contractions are non-peristaltic and infrequent (<10%)
- Primary and secondary peristalsis carry saliva which neutralizes acid

Esophageal Peristalsis

- Larger bolus induces stronger peristalsis
- Warm bolus augments peristalsis
- Cold bolus inhibits peristalsis
- Osmolality of food has no influence
- Not affected by age—'presbyesophagus'

Effects on LES Pressure By Various Agents

Increase LES pressure
- Gastrin
- Substance P
- Angiotensin 2
- Motilin
- Dopamine
- Metoclopramide
- Cisapride

Decreasing LES pressure
- Secretin
- Glucagon
- GIP/VIP
- CCK
- Atropine
- Nitrates
- CCB
- Morphine
- Progesterone

1.2 ESOPHAGEAL DIVERTICULA

- A result of primary motor disturbance of UES or LES
- Three types according to position
  - Pharyngoesophageal (Zenker's)
  - Parabronchial (Midesophageal)
  - Epiphrenic (Supradiaphragmatic)
- True vs False
  - Pulsion type are false diverticula

– Due to increased intraluminal pressure
– They only have mucosa and submucosa
– E.g.: Zenker and Epiphrenic

- Traction type are true diverticula
  – Mediastinal nodes cause—fibrosis and traction.
  – Mainly seen in mid-esophageal or carinal region.

Zenker's Diverticulum

- Described by Zenker and von Ziemssen
- Most common esophageal diverticulum
- Seen in elderly in 7th decade
- Due to loss of tissue elasticity and muscle tone with age
- Through Killian's triangle

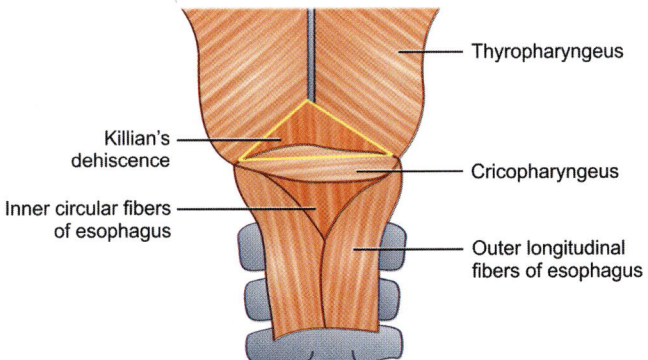

- Dissects through left side of esophagus into superior mediastinum and posteriorly along pre-vertebral space.
- Also called cricopharyngeal achalasia or posterio-lateral diverticula

Clinical Features

- Asymptomatic
- Food sticking in throat—most common
- Cough, RTI
- Halitosis
- Voice change
- Aspiration pneumonia, lung abscess

Diagnosis

- Barium esophagogram—lateral view
- Diverticulum is seen posteriorly, also called "Cricopharyngeal bar"
- Lateral view is better
- There is no role for manometry or endoscopy

Treatment
Surgical

- Diverticulectomy/diverticulopexy
- Myotomy of thyropharyngeus and cricopharyngeus is a must
- For diverticula <2 cm need only myotomy
- >5 cm needs excision
- Diverticulopexy—diverticulum is fixed to posterior pharynx and not to prevertebral fascia to allow free pharyngeal movements
- Patient can eat or drink after 2–3 days

Endoscopy
Dohlman's Procedure

- Division of common wall between diverticulum and esophagus is done
- Uses laser, cautery or stapler
- It is useful in larger diverticula
- Needs maximum extension of neck, so contraindicated in spondylosis
- Early feeds can be started

> Diverticula <3 cm surgery better
>
> >3 cm both surgery and endoscopic treatment have similar results
>
> Hospital stay less with endoscopic
>
> Results are equally good in both groups

Killian-Jamieson diverticulum

- Rare
- Discovered in 1983
- Occurs inferior to cricopharyngeus
- Anterolateral aspect of esophagus near the insertion of cricopharyngeus to cricoid

Treatment

- Diverticulectomy through cervical incision is done
- Myotomy for 3 cm

Laimer's Diverticulum

- Occurs through Laimer's triangle
- In the posterior midline
- Below cricopharyngeus

- Seen in younger associated with EMD unlike Zenker
- It is a true diverticulum
- Manometry is indicated
- It is broad/wide mouthed

Treatment

- Not transoral—due to varied position
- Trans cervical route is preferred diverticulectomy and myotomy below the diverticulum is done
- Side of surgery is based on side of presentation

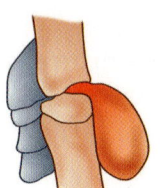
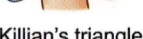
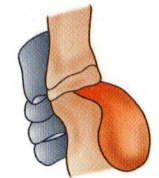

Killian's triangle   Laimer's triangle

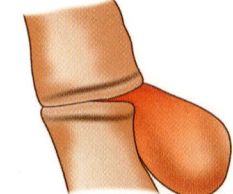

Killian-Jamieson triangle

- **Killian's triangle**
  - Region between the thyropharyngeus and cricopharyngeus
- **Laimer's triangle**
  - Region between cricopharyngeus and superior esophageal circular muscle
- **Killian-Jamieson's triangle**
  - Between the oblique and transverse fibres of the cricopharyngeal muscle

Mid-esophageal Diverticula

- Caused by mediastinal nodes
- Histoplasmosis—now common
- Traction diverticula
- Also due to motility disorders like achalasia, DES.

Clinical Features

- Asymptomatic usually
- Dysphagia, chest pain, regurgitation
- Chronic cough suggests B-E fistula
- Barium studies are the choice
- Occurs typically on right side, wide mouthed
- CT is done for evaluating LN enlargement
- Endoscopy for assessing mucosal pattern and fistula
- Manometry is done in all patients for assessing motility disorders
  - Treatment is guided by manometry
- Treat the LN enlargement
- <2 cm—may be observed
- Symptomatic or >2 cm surgery
- Diverticulopexy to prevertebral fascia is done
- Long esophageal myotomy is done in chest pain and motility disorders

Epiphrenic Diverticula

- Occurs within 10 cm of GEJ
- Pulsion type
- Associated with DES, Achalasia, Ehlers-Danlos syndrome
  - It is more common on right side
  - Wide mouthed
  - Asymptomatic
  - Sometimes incidental finding
  - Barium studies are the choice in diagnosis
  - Size, position, proximity to diaphragm can be delineated
  - Manometry can be done
  - Endoscopy for assessing mucosa to rule out cancer.

Treatment

- Similar to mid-esophagus diverticula
- For >2 cm surgery
  - Diverticulopexy to vertebral fascia
  - Myotomy is done from neck of diverticulum to LES
- Diverticulectomy can be done with stapler
- Long myotomy is done on opposite wall of diverticula
- Repair hiatus hernia, if present

Diffuse Intramural Pseudodiverticulosis

- They are multiple tiny outpouchings from lumen
- They are dilated excretory ducts of esophageal sebaceous glands
- Mainly asymptomatic

1.3 DYSPHAGIA AND ESOPHAGEAL MOTILITY DISORDERS

Dysphagia Causes

- Webs/strictures
- Motility disorder
- Cancer
- Achalasia
- Diffuse esophageal spasm
- Diagnosed when monomeric findings exceed two standard deviations from normal
- Manometry—the choice in all motility disorders

Chicago Classification

- Based on high resolution manometry
- HRM pr. Sensors 1 cm apart
- Up to 36 sensors used
- **Achalasia and OG junction**
- **Outflow obstruction**

Classic achalasia (Type 1)	Median IRP> 15 mmHg; 100% failed peristalsis (DCI< 100 mmHg × s × cm); premature contractions with DCI< 450 mmHg × s × cm
Achalasia with oesophageal compression (Type II)	Median IRP > 15 mmHg; 100% failed peristalsis, pan-esophageal pressurisation with 20% of swallows
Spastic achalasia (Type III)	Median IRP > 15 mmHg; no normal peristalsis, spastic contractions with DCI> 450 mmHg × s × cm with 20% of swallows
Achalasia in evolution (OG junction outflow obstruction)	Median IRP < 15 mmHg; sufficient evidence for peristalsis present not meeting above criteria

- **Major disorders of peristalsis**

Absent contractility Distal esophageal spasm	Normal median IRP 100% failed peristalsis Normal median IRP = 20% Premature contractions with DCI >450 mmHg × s × cm
Hypercontractile esophagus (jackhammer or nutcracker)	At least 2 swallows with DCI> 8000 mmHg × s × cm

- **Minor disorders of peristalsis**

Ineffective esophageal motility	= 50% ineffective swallows
Fragmented peristalsis	= 50% fragmented contractions with DCI > 450 mmHg × s × cm
Normal esophageal motility	None of above criteria satisfied

- **IRP:** Integrated relaxing pressure—mean relaxation pressure of 4 seconds with maximal deglutitive relaxation after swallowing in a 10s window.
- **DCI:** Distal contractile integral = Amplitude × Duration × Length—measures the pressure in esophagus from transition zone to LES.

> **EVALUATION**
> - Evaluate cardiac, esophageal causes
> - Connective tissue disorders
> - Endoscopy
> - CT
> - pH studies

Primary Motility Disorders

- Achalasia
- Diffuse esophageal spasm (DES)
- Hypertensive LES
- Nutcracker (jackhammer) esophagus
- Ineffective esophageal motility (IEM)

Secondary Motility Disorders

- Collagen vascular or neuromuscular disorders
- Scleroderma
- Dermatomyositis
- Polymyositis
- LE
- Chagas disease
- Myasthenia gravis

- Classification based on anatomy
  - Oropharyngeal
  - Disorders of esophageal body
  - Body and LES
  - LES
- Oropharyngeal or transfer dysphagia
  - Video fluoroscopic evaluation with high frequency digital recording—the choice
  - Penetration aspiration score
  - Functional Lumen Imaging Probe (FLIP)—to test the distensibility of lumen

Disorders of Esophageal Body

- **DES**
  - In Chicago classification: Distal esophageal spasm
  - Five times less common than achalasia
  - More in women with other medical complaints
  - Motor abnormality of esophageal body in lower two-thirds
  - Muscular hypertrophy and degeneration of vagal branches
  - Esophageal contractions are
    - Repetitive,
    - Simultaneous and
    - High amplitude

Clinical Features

- Chest pain—radiating to neck
- Dysphagia
- Related to eating or exercise—like angina
- Regurgitation of esophageal contents—not acid
- May have IBS, pylorospasm

Diagnosis—Radiography, Manometry

- Esophagogram shows 'Corkscrew' or 'pseudo-diverticulosis'
  - Caused by tertiary contractions in advanced disease
  - Distal bird beak and normal peristalsis also seen

DES-Manometry

- Simultaneous multipeaked contractions of high amplitude (>120 mmHg) of long duration (>2.5 seconds)

- Occur after >10% of wet swallows
- Spontaneous and intermittent normal contractions also occur
- So standard manometry may not be enough
- Subjective correlation and vagomimetic—bethenecol will help in diagnosis.

Treatment

- Can achieve partial relief only
- Nonsurgical—medical/endoscopic
- Evaluate psychiatric like depression, anxiety
- Eliminate trigger food
- Acid suppression—in case of reflux disease
- Peppermint may be useful
- Calcium channel blockers, nitrates, sedatives, anticholinergics
- Botox injection—no sustainable results
- Esophageal dilatation up to 50–60F

Surgery

- In incapacitating chest pain/dysphagia and failed medical treatment
- Long esophagomyotomy including all pathological segments
- Include LES—no need to include stomach
- Dor fundoplication is added
- Relief of symptoms will be seen in nearly 80%

Nutcracker Esophagus: Jackhammer

- In Chicago—hypercontractile esophagus
- Excessive contractility
- Hypertensive peristalsis with high amplitude peristaltic contractions
- Seen in all ages
- Most common esophageal hypermotility disorder
- Due to hypertrophic muscle and contractions
- Most painful EMD
- Produce chest pain, dysphagia, odynophagia
- Regurgitation and reflux—uncommon
- Esophagogram may show normal results—depends on the time of examination
- Subjective chest pain
- Distal contractile integral >8000 mm/s/cm

- LES pressure—normal—relaxes with each wet swallow
- Ambulatory monitoring—distinguishes from DES
- No role for surgery

Medical

- Ca channel blockers
- Nitrates
- Antispasmodics
- Bougie dilatation—no long-term benefit
- Avoid trigger food like caffeine, cold and hot drinks

Motility Disorders of LES

Hypertensive LES

- Chicago—EGJ outflow obstruction
- Median integrated relaxation pressure >15 mm Hg (hypertensive poorly relaxing sphincter)
- Has effective peristalsis unlike achalasia
- Manometry—LES pressure >26 mmHg

Treatment

- Endoscopic and surgical
- Botox injection
- Hydrostatic balloon dilatation
- Lap modified Heller—surgery of choice
- Dor or Toupet added if motility is normal
- POEM

Motility Disorders of Both Body and LES

Achalasia

- Achalasia = failure to relax
- More in young women
- Idiopathic/infectious
- Associated with Chagas, emotional stress, drastic weight reduction
- Destruction of nerves to LES is primary pathology and the effect on body of esophagus is secondary
- LES fails to relax on swallow which causes increased pressure and dilatation leading to progressive loss of peristalsis
- **Vigorous/spastic/type 3 achalasia**
  - Hypertensive LES fails to relax
  - Contractions simultaneous, nonperistaltic.
- **Achalasia: Clinical Triad**
  - Dysphagia
    □ First for liquids—later solids
    □ Drink large quantity of liquid
  - Regurgitation
    □ Undigested food—aspiration
  - Weight loss

- **Premalignant**
  - In 20 years—8% chance
  - SCC—most common—due to long-term contact with fermenting food
  - Adenocarcinoma can develop at midesophagus—below the air fluid level even after treatment—risk of cancer is high
  - **Diagnosis**
- Esophagogram
- Bird's beak appearance
- Dilated esophagus
- LES spasm
- Delayed emptying
- Lack of peristalsis in body and failure of LES relaxation
- Lack of gastric air
- Mega (sigmoid) esophagus

Manometry

Gold standard

- Two LES findings
  - LES hypertensive, pressure >35 mmHg
    □ Fail to relax with swallow
- Three body abnormalities
  - Pressure above baseline (pressurization)—incomplete air evacuation
  - Simultaneous, mirrored contractions that is non-progressive peristalsis
  - Low amplitude waveforms is due to lack of muscle tone.
- Endoscopy to evaluate the mucosa

Treatment

Most are directed at LES, does not address the motility—hence, palliative

- Nonsurgical
  - Medicines
- Nitrates
  - Ca channel blockers
  - Pneumatic dilatation
    □ Good relief
    □ Chance of perforation <4%
  - Inj. Botox
    □ Symptoms recur in >50% in 6 months
- Surgical
- Modified Heller's myotomy (myotomy is done on anterior wall only)
  - With Toupet or Dor

POEM

- Endoscopic
- Mucosa divided around mid to distal third

- Submucosal tunnel is created
- Muscle of lower esophagus, LES and cardia divided
- No fundoplication is done
- For achalasia type 1 and 2—short myotomy is done
- Type 3—long myotomy is done
- Mucosal incision is made 3–4 cm proximal to site of myotomy.
- Myotomy proceeds antegrade
- Circular muscles are cut, longitudial muscles are split and can visualise mediastinal structures through adventitia is called "mediastinal exposure"
- Myotomy continued on to stomach wall
- Extended myotomy—in
  - Noncardiac chest pain
  - Type 3 achalasia
  - Few cm distal to gastric cardia
- Esophagectomy in
  - Tortuous sigmoid esophagus
  - Failure of >1 myotomy
  - Reflux stricture not amenable to dilatation
  - Eliminates risk for cancer
    - □ Trans hiatal esophagectomy preferred
- Eckardt clinical score <3—indicates successful POEM

Score	Weight loss	Dysphagia	Regurgitation	Retrosternal pain
0	Nil	Nil	Nil	Nil
1	< 5 kg	Occasional	Occasional	Occasional
2	5–10 kg	Daily	Daily	Daily
3	>10 kg	Every meal	Every meal	Every meal

Hallmarks of End Stage Achalasia

Clinical—severe dysphagia or regurgitation

Radiographic—megaesophagus

Pathologic—reduction/absence of ganglion with fibrous replacement of myenteric plexus

- Incidence of perforation
  - During dilatation—4%
  - During myotomy—12%

Pseudoachalasia

- Achalasia like
- In adenocarcinoma of cardia
- Inability of sphincter to relax linked to loss of peristalsis
- Also seen in
  - Benign tumors in this region
  - Ca bronchus, pancreas

Ineffective Esophageal Motility

- Contraction abnormality of distal esophagus
- Associated with GERD
- Secondary to inflammatory injury
  - Dampened esophageal motility and poor acid clearance
  - Once motility is altered, it is irreversible
  - Best treatment is prevention and treatment of GERD

Feature	Normal	Achalasia	DES	Nutcracker esophagus
LES pressure	15–25 mmHg	Hypertensive >26 mmHg	N/slightly high	N
LES relaxation	Follows swallowing	Incomplete residual pressure (>5 mmHg)	N	N
Amplitude pressure	50–120 mmHg	Decreased	N	Hypertensive (>180 mmHg)
Contraction waves	Progressive	Simultaneous Mirrored Pressurised	Simultaneous Repetitive	Long duration (>6s)
Peristalsis	N	None	Hypertensive peristalsis	Hypertensive peristalsis

1.4 GERD

- Most common benign condition of stomach and esophagus

Endogenous Antireflux Mechanisms

- Spontaneous esophageal clearance
- LES—a high pressure zone

  LES—four anatomic structures
  - Intrinsic musculature of lower esophagus in tonic contraction
  - Within 500 milliseconds of swallow—LES relax

- Sling fibers of gastric cardia
  - Arranged diagonally from cardia—fundus junction to lesser curve
  - Situated at same depth as circular muscle
- Crura of diaphragm
  - During inspiration, intrathoracic pressure decreases—crura compress esophagus which increase pressure at LES
- GEJ firmly anchored to abdominal cavity—increased abdominal pressure transmitted to GEJ which reduce reflux

GERD: Basic Pathology

- Intragastric pressure >HPZ
- LES resting pressure too low (hypotensive)
- LES relaxes without peristalsis (spontaneous LES relaxation)
- Due to hypotensive LES, GEJ may be displaced to posterior mediastinum
- GERD is physiological
- GERD depends on
  - Total amount of acid exposure
  - Symptoms
  - Mucosal damage

Pathophysiology

- Primary barrier to gastroesophageal reflux is the lower esophageal sphincter
- LES normally works in conjunction with the diaphragm
- If barrier is disrupted, acid goes from stomach to esophagus

GERD: Clinical Features

- Heartburn
- Epigastric/retrosternal—caustic or stinging
- Does not radiate to back
- Not as a pressure sensation
- Regurgitation/reflux of digested food
- Reflux of undigested food seen in achalasia, diverticulum
- Waterbrash

Extraesophageal Symptoms

- Laryngeal symptoms hoarseness, dysphonia, globus, choking, throat pain
- Pulmonary symptoms—cough, shortness of breath wheezing

Mechanisms of Symptoms

- Reflux—micro aspiration of gastroduodenal contents and caustic injury to larynx
- Distal esophageal acid exposure leads to vagal reflex—bronchospasm and cough (due to common vagal innervation of trachea and esophagus)
- Typical symptoms—resolve with PPI
- If extra esophageal symptoms—may not resolve with PPI
- Only acid is suppressed by PPI
- Acid is not the only insult
- Bile salts and pepsin are there in refluxate
- So may need a mechanical barrier like fundoplication
- In extraesophageal symptoms—rule out primary laryngeal or pulmonary problems
- If no extra esophageal symptoms are there, consider LARS (lap anti-reflux surgery)
- If extraesophageal pathology is present, avoid LARS

Pulmonary Disease and GERD

- GERD and asthma: Improved by antireflux surgery than medication
- Idiopathic pulmonary fibrosis
  - Due to reflux and microaspiration of acid and nonacid contents
  - In IPF, incidence of GERD—94%
  - LARS is better than PPI

Other Features

- Frequent drinking water
- Leaning forward posture with lungs inflated which
  - Flattens diaphragm
  - Narrows AP diameter of hiatus
  - Increases LES pressure
- Erosion of dentition—yellow teeth—loss of dentin
- Injected oropharynx
- Chronic sinusitis

Diagnosis

- Mainly based on clinical improvement on PPI

4 Tests
- Ambulatory pH and impedance monitoring
- Esophageal manometry
- OGDscopy
- Barium studies

Ambulatory pH and Impedance Monitoring

- Quantifies distal esophageal acid exposure
- Stop PPI 1 week before

'Gold standard'

- 24-hour monitoring
- Dual probe catheter into esophagus through nares
- Two solid state electrodes 10 cm apart—detect pH 2 to 7
- First electrode is placed 5 cm proximal to LES

Data

- Total number of reflux episodes (<pH 4)
- Longest episode of reflux
- Number episodes lasting >5 minutes
- Percentage of time in upright and supine positions
- DeMeester score >14.7—is indicative of abnormal distal esophageal acid exposure

Ambulatory pH

- Also assess symptom related probability
- If a symptom occurs within 2 minutes of reflux, high temporal relationship

Esophageal Impedance Monitoring

- Identifies—episodes of nonacid reflux
- Flexible catheter through nares placed in esophagus 1 cm apart
- Detects resistance to flow of electric current (impedance)
- Impedance increases in presence of air and decreases with liquid bolus
- pH—impedance probes:
  - Can measure both acid and nonacid reflux
  - Determine direction of movement of acid
  - Antegrade (swallow) vs retrograde can be differentiated.
  - Proximal probe—detect pharyngeal acid reflux

Acid Reflux is More Significant Predictor

Esophageal Manometry

- Most effective way to assess function of esophageal body and LES
- Standard manometry is linear tracing of pressure waves
- High resolution manometry:
  - 32 channel flexible catheter
  - Pressure tracings at 1 cm intervals
- Can detect achalasia in GERD

OGDscopy

- To study mucosal injury like
  - Ulcer, stricture, Barrett esophagus
- LA (Los Angeles type) C and D, and peptic strictures—pathognomonic of GERD
- If type C and D strictures seen, ambulatory pH study is unnecessary
- In LA A and B, pH study is needed
- OGD—assess flap valve of GEJ
- Graded 1 to 4 according to length and tightness

Barium Studies

- Provide anatomic evaluation
- Hiatus hernia, diverticula, motility, stricture

Anatomical road map achieved by

- Video esophagography, fluoroscopy

Esophagitis

Eosinophylic Esophagitis

- Food allergy—allergic esophagitis
- Personnel and family history of allergy, asthma—esophageal asthma
- Ringed esophagus—trachea like
- Vertical furrows
- White specks (1–3 mm eosinophilic infiltrates)
- Small caliber esophagus and strictures
- Fragile mucosa
- OGD dilatation can cause tear
- Treat the allergy
- Immunotherapy against IL-6

Other names

- Feline esophagus
- Ringed esophagus
- Corrugated esophagus
- Small caliber esophagus
- Stiff or non-compliant esophagus
- Trachealisation
- Linear furrows

Clinical Presentation

- At any age
- In adults most common symptom is dysphagia to solid, intermittent type and rarely with odynophagia, may be confused with GERD.
- May lead to malnutrition

- Heartburn, chest pain
- Food impaction—needing intervention

Clinical Presentation in Children

- Most common is heartburn and abdomen pain with vomiting
- Growth failure
- Hemetemesis
- In infants—"gagging" or "choking"
- Can progress to stricture
- There is rise in incidence
- 'Hygiene hypothesis' due to decreased infection leading to more atopic diseases.

EoE: Diagnosis

1. Clinical
2. Pathological: Eosinophilic inflammation esophagus—at least 15 eosinophils/HPF
3. Other causes for eosinophilia
4. Mucosal eosinophilia persist after PPI therapy
5. Response to allergy treatment
   - pH study—not mandatory
   - **"GERD refractory to PPI"**
   - **"GERD refractory to surgical Rx"**

Treatment

- Dietary modification—avoiding allergans
- Dilatation for stricture

Feline Esophagus

- Seen in eosinophilic esophagitis
- Fine evenly spaced transverse folds
- More seen in GERD
- Occurs immediately after an episode of GERD
- Also seen in asymptomatic
- Due to contraction of longitudinal muscle

Stricture

- Stricture is pathognomonic of GERD—no need of pH study
   - Biopsy is indicated
   - Stricture is mucosal in nature
   - Occurs at GEJ
   - Eccenteric and transversely placed stricture
- Schatzki ring—may be seen

Schatzki Ring

- Submucosal fibrotic bands
- Occurs at distal esophagus near squamocolumnar junction
- Idiopathic
- Not pathognomonic but associated with GERD

- So need pH studies to confirm
- Simultaneous dysphagia for solid and liquids so neuromuscular or autoimmune
- *Causes intermittent/episodic dysphagia*
- Schatzki ring—squamous epithelium above and columnar epithelium below
- In peptic stricture, mucosa is columnar both above and below it.
- Treatment—balloon dilatation

GERD: Treatment
Medical

- PPI—for 8 weeks after excluding other causes
- No improvement—further evaluation
- PPI—irreversibly blocks the proton pump of parietal cells
- Maximal effect in 4 days
- Lasts throughout the life of parietal cells
- Long-term PPI treatment can cause hypergastrinemia and proliferation of enterochromaffin cells leads to carcinoid

GERD: Surgery in

- Not relieved by medical means
- Extraesophageal symptoms
- Ulceration, stricture
- Barrett

Partial Vs Complete Fundoplication

- GERD with dysmotility—partial fundoplication is better
- Nissen—360° wrap is associated with more dysphagia
- Anterior (90°/180°) has more recurrence: Thal or Dor
- Partial posterior (180°/270°) better symptom control and less side effects: Toupet
- Watson—anterior 90° degree
- Belsey mark IV—intrathoracic posterior 270° degree

Nissen

- Wrap of 2.5 to 3 cm length
- Associated with posterior crural repair
- Pass bougie of 52F
- Fundoplication is done with fundus

In Partial Posterior

- Most cephalad sutures include fundus, crus of diaphragm and esophagus

In Anterior

- Fundus of stomach is anchored to esophagus and hiatus

Complications of Peptic Reflux

Peptic Stricture

- Evaluated by endoscopy
- Bougie, in French = wax candle
- 1 mm = 3 French

Peptic stricture treatment

- Dilatation
- PPI
- Intralesional steroid injection
- Esophageal stents currently not recommended
  - Most important complication—stent migration

Surgery considered if dilatable stricture

Short Esophagus

- Means <3 cm of intra-abdominal esophagus
- Need 3–4 cm intra-abdominal esophagus
- Achieved by
  - Extensive posterior mediastinal mobilisation
  - Single vagotomy—1 to 2 cm extra length
  - Both vagotomy—3 to 4 cm
- **Stapled wedge gastroplasty**

  #### For esophageal lengthening

  - Wedge gastroplasty with 46F bougie and
  - Collis gastroplasty

Collis Gastroplasty

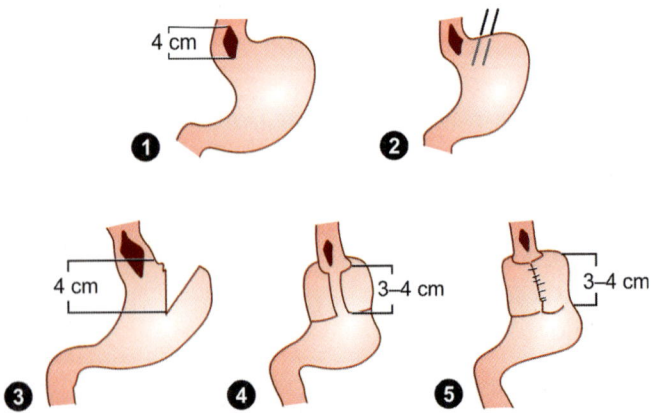

Vagal Sparing Esophagectomy

- Esophagus stripped out of mediastinum with simultaneous mucosal inversion

- Nerves are sheared off muscularis propria
- Esophageal plexus will be intact

Failed Antireflux Surgery

- Persistent symptoms beyond 2–3 months
- Very rarely only need intervention—5.6%
- Reasons
  - Recurrent hiatal hernia
  - Slipped fundoplication
  - Incorrect fundoplication
- Evaluate by manometry, 24-hr pH monitoring
- If abnormal—esophagogram and OGD
- PPI usually resolve
- Consider resurgery
- Late onset dysphagia—usually due to failure and need surgery

Not Improving/Worsening

Obstruction due to gastric body wrap—leads to recurrence of hiatal hernia—resurgery may be indicated

Other Methods

- RF energy
- Injection of bioinert polymers
- Endoscopic gastroplication
- Transoral Incisionless Fundoplication (TIF) (EsophyX)
- Magnetic Sphincter Augmentation Device (MSAD)—LINX

EsophyX

- Multichannel endoluminal device: Fasteners—full thickness gastric plication—antireflux valve at GEJ
- Can create plication of 4 cm and 270 degree
- Through gastroscope
- Reduces acid exposure—not abolish
- But not completely avoiding PPI use

LINX

- Through laparoscope
- Magnetic beads implanted near LES
- Closes the sphincter
- Allows swallowing and belching
- Late onset dysphagia—needs dilatation—improves which may be due to fibrous bands near beads

Para Esophageal Hernia

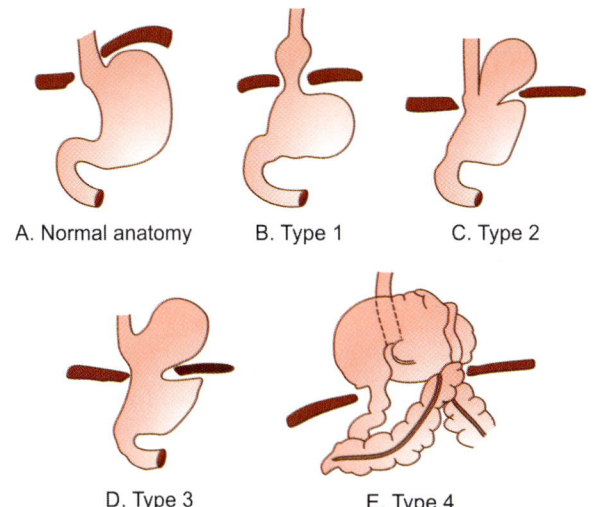

A. Normal anatomy   B. Type 1   C. Type 2

D. Type 3   E. Type 4

PEH: Pathophysiology
- Widening of esophageal crura
- Stretching of phrenoesophageal membrane
- Most common structure herniated: Fundus of stomach
- Later gets incarcerated—irreducible
- Volvulus/gangrene of stomach—can happen
- Risk of strangulation—1% per year
- Large hernia in young may be asymptomatic needs surgery

Clinical Features
- Dysphagia
- Odynophagia
- Epigastric, chest pain

Diagnosis
- Barium
- Endoscopy
  - Barrett
  - Cameron ulcers
- Manometry
- Ambulatory pH measurement

Cameron Ulcers
- **'Riding ulcers'**
- Due to constant rubbing movement of stomach against hiatus
- Swallowing movements compounds this pathology
- Most common on lesser curvature at diaphragmatic hiatus
- Seen in 5% in PEH
- Risk increases with size of hernia

- Can cause bleeding and anemia
- Resolves after surgery

Surgery: 4 Components
- Reduction of contents into abdomen
- Complete excision of hernia sac from mediastinum
- Mobilisation and achieve minimum 3 cm intra-abdominal length of esophagus
- Antireflux procedure
- Lap or open
- Sac excision taking care of aorta, pericardium, inferior pulmonary vein.
- Closure of crura
  - Primary
  - Can place mesh at the incision
  - Synthetic mesh is not preferred as it causes erosion of esophagus
- Nissen or Toupet fundoplication is added
- Volvulus, incarceration and strangulation—please refer to miscellaneous section of stomach
- Most serious complication of PEH

Barrett Esophagus
- Macroscopically—presence of any length of columnar epithelium proximal to GEJ
- Microscopically—presence of true goblet cells, establishing presence of intestinal metaplasia (IM)
- Due to long standing acid/alkaline exposure esophageal squamous mucosa turns to columnar—intestinal metaplasia (Barrett)—goblet cells
- >3 cm—classic long segment
- <3 cm short segment
- Cardia metaplasia—intestinal metaplasia at GEJ without any macroscopic change—ultra short
- Biopsy, if shows dysplasia, more chance of adeno ca
- Barrett—25–40 times more chance of carcinoma (.5% per patient per year)

Stains in Barrett—to Diagnose Intestinal Metaplasia
- H and E
- Alcian blue at pH 2.5—more definite in staining goblet cells—due to high mucin content—strong vacuolar staining
- Pseudogoblet cells—mucous cells lining surface with cytoplasmic vacuoles containing neutral mucin
- IM distal to GEJ is **gastric type—related to** *H. pylori*—not GERD
- To diagnose IM—most proximal columnar segment should be biopsied. IM will be just distal to squamous epithelium.

- Non-intestinalised mucosa will be distal to that, this is called zonation
- IM in cardia mucosa with endoscopically normal GEJ without a columnar segment—cardiac intestinal metaplasia (CIM)

Subsquamous Barrett (Burried Barrett)

- IM develops under squamous epithelium—so endoscopic appearance is normal. Happens following ablative procedures, these are dysplastic and there is increase chances of cancer
- Lowest following RFA
- Occurs within 5 mm from neo squamocolumnar junction
- 3D OCT—optical coherence tomography on endoscopy—can assess depth of 1–2 mm

Barrett Pathophysiology: Two Steps

- Fatty food causes effacement of stomach and more exposure of lower esophagus to acid, this causes porous epithelium and nerve endings are exposed producing heartburn
- Columnar metaplasia develops
- Later inflammatory infiltrate leads to shortened esophagus
- More acid exposure—columnar segment progresses

Second Step: Goblet Cells

- In this step three changes are happen:
  1. They remain as cardiac cells
  2. Acquire parietal cells and form oxyntocardiac cells—having no malignant potential
  3. Form goblet cells (intestinal metaplasia) which has malignant potential
- So Barrett esophagus develops when squamous epithelium on chronic exposure to gastric juice will be converted to cardiac mucosa which takes several years
- Second step cardiac mucosa—intestinal metaplasia and acquiring goblet cells which can turn into Barrett dysplasia and cancer

Two Steps

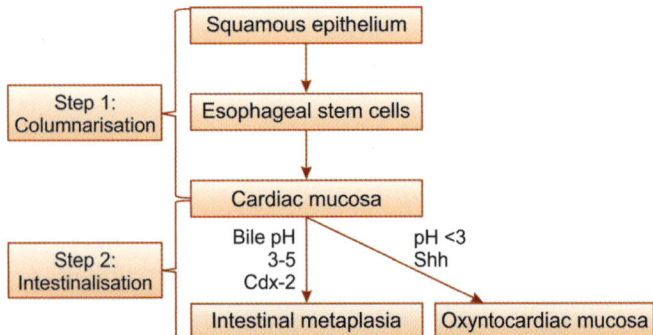

- BMP4: Bone Morphogenic Protein 4
- Cdx-2 gene: Caudal type homeobox 2
- Shh gene: Sonic hedgehog gene

Metaplasia in Three Layers

- Intestinal metaplasia on top near neo squamo-columnar junction
- Pure cardiac mucosa in the middle
- Oxyntocardiac mucosa near GEJ

Prague Criteria

- For endoscopically suspected columnar metaplasia/Barrett, esophagus
- Prague C: Circumferential metaplasia
- Prague M: Proximal extent of metaplasia

Decreased Risk for Barrett

- Tall people
- *H. pylori* infection—exact reason unclear
- Atrophic gastritis—reduced acid
  - Generate ammonia—reduced acid
- NSAIDs—COX2 inhibition
- Statins
- PPI, antireflux surgery
- Nutrition—fibers, vegetables, proteins
  - Trans fat—increases risk

Risk factors for progression of BE to cancer
- Men—more risk
- Advanced age
- Duration—more risk—>10 years
- Obesity and smoking
- Alcohol—not found a risk
- Recurrent GERD
- Barrett >3 cm more risk
- Stricture, nodule
- Dysplasia—high grade
- Molecular
  - TP53 mutation
  - Aneuploidy
  - Transcriptomic, methylomic and proteomic profiles

Seattle Protocol for Endoscopic Biopsy

- 4 quadrant biopsies
- 1 cm apart
- Beginning at the proximal gastric folds
- To the most proximal extend of IM

Antireflux Surgery

- Choice: Nissen
- May prevent progression of disease
- May regress dysplasia
- Cannot completely prevent development of adenocarcinoma

Endoscopic Ablation

Not indicated in non-dysplastic BE

- EMR in high grade dysplasia
  - In lesions <1.5 cm

Vienna classification is used for Barrett's esophagus classification. Classified from category 1 to category 5.2 which ranges from no dysplasia to submucosal cancer

For larger lesions—SRER (stepwise radical endoscopic resection)

Management guidelines by American College of Gastroenterology

No dysplasia—repeat biopsy in 3–5 years interval

Indefinite for dysplasia—confirmation by two experienced pathologists, endoscopy in six months interval.

Low grade dysplasia
- **Flat mucosa**—confirmation by two pathologists, offer RFA and yearly surveillance. If no treatment is offered, need six monthly surveillance
- **Nodular**—EMR for staging, give RFA, then yearly surveillance

High grade dysplasia
- **Flat** mucosa—two pathologists confirmation and RFA indicated
- **Nodular**—EMR of nodule, RFA for rest of the Barrett's lesion

1.5 ESOPHAGEAL PERFORATION

Causes
- Endoscopy—59%
- Trauma, FB—10%
- Rigid endoscopy—0.1% risk
- Flexible—0.03% risk
- EMR, RFA—<1% risk
- Blunt trauma—very rare—0.001%
- Penetrating trauma—6%—mostly cervical esophagus
- FB perforation—most common cricopharyngeus
- 75–90% of perforations during endoscopy occur just above or directly through a stricture

Clinical Features
- Pain—most common
- Fever
- Dyspnea
- Crepitus
- **Cervical esophagus**
  - Neck pain, crepitus, odynophagia, dysphagia
- **Proximal/mid-esophagus**
  - Fever
  - Right-sided pleural effusion

- **Mid-thoracic**
  - Substernal/epigastric pain
  - Mediastinal air
  - Mediastinal crunch on auscultation
- **Spontaneous lower eso perforation**
  - Left pleural contamination
  - Mackler triad
    - Thoracic pain
    - Vomiting
    - Subcutaneous emphysema

Abdominal Esophagus
- Epigastric pain—radiating to left shoulder
- Peritoneal signs
- **Hemetemesis—not feature of perforation**

Pittsburgh Severity Score

Esophageal perforation severity score	
Variable	*Score (range 1–3)*
Age >75 yrs	1
Tachycardia >100 b/min	1
Leucocytosis >10,000 WBC/ml	1
Pleural effusion	1
Fever >38.5°C	2
Uncontained leak (CT or Ba swallow)	2
Resp. rate >30/mechanical ventilation	2
Time to diagnose >24 h	2
Cancer	3
Hypotension	3
Total potential score	**18**

Diagnosis
- Suspected endoscopic injury—contrast esophagogram—choice (Gastrografin followed by thin Barium)—can plan treatment
- As there is high risk for aspiration in tracheoesophageal fistula—Barium study is preferred over Gastrografin study, as Gastrografin, if aspirated has a higher risk of pneumonitis
- Contrast esophagogram—right lateral decubitus and left lateral decubitus views are better because upright position causes rapid transit
- False negative esophagogram—10–38%

- CT—cannot localise and see luminal pathology
- Endoscopy in OT—can aggravate pneumomediastinum
- Accurate localisation of perforation and extend of extraluminal contamination is necessary before intervention
- May need a combination of investigations

Endoscopy Perforation

- Incidence 1 in 4000
- Causes
  - Large anterior osteophytes
  - Pharyngeal pouch, obstructions
  - Malignancy
- In therapeutic scopy—10 times more common
- X-ray chest shows air in mediastinum
- CECT is the choice
- If no CT—Gastrografin—followed by Barium

Instrumental perforation

- Intrathoracic and intra-abdominal more common

Management of esophageal perforation	
Favouring non-surgical management	*Favouring surgical repair*
Low septic load	High septic load
Minimal cardiovascular upset	Septic shock
Perforation contained within mediastinum	Breach of pleura
Perforation by flexible endoscope	Boerhaave's syndrome
Cervical esophageal perforation	Abdominal esophageal perforation

Treatment

- Conservative
- Endoscopic
- Surgical
- **Endoscopic**
  - Endoluminal suturing (overstitch)
  - Through the scope (TTS) clips
  - Over the scope clips (OTSC)
  - Endoscopic vacuum therapy (EVT)—can use in any location
  - Covered metallic stents—most commonly used

- **Surgery—gold standard**
  - In early perforation <24 hours
  - Direct repair—if within 4–6 hours
  - Cervical injury—left-sided approach
  - Thoracic esophagus—right 6th intercostal space approach
  - Distal thoracic—above 8th rib left side
  - Abdominal esophagus—laparotomy
- **In surgery repair**
  - Defect primary suture—in two layers
  - With pleural flap, pericardium

In Selected Cases

- T tube drainage
- Cervical esophagostomy
- Gastrostomy
- Esophagectomy
- **T-Tube Intubation**
  - Partial repair over 6–10 mm T-tube
  - Controlled esophagocutaneous fistula
  - 3 weeks to form mature tract
- In achalasia associated with esophageal perforation, repair of perforation and myotomy on opposite wall of lower esophagus is done

Principles

  - Control infection
  - Drainage
  - Source control
  - Enteral feeding access
- Malignant perforation if unfit for surgery—metallic stent
- Benign disease should use stent with caution—reasons
  - Tissue reaction
  - Inability to remove later
- Biodegradable stents can be considered if perforation is accompanied by obstruction and can act as bridge to later treatment

Benign Perforations

Indications for Non-operative Management

Cameron's **Altorjay** *Criteria*

- Low grade fever/leucocytosis
- Mild pain controlled by opiates
- Absence of systemic sepsis/shock

- Cavity confined to mediastinum
- Drains back into esophagus on contrast radiography

Barotrauma (Spontaneous Perforation, Boerhaave's Syndrome)

- In vomiting against closed glottis or failure to open glottis
- Pressure rises and ruptures at its weakest point at lower third.
- Large volume of material released under pressure.
- Can cause chemical pleuritis—infection and left side effusion

Clinical Features

- Can cause pain in chest and abdomen—DD-MI, DU perforation, pancreatitis
- Dyspnoea
- Abdomen guarding may be there but there may not be any peritoneal contamination
- X-ray chest—pneumomediastinum, pleural effusion, pneumothorax
- CECT
- Mackler triad
  - Thoracic pain
  - Vomiting
  - Subcut emphysema
- Naclerio V sign—pneumomediastinum associated with Boerhaave syndrome, one limb of the V is along the mediastinal border and the other limb along lateral hemidiaphragm
- Treatment: Surgery
  - <24 hours—primary closure
  - >24 hours—resection—cervical esophagostomy—FJ—later reconstruction

Corrosive Injury

- Substances with pH <2 and >12 cause significant damage
- Alkalies are ingested in large quantity as they are tasteless, odourless

Alkalies Cause

- Liquefaction necrosis
- Saponification of fat
- Dehydration of tissue
- Thrombosis of vessels
- Fibrous scarring

Acid Causes

- Coagulative necrosis with eschar
- Coagulant limit deeper penetration in esophagus
- Hydroflouric acid causes liquefactive necrosis—deeper injury.
- Acid causes more gastric damage than alkali because of intense pylorospasm and pooling.
- Electrolyte abnormalities
  - Hypocalcemia (phosphoric, hydrofluoric)
  - Hyponatremia (strong acids, alkalies)
  - Hypokalemia
  - Acidosis
- Injury depends on pH, volume, duration of exposure
- In airway compromise—intubation under bronchoscopic guidance
- Cricothyroidotomy may be needed
- NGA or orogastric tubes—should not be done blindly
- CECT—the choice

Grading for CT findings	
Grade	CT findings
Grade I	No swelling of esophageal wall (<3 mm)
Grade II	Edematous wall thickening (>3 mm) without perioesophageal soft tissue infiltration
Grade III	Edematous wall thickening + perioesophageal soft tissue infiltration + well-demarcated tissue interface
Grade IV	Edematous wall thickening + perioesophageal soft tissue infiltration + blurring of tissue interface OR localised fluid collection around esophagus or descending aorta

- Barium—cause less pneumonitis—if aspirated—but more irritation of pleura and peritoneum
- Water soluble (Gastrografin) more pneumonitis and less pleural and peritoneal irritation.
- Alkali injury phases
  1. Acute necrosis—1–4 days—coagulation of proteins
  2. Ulceration and granulation tissue onset 3–5 days and duration 3–12 days—tissue sloughs
  3. Cicatrization—onset in 3 weeks and duration 1–6 months—adhesion and sloughing—fibrosis

Zargar's Endoscopic Grading

Classification for Caustic ingestion	
Endoscopic finding	*Grade*
Normal	0
Superficial edema/erythema	1
Mucosal/submucosal ulceration	2
Superficial edema/erythema	2A
Deep or circumferential	2B
Transmural ulceration with necrosis	3
Focal	3A
Extensive	3B
Perforation	4

- EUS—limited role in acute injury
- Sucralfate labelled Tc99m—in children
- CECT
  - Suspicion of perforation

Chirica et al—radiological classification

- **Grade 1—normal, correspond-(0-2A)**
- **Grade 2—edema, wall enhancement-(2B-3A) without transmural necrosis**
- **Grade 3—absence of contrast enhancement— transmural necrosis-3B**

- **Corrosive injury—management**
  - Evaluation in OT
  - Early endoscopy is considered in all cases
  - After 48 hours—risk of perforation high
  - Pediatric endoscopes better
  - Endoscopy of esophagus and stomach—not to stop at first sign of injury. Should try to complete the endoscopy
  - Repeat endoscopy 48–72 hours, if needed

Treatment

- No antiemetics
- No early NG tube
- No neutralizing agents
- Steroids only for respiratory injury—no other role— may mask signs of peritonitis/mediastinitis
- PPI—IV—indicated
- Nutrition: Enteral vs TPN

- **Grade 1 and 2a—trial oral, observation**
- **Grade 2b, 3a—NPO, ICU, follow-up endoscopy in 5–7 days**
- **Grade 3b, 4—urgent surgery**

- **Treatment: Chronic phase**
  - Dilatation may have to be repeated
  - Bypass—leaving stricture *in situ*
    - May produce cystic dilatation of esophagus
    - More acid reflux
    - Doubtful cancer
- Antibiotics
- Varies from conservative to surgical
- Jejunostomy, gastrostomy
- Esophagectomy—elective deferred for 3 months— difficult with fibrosis
- >1000 times chance of cancer (lifetime risk <5%)
- 30% of cases develop cancer in injured and non-injured segments, latent period 15 to 40 years
- **Systemic steroids have doubtful role in preventing stricture—may even aggravate injury**

Emergency Surgery—in Peritonitis, Perforation, Hematemesis

- Esophagectomy—transhiatal
- Total gastrectomy
- FJ
- Reconstruction later

Complications

- Bleeding
- Fistula
- Aspiration
- Stricture
  - Most important complication—in 50%
- Endodilatation started about 6–8 weeks after injury
  - Should not wait for symptoms
  - Done every 2–3 weeks
  - Target lumen—14 mm (40F)

Indications for Surgery

Failure to pass guidewire

Refractory stricture—inability to achieve dilatation 14 mm even after 5 sessions 2 weeks apart

Recurrent stricture—inability to maintain luminal diameter for 4 weeks after achieving 14 mm dilatation Long >10 cm stricture

Multiple strictures

- Wait until all strictures have developed to avoid anastomotic stricture

  Ideally 6–12 months

Choice of Conduit

- Stomach:
  - Based on RGA, RGEA
  - Only one anastomosis

Colon

- Right colon
  - Based on MCA
  - Terminal ileum used—isoperistaltic
- Left colon
  - Based on ascending branch of LCA
- Mid-colon
  - Based on LCA
  - Mobilise ileum, right colon, transverse colon and left colon
  - Excess colon excised
  - No tension at anastomosis
- Stomach
  - One anastomosis
  - Results deteriorate with time—reflux, stricture, intestinal metaplasia
- Colon—three anastomosis
  - Function improve with time
  - Lower stricture rate
- Jejunum—when stomach and colon not available
  - Jejunal conduits can reach up to middle or upper mediastinum, then may require free jejunal flaps for anastomosis to pharynx based on ECA and IJV.

1.6 CARCINOMA ESOPHAGUS

- Pathology
  - SCC
  - Adenocarcinoma
  - Leiomyosarcoma
  - Melanoma
  - Metastatic lesions
- Decline in incidence of SCC and increase in adenocarcinoma
- There is a protective role of *H. pylori* for Barrett's and reflux diseases

Adenocarcinoma

- Adenocarcinoma—most common type in West
- Infiltrative type—most common
- Arise in Barrett's

More in

- Males
- Smoking, obesity, GERD
- Familial Barrett's
- GEJ tumors
- Common in achalasia—near air fluid level

Barrett's Esophagus

- Absolute risk of developing Ca in a year—0.12–0.33%

Tylosis

- Also known as focal nonepidermolytic palmoplantar keratoderma
- Autosomal dominant
- Keratosis of palms and soles and esophageal papillomas
- Tylosis esophageal cancer gene—17q25

SCC

- **Most common malignancy type worldwide**
- Can develop in any part of esophagus
- Most common site of Ca—middle third
- Exophytic—fungating—most common

High risk in

- Radiation, achalasia alcohol, smoking, Plummer-Vinson

Other Tumors

- Most common mesenchymal tumor—leiomyosarcoma—<1% of esophageal cancers
- Occurs at lower third
- Bulky with necrosis

Risk factors for the development of esophageal adenocarcinoma and squamous cell carcinoma		
	Adenocarcinoma	*SCC*
Age	High	High
GERD/Barrett's	High	–
H. pylori	Low	?
Male	High	High
NSAIDs	Low	Low
PPIs	High	–
Tobacco	High	High
Caucasian	High	Low
Obesity	High	Low
Low socioeconomic status	Low	High
Fruits and vegetables intake	Low	Low
Alcohol	–	High
Achalasia	High	High
LES relaxants	High	–

- *H. pylori* and Ca esophagus
  - *H. pylori*—reduced gastric acid—reduced reflux
  - *H. pylori*—reduced Ghrelin—reduced appetite—less obesity
  - *H. pylori* especially Cag A protects against adenocarcinoma

Clinical Features

- Progressive dysphagia with food sticking
- Odynophagia/chest pain
- Weight loss
- Hematemesis/melena
- Advanced tumor
  - Hoarseness
  - Diaphragmatic palsy
  - Horner's
  - TEF
  - Spine pain
- Adeno and SCC—together constitute >90%
- Metastasis from melanoma, breast, lung in ca esophagus
- Diagnosis
  - Barium—Apple core
  - Endoscopy
    - Friable ulcers
    - Multiple biopsies taken
    - Note relation with incisor, GEJ
    - Look for Barrett
    - Small lesion—EMR—to assess depth
    - Tumor <5 cm length—likely T1/T2
    - >5 cm length likely T3
    - Stenosis suggestive of advanced stage

EUS: Seen as 5 Layers

- 1: Epithelium and lamina propria (mucosa)—hyperechoic—white
- 2: Muscularis mucosa—hypoechoic—black
- 3: Submucosa—hyperechoic—white
- 4: Muscularis propria—hypoechoic—black
- 5: Periesophageal—hyperechoic
- Tumor—hypoechoic—black
- **Deeper lesions are better delineated**
- Accuracy
  - T_1—75–82%
  - T_2—64–85%
  - T_3—87–94%
  - T_4—100% shows involvement of adjacent structures
  - Accuracy in T1a and T1b cancers is only 20%, where EMR may be better
- **EUS LYMPH NODE ENLARGEMENT**
  1. Poorly defined, diffuse homogenous—benign
  2. Well defined, weak sonoluscent—malignant

3. Well defined with strong internal echoes and notching—malignant

- Hypoechoic, round, width >5–10 mm—malignant

CT

- Normal thickness of **esophagus**—5 mm or less
- For depth of invasion—EUS better
- Better to distinguish T4 from early lesions

CT criteria

- Loss of fat planes
- Adjacent tissue thickening
- Aorta—area of contact >90
- Infiltration
- CT in prone position—better accuracy
- LN assessment—less accurate than EUS
- For small lesions—EMR for further T staging
- EUS has less accuracy for superficial disease

For Larger Lesions

- CECT chest/abdomen
- PET CT for metastases

Staging

Siewert	Description In relation to cardia	Approach
I	Tumor center located between 5 and 1 cm proximal to cardia	Esophageal or EGJ cancer
II	Between 1 cm proximal and 2 cm distal	Esophageal or EGJ cancer
III	Between 2 and 5 cm distal	Stomach cancer

- Siewert and Stein's classification of adenocarcinoma of GEJ

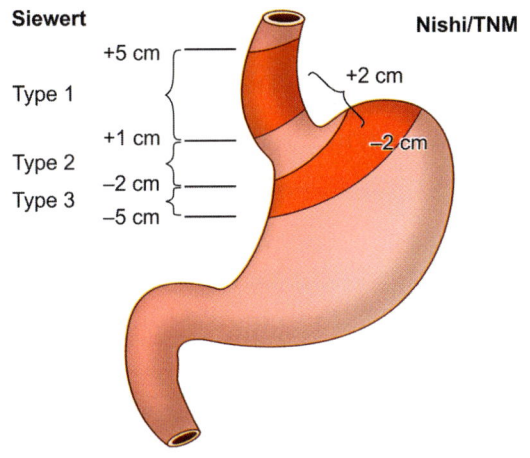

Nishi classification—subclassification of Siewert II

Epicenter 2 cm on either side of EGJ, tumor diameter 4 cm or less, any histology

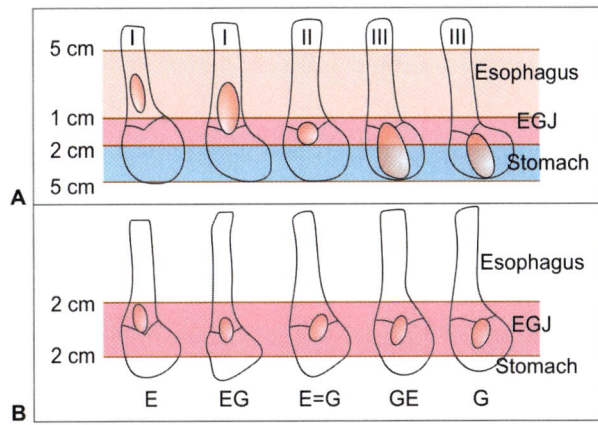

A—Siewert, B—Nishi, E—mainly esophagus

EG—esophageal involving stomach

E = G—Equal, GE—stomach involving esophagus

G—Gastric

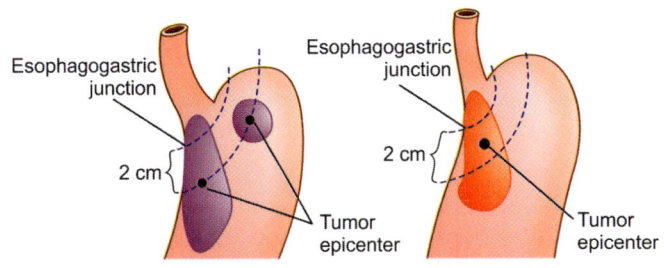

A. Tumor with epicenter located >2 cm from EG junction or a tumor located within 2 cm from EG junction but not involving EG junction classified as stomach cancer. (AJCC)

B. Tumor with epicenter located within 2 cm of EG junction and involves the EG junction is classified as esophageal cancer.

(AJCC 8th Edition)

- SCC and adenocarcinoma—LN mets
  - Confined to mucosa T1a LN mets—0–7%

- Submucosa—T1b 24–50%
- Muscularis propria—T2 >50%
- Transmural T3, T4—72%
- LN involvement—not segmental—but longitudinal

Locoregional nodes include
- **Celiac nodes**
- **Left gastric, CHA, proximal splenic artery nodes**
- **Level 6 and level 7 neck nodes—periesophageal**
- **Anything beyond these—metastatic**

Japanese Esophageal Society—Division of T1 Tumors	
Tx	Depth of invasion (DOI) cannot be assessed
T0	No evidence of primary tumor
T1a	Invades mucosa
T1a-EP	Carcinoma *in situ* (Tis)—formerly corresponds to M1
T1a-LPM	Invades lamina propria mucosa (LPM)—formerly M2
T1a-MM	Invades muscularis mucosa (MM)—formerly corresponds to M3
T1b	Invades submucosa
SM1	Invades upper 3rd of submucosal layer
SM2	Invades middle 3rd of submucosal layer
SM3	Invades lower 3rd of submucosal layer

- T1b SM1 <200 micrometer into submucosa
- T1b SM2 >200 micrometer deep

SCC Grading
- G1: Well differentiated
  - Prominent keratinisation
  - Minor component nonkeratinising basal-like cells
  - Keratin pearls seen
  - Low mitotic count
- G2-MD—most common type
  - Parakeratotic—poorly keratinising
  - Squamous pearls absent
- G3-PD
  - Basal cell like with central necrosis
  - Nests have pavement like arrangement

- Staging investigations
  - Clinical
    - Neck nodes, hoarseness
  - X-ray chest—solitary lesion primary lung
  - Barium studies
  - Endoscopy
  - EMR, ESD—in T1a
    - Limited to epithelium and lamina propria
    - Muscularis mucosa and SM1—relative indications
  - Bronchoscopy
  - CT criteria for evaluation
    - Area of contact with aorta >90–80%—infiltration
    - Thoracic and abdominal LN >1 cm
    - SCLN short axis >.5 cm
    - Retrocrural LN > .6 cm
  - Main use of CT—distant mets
  - EUS—3 probes
    - Radial 360 degree 5–20 MHz
    - EUS microprobes 360 degree, at 12, 20, 30 MHz
    - Curved linear array—for FNAC
    - For celiac nodes—better than CT
- PET scan
  - No value in T staging
  - Adenocarcinoma GEJ and prox stomach—non-avidity (especially poorly differentiated, non-intestinal, mucus containing)
  - SCC—accumulate FDG
  - Juxtatumoral metastasis—poor sensitivity
  - If CT/EUS show no metastais seen, do PET
  - Role of PET is to identify occult metastasis in apparent early disease
  - No value in lesions which have already metastasized
  - In assessing response to therapy—role of PET not clear

- Thoracoscopy—rarely done
- Laparoscopy done for GEJ tumors
- **Post-neoadjuvant Chemo**
  - PET is better than CT or EUS
  - EUS is not recommended

High Grade Dysplasia and Superficial Ca

- Dysplasia—atypical nuclei, mitoses and lack of surface maturation
- More cytological changes—high grade
- Limited to epithelium without invasion of BM, carcinoma *in situ*
- Barrett without dysplasia—annual risk of ca—0.39%
- With low grade dysplasia—0.77%
- Superficial cancers—Ca limited to submucosa
- Early stage cancer—Ca within mucosa without metastasis (TisN0M0, T1aN0M0)

Endoscopic Management

- SCC: High resolution/magnifying endoscopy
- 1–3% Lugols iodine applied—forms glycogen in normal tissue—turns brown, if unstained—pathologic—go for biopsy
- **Early adenocarcinoma in Barrett's**

> **Methods of diagnosis**
> - **High definition white light endoscopy**
> - **Chromoendoscopy**
> - **Narrow band imaging**
> - **Autofluoresence imaging**
> - **Confocal laser endomicroscopy**
> - **Endoscopic optical coherence tomography**

- Seattle biopsy protocol in Barrett
  - 4-quadrant biopsy at 1 cm interval along the whole length of Barrett
  - Also biopsy of any lesions
- **Therapy**
  - RFA: In Barrett and dysplasia
  - Using circumferential balloon or electrical plate using bipolar electrode
  - Transmits RF energy—heat

- Depth of ablation 500 to 1000 micro m
- Ablate epithelium and lamina propria
- Most common complications
  - Chest pain >1 week
  - Stricture (6–8%)
  - Bleeding 1%
- Poor response—<50%
- Regression of Barrett occurs 3 months after circumferential ablation
- **Cryotherapy**
  - Less pain and stricture
  - Probe need not be in contact with tissue
  - Needs close surveillance
  - Acid suppression is needed prior to therapy
  - Repeat endoscopy after 3 months
  - New epithelium develops
  - Small areas can be treated corresponding to 2–3 cm **OR** from one-third to half the circumference.
  - Uses liquid nitrogen or CO_2 gas
  - Most common complication—stricture 3%
- **Early Ca other options**
  - Laser
  - Electrocautery
  - Photodynamic therapy
  - Argon plasma coagulation
- **Disadvantages of ablative procedures**
  - Limited depth
  - No biopsy
- **Endoscopic Mucosal Resection**
  - In nodular raised Barrett and superficial Ca—preferred diagnostic and therapeutic tool
  - Resects whole mucosa down to submucosa
  - T1a—risk of LN mets (depends on size, lymphovascular invasion, differentiation)
  - T1a—lamina propria, muscularis mucosa
  - T1b—more chance of LN involvement so not ideal

- SCC—more LN metastasis
- T1a—with good surgery risk and high risk features—surgery is better
- T1 lesions EUS—not accurate—EMR better
- Larger lesions removed piecemeal
- High dose PPI for healing
- May need multiple procedures
- Endoscopy after 3 months
- FDG PET—no value in follow-up
- Lymph node metastasis in superficial cancer

- T1aEP—Nil
- T1aLPM—3%
- T1aMM—12%
- T1bSM1—30%
- SM3—>50%

EMR recommeneded in
- T1aEP, T1aLPM
- T1aMM and T1bSM1
- T1bSM2, T1bSM3—LN metastasis high, so treated as advanced and surgery preferred
- **EUS not showing LN mets—EMR**

EMR/ESD INDICATIONS		
	EMR	ESD
SCC	Moderate/well differentiated Less than 2/3rd mucosal invasion (M1/M2) Less than 2/3rd esophageal circumference <2.0 cm	Moderate/well differentiated Mucosal invasion at least avoided in circumferential involvement
Adenocarcinoma	Moderate/well differentiated Mucosal invasion T1a <2.0 cm	Moderate/well differentiated Mucosal invasion avoided in circumferential involvement

- **Vagal sparing esophagectomy**
  - In intramucosal T1a
  - Alternative to standard surgery
  - HSV is done in shortened esophagus and stricture

Surgical Treatment of Ca Esophagus

- First resection for Ca esophagus, 1913, Torek—used extracorporeal tube
- First esophagogastrostomy following resection: Oshawa, 1932, Japan

- **Esophagectomy is preferred in**
  - T1b Tumors and above
  - High risk T1a
  - Extensive, multifocal
  - Ulcerated

Conventional approaches to esophageal resection for cancer
Transhiatal (Orringer)
• Laparotomy + cervical approach
• En bloc resection possible in distal tumors
• Peritumoral/2 field nodal dissection
• Cervical anastomosis
Transthoracic
• **Ivor Lewis**
– Right thoracotomy + laparotomy
– Peritumoral or 2-field nodal dissection
– En bloc resection possible for middle/distal thoracic tumors
• **McKeown** or 3 hole
– Right thoracotomy + laparotomy + cervical approach
– Peritumoral, 2 or 3 field nodal dissection
– En bloc resection possible for middle/distal thoracic tumors
• **Left thoracotomy**
– With or without cervical approach
– Peritumoral lymph nodes dissection
– Intrathoracic/cervical anastomosis
• **Left thoracoabdominal**
– Peritumoral/2 field nodal dissection
– Intrathoracic anastomosis

- Extended esophagectomy
  - Mid and lower third lesions—esophagus, adjacent pleura, pericardium, esophageal hiatus, azygos vein, thoracic duct with two or three field lymphadenectomy dissection
- Optimum lymphadenectomy
  - No agreed consensus on optimal number LN to be resected
  - T1—optimum 10 LN
  - T2—20 LN
  - T3 or T4 >30 LN
  - Three field—cervical, thoracic and abdominal
- Two field lymphadenectomy
  - Standard—abdominal and thoracic up to carina
  - Extended—also dissection around recurrent laryngeal nerve on one side
  - Total—dissection around both recurrent laryngeal nerves

- Tumor location
  - Upper and mid-thoracic tumor—cervical LN dissection
  - In lower thoracic esophageal Ca—involvement of RLN nodes—indication for cervical LN dissection. Otherwise—two fields
  - In palpable cervical LN: Neck dissection not recommended
  - GE junction tumor extending more on to esophagus—abdominal and mediastinal nodes dissected
  - Extending more on to stomach—mediastinal nodes are not dissected
- In SCC—two-field dissection—upper abdomen + dissection of inferior and superior mediastinum along RLN
- In adenocarcinoma—two fields—upper abdomen celiac + inferior mediastinum up to carina
- Abdominal lymph node dissection—superior gastric, celiac (LGA, SplA) and common hepatic beyond this considered as metastatic nodes
- Intramural spread distally to abdominal nodes greater for adenocarcinoma (54%)
  - SCC—10%
- Cervical dissection
  - Along both RLN
  - Deep external—lateral to IJV
  - Deep internal—RLN
  - Deep lateral—along spinal accessory—rare
  - RO resection should be the aim
  - R1—microscopic transection or within 1 mm
  - *Marginal or apical node*—LN near resection margin most distant from tumor

Conduits

- Stomach—most commonly used
- Left colon based on ascending branch of LCA—iso-peristaltic
- Jejunum is used if short segment
- Gastric tube—vascularity 60% based on RGE and remaining on collaterals
- Cervical anastomosis higher leak 2–26%
- Thoracic leak—0–9.3% but higher mortality

Lerut Classification of Anastomotic Leak

Leak	Definition	Treatment
Major clinical	Severe disruption on endoscopy/sepsis	Change management: CT guided drainage
Minor clinical	X-ray contained leak (thoracic anastomosis)	Delay oral intake
	Fever, leucocytosis, raised CRP	Antibiotics
	Cervical wound inflammation	Drain wound
Radiological	No clinical signs	No change in treatment
Conduit necrosis	Endoscopic confirmation	Reintervention necessary

- For leaks
  - Covered metallic stents
  - Intracavitary vacuum therapy
- Stricture
  - 10–40% incidence
  - Two-layer anastomosis—more stricture
  - Circular stapler—more stricture

Right vs left colon grafts		
	Right colon graft	*Left colon graft*
Advantages	Caecum—large capacity	Smaller diameter
	Ileum and esophagus have similar diameters	Better blood supply
	Bauhin valve prevents regurgitation	Good length
Disadvantages	Variable anatomy of blood vessels Increased regurgitation frequency Large, bulky caecum	Chance for inferior Meseneteric artery atherosclerosis

Routes of conduit anastomosis

- Posterior mediastinal—shortest route
- Transhiatal—no chest opening
- Left or right transthoracic by VATS—more lung problem

- Substernal—long route and angulation
- Subcutaneous—easy dissection but cosmetically not good

Locally Advanced Ca

- Majority have dysphagia and are T3 lesions and LN metastasis in 80%
- For GEJ adenocarcinoma—LN from celiac axis to paratracheal are regional. Outside this considered distant
- For SCC of midesophagus—periesophageal cervical lymph nodes considered regional

Radiation

- Neoadjuvant—20–40 Gy
- Adjuvant—40–60 Gy

Chemotherapy

- Platins with 5 FU

Neo Adjuvant CT/CRT

- North American Intergroup Trial (INT 0113)—showed no benefit
- Medical Research Council (MRC), UK showed benefit in CT with surgery
- MAGIC (MRC Adjuvant Gastric Infusional Chemotherapy)—showed benefit

Chemoradiation Alone

- T3, T4 tumors
- 50.4 Gy concomitantly with chemo—definitive dose

CRT with Surgery

- CROSS trial (Chemo Radiotherapy for Oesophageal Cancer followed by Surgery Study)—showed benefit in CRT group

Target Therapy

- Trastuzumab
- Bevacizumab

Treatment Recommendations

- Stage T1a and limited T1b—EMR, ESD
- Stage 1, 2, 3—esophagectomy is appropriate
- Stage 2 and 3—definitive chemo RT an option
  - In unfit patients
  - SCC at or above carina
  - May be followed by surgery
- Stage 2B and 3—preop chemo RT beneficial
- Postop chemo RT—reserved for adenocarcinoma of GEJ
- Stage 4—clinical trials, chemotherapy

1.7 BENIGN TUMORS AND CYSTS

- Sussius 1559—first description about leiomyoma
- First pathologic description of same Virchow, 1863
- First open surgical removal—Oshawa, 1933

Clinical Features

- Asymptomatic
- Intraluminal obstruction
- Extraluminal extension with involvement of other structures
- Regurgitation of pedunculated polyp
- Ulceration and bleeding
- Dysphagia most common symptom—still rare
- Dysphagia incidence—0.075 to 0.14%
- Cysts—rarely symptomatic
- Cough, wheezing, infection, bleeding
- Benign—18%
- Malignant—82%
- **Diagnosis**
  - Barium
  - X-ray chest
  - Endoscopy
  - CT
  - EUS
- **Intramural/Extramucosal**
  - Mesenchymal tumors

- Leiomyoma
- GIST
- Schwannoma
- Common cell of origin

Esophageal mesenchymal tumors			
Features	Schwannoma	Leiomyoma	GIST
Histology	Moderate cellularity with peripheral lymphoid cuff Presence of spindle cells	Eosinophilic cytoplasm	High rate of cellularity
Molecular genetic markers	+S–100, GFAP –CD117, CD34, SMA	+ Desmin, SMA-CD117, CD34	+ CD117, CD34
Sex M:F	1:1	2:1	2:1
Mean age (y)	55	36	62
Malignant potential	Lowest	Mixed	Highest

GFAP—Glial Fibrillary Acidic Protein

- Leiomyoma—most common
- Schwannoma—least common
  - Lowest malignant potential
- GIST: Highest malignant potential
  - Large tumor—more malignant
- Origin—interstitial cell of Cajal

Leiomyoma of Esophagus

- Two-thirds of all benign tumors (60–70%)
- Esophageal cancer is 50 times more common than leiomyoma
- Age—30–50
- M:F 2:1
- Most common site lower third—intramurally (46%)
- Can occur as intraluminal and extraluminal mass
- Firm, rubbery encapsulated, intact mucosa
- Usually 5–10 cm
- >1000 g—termed giant
- Histology—spindle cells in whorls or fascicles
- Mostly single—97%
- Rarely leiomyomatosis
- Can originate from muscularis mucosa, muscularis propria or submucosa

- 0.2% malignant transformation—sarcoma
- Conditions associated
  - Hiatal hernia
  - Diverticulum
  - Achalasia
- Motility disorders due to Cajal cell
- 12% of all GIT leiomyoma in esophagus
- 0.4 to 1% of all esophagus tumors

Syndromes and Leiomyoma

- Li-Fraumeni—p53 mutation
  - Sarcoma, breast cancer, brain cancer, esophageal leiomyomas
- Alport's syndrome—X-linked recessive
  - Sensory neural deafness, ocular abnormalities, multiple site leiomyomas

Diagnosis

- Plain X-ray:
  - Mediastinal mass
  - Punctate calcification in posterior mediastinum

Barium

- Crescent shaped—half in wall—half in lumen
- Mass—wall junction—sharp—90 degree
- No obstruction
- Overlying mucosa intact smooth, stretched
- Mucosa of opposite wall—intact
- Proximal dilatation—unusual
- Near GE junction may impair emptying
- May cause dilatation—like achalasia
- CT eccentric tumors
- FDG PET—abnormal uptake—still benign
  - Only 8.3% PET avid esophageal lesions are malignant
- **Endoscopy**
  - Segmental
  - Intact mucosa
  - Narrowing of lumen without obstruction
  - Movable mass
  - Rarely ulceration

- **EUS**
  - Leiomyoma from 4th layer—muscularis propria
  - Rarely 2nd layer—muscularis mucosa
- EUS pattern
  - Hypoechoic
  - Homogenous
  - Well demarcated
  - No LNE
  - >4 cm—atypical
- EUS-FNA
  - Indicated
    - \>2 cm
    - Rapid growth
    - PET avid
    - Sensitivity—95%, specificity—100%

RICE Classification

Correlation between endosonographic layer and pathology		
EUS layer	*Esophageal tumor*	*Esophageal cyst*
1st/2nd layer (mucosa and deep mucosa)	Fibrovascular polyp Squamous papilloma Granular cell tumor	Retention cyst
3rd layer (submucosa)	Fibroma Neurofibroma Granular cell tumor Lipoma	
4th layer (muscularis propria)	Leiomyoma	Cysts and duplications
5th		Cysts and duplications

Leiomyoma of Esophagus

Treatment

- Observation
  - <2 cm
  - Extramucosal—intramural
  - No LNE
  - Asymptomatic
- EUS every 1–2 years
- CT as indicated
- Resection is considered when
  - Symptomatic
  - Larger size
  - Mucosal erosion

  - LNE
  - Tumor growth

Surgery

- Lower third lesion—left thoracotomy
- Proximal lesion—right thoracotomy
- GE junction laparotomy/transhiatal
- After splitting the muscle, enucleation is done. Mucosa is not opened.
- Lap/thoracoscopic
- Robotic
- Combined endoluminal intracavitary thoracoscopic enucleation
- Laparoscopic—transgastric or intragastric
- Balloon push out technique
  - Thoracoscopy done with endoscopy and balloon inflated from inside
- Intraluminal—endoscopy-polypectomy
- Banding of tumor
- Electrocautery
- Esophagectomy in 10% indicated in large (>8 cm), multiple
- In children
  - Rarely before 10
  - Common in girls
  - Diffuse in 91%
  - Dysphagia—most common symptom
  - Treatment—esophagectomy
  - Mortality high—21%
- **GIST**
  - Age >40
  - Slightly more common in males
  - Stomach—most common site
  - <5% in esophagus (1%)
  - Most are benign
  - Most common site—lower third since more cells of Cajal present.
  - If >2 cm—prompt staging work up is required—
    - CT chest, abdomen, pelvis
    - PET
    - EUS-FNA
  - Malignant
    - Mitoses 5–10/HPF
    - Size >10 cm
- **Surgery indications**
  - >2 cm

– Symptomatic patients

– Growth occurring under observation

– In high-risk cases—surgery even if <2 cm

– Small are enucleated

– Larger—adherent to mucosa—esophagectomy

– Imatinib/sunitinib—experience limited in esophagus

– **Prognosis of GIST esophagus worse than other organs**

- **Organ sparing surgery preferred**
- **Lymphadenectomy—not indicated—unless pathologically positive nodes**
- **If multiple organs involved—multiorgan resection—not the first line of treatment**
- **Re-resection of microscopically positive margins—not indicated**
- **Resection of metastasis—not indicated—except for palliation**

Schwannoma

- Age 47–62
- No gender predominance
- Tan masses, firm, rubbery
- Cajal cell origin
- Histology—cellular, peripheral rim of lymphoid cells
- Some have melanin pigmentation
- Stomach—60%—most common among GIT
- Esophagus: 5%
- In esophagus—occur proximally—can cause tracheal compression if large
- Benign lesions also uptake PET
- Treatment
  – Observation
  – Resection of tumor
  – Similar to leiomyoma
  – Larger size—more malignant

Granular Cell Tumor

- Also known as granular cell myoblastoma
- Rare submucosal tumor
- Most commonly in submucosa of tongue (40%), GIT (5%)

- Of GIT—one-third in esophagus
- Most are benign, isolated
- Malignant 2–3%
- Cell of origin—neural cells
- Stain for S-100 and neuron-specific enolase
- Only 1–2% found in esophagus
- Of this, 60% are seen in distal esophagus
- When esophagus is involved that is the only organ in most cases.
- Mucosa intact and translucent, therefore, appears as if it is absent
- Mucosa shows pseudoepitheliomatous hyperplasia
- Features of malignancy
  – >4 cm, rapid growth, recurrence
  – Local invasion and mets seen in malignant
- Clinical features—similar to leiomyoma
- Investigations
  – Barium
  – Endoscopy—yellow molar-shaped polypoid lesion
  – EUS—hyperechoic solid mass surrounded by hypoechoic submucosa without continuity to muscularis propria
- Treatment
  – Similar to leiomyoma
  – Observation, endoscopic, laser

Hemangioma

- Rare 3% of all benign esophageal tumors
- In Rendu-Osler-Weber syndrome—multiple lesions are seen
- Submucosal
- Middle or lower third
- Non-circumferential
- May cause dysphagia, pain and bleeding
- Barium—submucosal lesions
- Endoscopy—bluish lesions
- Biopsy is not done
- CECT—useful

- Treatment
  - Endoscopic resection
  - YAG laser
  - Sclero/RT
  - Surgery

Other Rare Tumors
- Lipomas and fibroma
  - Usually intraluminal
  - Submucosal also
- **Pseudotumors**
  - Due to submucosal inflammation
  - Any where in esophagus
  - Due to perforation, postop healing, autoimmune, subclinical infection
  - Submucosal location
  - Contain fibroblasts and blood vessels
  - Treatment: Steroids and surgery
- **Intraluminal/mucosal lesions**

  Fibrovascular polyp

  - Second most common benign esophageal tumor
  - Most common intraluminal tumor
  - Fibromas, fibrolipomas, myomas, myxofibromas
  - Origin—arise as thickening in submucosa—elongate into lumen due to peristalsis and form polyp
  - Most common site proximal just distal to cricopharyngeus (80%)
  - May reach stomach
  - Pathology
    - Esophageal dilatation
    - More in males—older
    - Contain fibrous tissue, fat, and vascular tissues
    - Covered by mucosa
    - No malignant change
- Clinical features
  - Dysphagia
  - Regurgitation—asphyxia
  - Bleeding into stomach—anemia

Investigation
- Barium—filling defect moving in the lumen
- Endoscopy may miss the lesion
- EUS—echodense lesion
- CT indicated

Treatment
- Resection—open surgical/endoscopic—fear of airway compromise
- Esophagotomy on opposite wall of tumor
- If polyp base not removed—recurrence possible

Squamous Papilloma
- Rare
- Males
- Associated with GERD, HPV
- Solitary in distal esophagus
- Most are <1 cm
- Asymptomatic
- Treated by endoscopic resection
- Can recur/spread after endoscopic fulguration—extreme care must be taken

Cysts and Duplications
Arbona et al

Classification of esophageal cysts
Acquired
• Retention (single/multiple)
Congenital
• Duplication
• Bronchogenic
• Gastric
• Inclusion
Other
• Neuroenteric

- 10–15% of GI duplications occur in esophagus
- More diagnosed in males and children
- Account for 0.5 to 3.3% of all benign tumors of esophagus.

Congenital origin
- Foregut lined by ciliated columnar epithelium—filling lumen—later vacuoles develop—canalize—some vacuoles form cysts/duplication

Hutchinson and Thomson Theory
- Endodermal tube destined to form foregut is part of yolk sac or archenteron

- Archenteronic cysts—some part may get separated
- **Palmer's pathologic criteria for duplication cysts**
  - Localised within esophageal wall
  - Covered by two muscular layers
  - Lined by squamous epithelium or embryonic (pseudostratified, ciliated columnar)
- **Duplication cysts**
  - More common on right side—due to elongation of viscera and dextrorotation of stomach
  - More commonly of cystic form (80%)—without communication to lumen
  - Tubular form (20%)—communicate with lumen
  - Wall contains only smooth muscle—no cartilage unlike bronchogenic cysts
- **Clinical features**
  - Cough, wheezing
  - Dysphagia, substernal pain
  - GERD
- **Investigations**
  - Barium and OGD—submucosal mass
  - CT/MRI
- **Treatment**—observation, aspiration, resection
  - Resection:
    - □ To control symptoms
    - □ Increase in size
    - □ To exclude malignancy
  - Open/thoracoscopic/lap
  - Tc 99 scan may be positive in duplication cysts if they contain gastric mucosa
  - Rarely can turn malignant
  - EUS FNA—avoided in anechoic, may be considered in hypoechoic lesions
- **Bronchogenic cyst**
  - Abnormality of lung bud separation
  - Sequestration
  - In esophageal wall
  - Contains cartilage
  - Middle and lower thirds

- Not associated with vertebral anomalies
- No neoplastic changes
- **Gastric cysts**
  - Cells forming stomach fail to descend
  - Located in esophageal wall
  - Contain muscular wall
  - Lined by gastric mucosa
  - Can produce ulceration—bleeding
- **Inclusion cysts**
  - Contain respiratory or squamous epithelium
  - Intramural
  - Do not contain cartilage or muscle compared to duplication cyst/bronchogenic
- **Neuroenteric cysts**
  - Also known as posterior mediastinum duplication cysts
  - Arise during notochord separation from foregut
  - Endodermal diverticulum remain attached and develop into cyst
  - Covered by muscle
  - Lined by GI mucosa
  - 'Split notochord syndrome'—neuroenteric cyst with vertebral anomalies—may not be at the same level as cyst
- **Other cystic lesions**
  - Mucosal and submucosal glands—coalesce—acquired cyst—if multiple—esophagitis cystica
  - More common in upper esophagus
  - Size varies from few mm to 3 cm

Investigations of Choice
- Motility disorders—manometry
- GERD—24-hour pH, manometry
- Diverticula—barium swallow
- Perforation—thin barium emulsion
- Corrosive poison—esophagoscopy and stent
- Caustic stricture—EUS
- Cancer—endoscopy

Stomach

2.1 ANATOMY

- Following birth—stomach is the most proximal abdominal organ
- Most proximal portion of stomach—cardia
- Incisura on lesser curvature—junction between body and antrum
- Angle between fundus and left margin of esophagus—angle of His
- Anteriorly covered by—left lateral segment of liver

Stomach has Three Muscle Layers

- Outer longitudinal—incomplete and present near lesser and greater curvature
- Middle circular—*only complete layer*—blends with LES and pylorus—forms pyloric sphincter
- Innermost—oblique—incomplete along anterior and posterior walls
- Strongest layer—submucosa
- At body and fundus—dominated by acid secreting oxyntic glands
- Oxyntic glands contain
  - Surface epithelial cells
  - Mucous cells
  - Parietal cells: HCL
  - Zymogenic (chief) cells: Intrinsic factor and pepsinogen
  - Enterochromaffin like cells (ECL)
- Distal antrum and cardia lack acid producing cells
  - Antrum—contains gastrin secreting (G) cells

Types, location and function of gastric cells

Cell type	Function	Location
Parietal	Secretes acid and intrinsic factor	Body
Mucus	Mucus	Body, antrum
Chief	Pepsin	Body
Surface epithelial	Mucus, bicarbonate, prostaglandins	Diffuse
Enterochromaffin like	Histamine	Body
D	Somatostatin	Body, antrum
G	Gastrin	Antrum
Gastric mucosal interneurons	Gastrin releasing peptide	Body, antrum
Enteric neurons	Calcitonin gene-related peptide	Diffuse
Endocrine	Ghrelin	Body

Gastrin

- From G cells antrum
- G34: Big gastrin—predominates in circulation—long half life
- G17: Little gastrin—90% of the released gastrin
- G14: Mini gastrin
- Gastrin and CCK similar, differ by tyrosine sulfation site
- Has trophic effect on parietal and ECL cells

Hypergastrinemia, cause

Nonulcerogenic causes	Ulcerogenic causes
Antisecretory agents (PPIs)	Antral G cell hyperplasia hyperfunction
Atrophic gastritis	Retained excluded antrum
Pernicious anemia	Zollinger-Ellison syndrome
Acid-reducing procedure (vagotomy)	Gastric outlet obstruction
Helicobacter pylori infection Chronic renal failure	Short-gut syndrome

Somatostatin

- 14 or 28 amino acid peptide
- In stomach 14 amino acid predominate
- Produced by neuroendocrine cells from fundus and antrum
- Paracrine actions on secretion of acid and gastrin
- Action
  - Direct inhibition of parietal cell
  - Through gastrin
- Through ECL—histamine

Gastrin Releasing Peptide

- Bombesin prepared from skin of *Bombina bombina* (European fire bellied frog)
- Mammalian counterpart GRP

- Prominent in nerve endings in acid secreting portions
- Stimulate gastrin release by binding to G cells
- Stimulate somatostatin and D cells
- Peripheral administration—increases acid secretion
- Central administration—reduces acid

Blood Supply

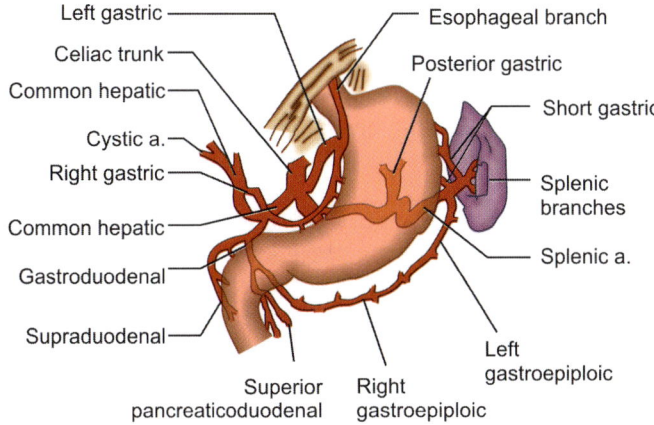

- Also by inferior phrenic artery—proximally
- Short gastric arteries—from splenic artery
- Largest branch—left gastric artery
- Aberrant left hepatic artery from LGA—in 15–20%
- Stomach survives even if 3 of the 4 arteries ligated but arcades must be preserved.
- Left gastric vein (coronary vein) and right gastric veins—drain into portal vein
- Right gastroepiploic vein to SMV
- LGEV to splenic vein
- Major named arteries of stomach travel longitudinally within peritoneal leave except **short gastric arteries.**
- **Posterior gastric A—a branch of splenic artery**

Lymphatics

Station description of lymph node location	
1	Right cardia
2	Left cardia
3	Lesser curvature of stomach
4sa	Short gastric vessels
4sb	Left gastroepiploic vessels
4d	Right gastroepiploic vessels
5	Supra-pyloric
6	Infra-pyloric
7	Left gastric artery
8a	Common hepatic artery (anterosuperior group)
8p	Common hepatic artery (posterior group)
9	Celiac artery
10	Splenic hilum
11p	Proximal splenic artery
11d	Distal splenic artery
12a	Hepatoduodenal ligament (along the hepatic artery)
12b	Hepatoduodenal ligament (along the bile duct)
12p	Hepatoduodenal ligament (behind the portal vein)
13	Posterior surface of pancreatic head
14v	Superior mesenteric vein
14a	Superior mesenteric artery
15	Middle colic vessels
16a1	Aortic hiatus
16a2	Abdominal aorta (from celiac trunk to left renal vein)
16b1	Abdominal aorta (from left renal vein to inferior mesenteric artery)
16b2	Abdominal aorta (from inferior mesenteric artery to aortic bifurcation)
17	Anterior surface of head of pancreas
18	Inferior margin of pancreas
19	Infra-diaphragmatic
20	Esophageal hiatus of diaphragm
110	Paraesophageal in lower thorax
111	Supra-diaphragmatic
112	Posterior mediastinal

- They follow the blood vessels and extensive submucosal plexus

Innervation

- Para sympathetic—via vagus
- Sympthetic—via-celiac plexus
- Left vagus—anterior, right posterior (LARP)
- Left vagus (anterior) gives off hepatic branch and then continues as anterior nerve of latarjet.
- Right vagus (posterior)—first branch criminal nerve of grassi
  – Gives off celiac branch
- Most vagal fibers (90%)—are afferent
- Efferent fibers from dorsal nucleus of medulla—synapse with neurons in myenteric and submucosal plexus
- Acetylcholine is the neurotransmitter
- Influences gastric motor and secretory function
- Sympathetics from T5 to T10—splanchnic nerve—celiac ganglion—efferents
- Auerbach and myenteric plexuses—intrinsic nervous system

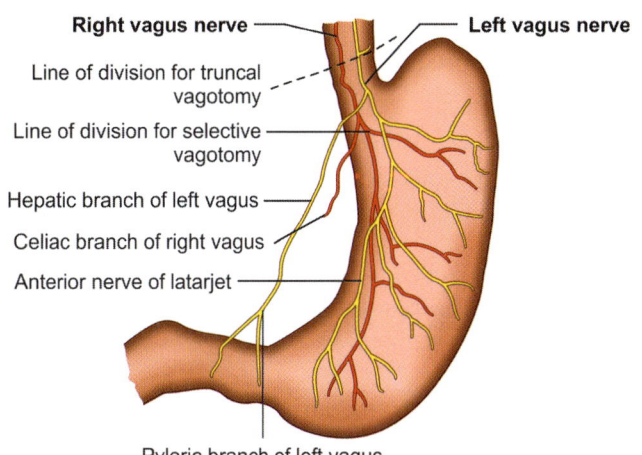

Histamine
- Stored in acid granules of ECL and mast cells
- H2B—completely abolishes gastric acid secretion in response to gastrin and A choline
- Release is stimulated by gastrin. Acetylcholine, epinephrine
- Somatostatin inhibits: Gastrin stimulated H2 release

Ghrelin
- 28 amino acid peptide—'hunger hormone'
- Also known as 'lenomorelin'
- Orexigenic (appetite stimulating)
- From endocrine cells of oxyntic mucosa (fundus and body)
- Anabolic hormone
- Upregulated in times of negative energy
- Downregulated in positive energy balance
- Role in obesity surgery
- Induces release of GH from pituitary

Acid Secretion
- Basal secretion—10% of maximal output
- Basal—1 to 5 mmol/hr of HCl
- H2B and vagotomy reduce basal output

Cephalic Phase
- Mediated by vagus and acetylcholine.
- Responsible for 20–30% acid secretion

Gastric Phase
- Due to—distension and gastrin
  - Food in antrum—distention—gastrin release—pyloro-oxyntic reflex
- Total acid in gastric phase—60–70%
- Distension causes 30–40% of maximum acid output
- Remainder—gastrin related

Intestinal Phase
- Not gastrin mediated
- Mediated by entero-oxyntin-peptide hormone
- Contributes 10% acid secretion
- *Parietal cell has the largest mitochondrial area among all mammalian cells—34% of cell volume*
- This is due to the need for high energy ATP for the H-K ATPase pump
- There are more than 1 billion parietal cells in stomach
- Each parietal cell secretes 3.3 billion H^+ ions/sec

Gastric Acid Secretion
- More in DU, gastrinoma
- Reduced in GU, pernicious anemia, atrophic gastritis, cancer
- Reduced secretion seen in proximal GU
- Distal antral and prepyloric ulcers—secretion similar to DU

Acid: Functions
- Helps digestion
- Converts pepsinogen to pepsin
- Causes release of secretin from duodenum
- Limits colonization of bacteria

Drugs
- H2 blockers
  - Most potent—famotidine

PPI
- Cause irreversible inhibition of proton pump
- For recovery—new pumps to be formed
- They are weak acids
- They increase serum gastrin and can cause carcinoids.

Gastric Juice
- Mixture of secretions of parietal cell, chief cell and mucus cells, duodenal secretions and saliva
- Parietal cell solution pH 0.8
- Lowest intraluminal pH in stomach is 2
  - Due to mixture of secretions

Intrinsic Factor
- 60 kDa mucoprotein
- Secreted by parietal cells
- For absorption of vitamin B_{12} in terminal ileum
- PPI do not block IF secretion
- Deficient in pernicious anemia and total gastrectomy

Pepsinogen
- Pepsinogen 1
  - From chief cells and mucous neck cells in the acid secreting portion
- Pepsinogen 2
  - From surface epithelium of acid secreting stomach, antrum and duodenum and also gastrin secreting mucosa.
- Converted to pepsin with acid
- Inactivated at pH>5
- Group 2 is active over a higher pH—involved in stress GU

Mucus and Bicarbonate
- Neutralise acid
- Secreted by surface mucous cells and mucous neck cells of acid secreting and antral portions
- Mucus
  - Mechanical barrier
  - Impediment to ion movement
  - Impermeable to pepsin
  - Secretion stimulated by vagus, cholinergics, PG
  - Inhibited by NSAIDs.
- *H. pylori* produces proteases and lipases—breakdown mucous layer

Gastric Motility
Fasting State
- Pacemaker—situated at mid-body greater curvature
- Slow wave 3 cycles/minute

- Also electrical spikes
- Both together constitute myoelectric migratory complex
- Lasts 90–120 minutes
- Clears stomach
- These activities are intact after vagotomy

Postprandial State
- Receptive relaxation and accommodation
- Mediated via vagus
- Mixes food to less than 1 mm size
- Liquids empty faster
- Carbohydrate empty faster than fat
- Hot and cold food empty slower than ambient temperature
- Increased concentration or acidity of liquid meals cause slower emptying
- These responses of luminal stimuli are regulated by enteric nervous system
- Also by the pH sensitive receptors of SI which cause feedback inhibition of gastric emptying
- Gastric emptying inhibitors are
  - CCK, glucagon, VIP, GIP

2.2 PEPTIC ULCER DISEASE
- Peptic ulcer—erosion in gastric or duodenal mucosa that extends into the muscularis mucosa
- Prevalence—4%
- 20% having asymptomatic ulcers
- Reduced incidence—due to better *H. pylori* treatment
  - DU reduction in incidence is more

Pathogenesis
- **Increased aggressive factors**
  - HCl, pepsin, ethanol, NSAID, bile reflux, ischemia
  - *H. pylori*
- **Reduced defensive factors**
  - Bicarbonate mucin, blood flow, PG, growth factors, cell renewal

H. pylori
- Associated with 80–95% DU
  - 75–80% GU
- Spiral/helical gram negative, micro aerophilic rod with 4–6 flagella (lophotrichous—multiple flagella on one side)
- Resides in gastric type epithelium, beneath mucuos layer—protected from acid
- Produces urease—splits urea into ammonia and bicarbonate and creates microalkaline environment
- *Campylobacter pylori* renamed *H. pylori* in 1989
- They can live only in gastric mucosa
- Also in heterotopic gastric mucosa in Barrett's esophagus, Meckel's diverticulum, gastric metaplasia duodenum, ectopic gastric mucosa in rectum

Mechanisms of *H. pylori* Injury
1. Production of toxic products ammonia, cytotoxins, phospholipase, platelet activating factor
2. Local immune and inflammatory reaction
3. *H. pylori* induced reduction in D cells and somatostatin which causes increased gastrin and acid secretion
4. Hyperacidity in duodenum—gastric metaplasia—further colonisation with *H. pylori* causing duodenitis and ulceration
5. Inflammation causes cytokine production: IL-8, IL-17, IL-18.

- Associated with antral gastritis
- Marshal and Warren won Nobel Prize in 2005 for their work on *H. pylori*
- Infection acquired in childhood
- More in low socioeconomic group
- Weak association with nonulcer dyspepsia
- Association with Ca stomach and MALTomas
- Eradication drastically reduces ulcer recurrence
- For diagnosis—evaluation for serum antibodies is test of choice if endoscopy is not done but remains positive after eradication
- To monitor treatment efficacy—serum antigen or urea breath test will be better
- In DU—maximum inflammation in antral region
- GU inflammation in body and antrum and acid secreting parietal cells are affected, thereby causing reduced acid

NSAIDs
- Risk of bleeding and ulcer—proportional to daily dosage
- Higher age, anticoagulants—more risk
- Absorbed through stomach and SI

- Systemic inhibition of cyclo-oxygenase—the rate limiting step in PG synthesis
- Ulcers are more in stomach, which are not associated with chronic gastritis
- When discontinued—ulcers do not recur
- Low dose aspirin (75 mg) can cause GU (dose dependent)
- PPI can reduce the ulcer

Acid

- Noncausative in ulcer
- 70% DU have normal acid range
- Types I and IV GU—no acid excess
- Types II and III GU—acid hypersecretion seen—behave more like DU

Duodenal Ulcer

- Caused by:
  - Acid, pepsin
  - *H. pylori*—>90% association
  - NSAIDs
- Pain—episodic, seasonal
- Relieved by food
- Radiation to back due to penetration of pancreas

DU: Diagnosis

- GI contrast study
- Single contrast—50% ulcers missed
- Double contrast—80–90% detected
- Endoscopy—gold standard
- *H. pylori* testing
- Invasive
  - Urease in biopsy
  - Sensitivity 90%
  - Specificity: 95–100%
  - Almost never false positive
- Sensitivity changed by H2B, PPI, antibiotics
- Rapid urease—result in 1 hour
- Histology
  - Visualising bacteria
  - Stains—H and E
  - Special stains—silver, giemsa, genta
  - sensitivity 95%, sp—99%
  - More accurate
- Culture—Skirrow's medium—takes 3–5 days

Noninvasive Tests

- Serology—IgG antibody tested—ELISA
  - Remains high for 1 year
  - So not good to assess treatment efficacy

- Urea breath test
  - Carbon labelled urea
  - performed 4 weeks after treatment
- Stool antigen
  - Most cost effective method to assess treatment efficacy

- Best noninvasive investigation to diagnose—ELISA
- Best to diagnose eradication—C13, C14 urea breath tests—after 4 weeks of therapy
- Best invasive test—after endoscopy—rapid urease
- Fecal antigen test—to confirm cure

Treatment

- Antacids are best taken 1 hour after a meal
  - On empty stomach antacids are emptied fast
- Sucralfate
  - Structurally similar to heparin—no anticoagulant action
  - Binds with protein and produce coating
  - Induce fibroblast growth
  - Action lasts 4–6 hours
- PPI
  - Work in acidic environment
  - Don't use H2B or antacids with PPI

Treatment of *H. pylori*

- *H. pylori* associated with DU >95%
- Antibiotics with antacids
- Antacids promote early healing.
- *H. pylori* eradication—eradicate recurrence
- Resistance to therapy seen in 20%
- Evaluation after 4–6 weeks with urea breath test/endoscopy

DU Complications

- In 20% PUD—complications
  - Hemorrhage
  - Perforation
  - Obstruction
  - Intractable ulcer (rare)

Hemorrhage

- Most common complication of PUD
- 70% nonvariceal hemorrhage due to—PUD

- Most bleeding stops by itself—80 to 85%
- Persistent bleeding—6–8% mortality

Blatchford score
- Predict need for intervention
- Blood transfusion
- Endoscopy
- Surgery
- Score> zero—99% sensitivity to predict intervention

Parameters considered are
- Blood urea
- Hb
- Systolic BP
- Others—pulse rate, melena, syncope, liver disease, heart failure
Scores—0, 1, 2, 3, 4, 6

- Uses clinical variables and upper GIscopy
- Predicts risk of rebleeding and mortality

Rockall clinical prediction score (0–3)
Variables are:
- Age
- Systolic bp
- Comorbidities
- Diagnosis
- Stigmata of recent hemorrhage

Forrest Classification: Endoscopic findings, rebleeding risks	
Classification	Rebleeding risk
Grade 1a: Active, pulsatile bleeding	High
Grade 1b: Active, nonpulsatile bleeding	High
Grade 2a: Nonbleeding visible vessel	High
Grade 2b: Adherent clot	Intermediate
Grade 2c: Black dot	Low
Grade 3: No signs of recent bleed	Low

Management
- IV access
- NG tube lavage
  - As a predictor for high risk patients
  - Aids for later OGD by removing blood
  - Bright red blood indicates high risk for rebleeding which warrants endoscopic intervention
  - Coffee ground caries less risk
- Upper GIscopy is done within 24 hours
- Endoscopic hemostasis achieved in 90% methods:
  - Epinephrine with thermal or clips or monotherapy with clips or thermal therapy
  - Epinephrine as a mono therapy is not advisable
- If rebleeding occurs in stable patients, re-endoscopy is done
- **High dose PPI** useful

Angiographic Management
Has a higher rate of rebleeding as compared to endoscopic
- Mortality, hospital stay, transfusion requirements are the same
- Indicated in rebleeding after endoscopy for those who are poor surgical candidates

Bleeding PUD
- Surgery—indications
  - Hemodynamically unstable
  - Blood transfusion >6 units of packed cells
  - Failure of endoscopy
  - Shock with recurrent bleeding: Continued slow bleeding with daily requirement of >3 units of blood
- Threshold is lowered in elderly—cannot tolerate transfusion

Surgical Management
- 5–10% have persistent bleeding
- Most common: Gastroduodenal artery
- Duodenotomy is carried to pylorus
- 'U' stitch is done
- Stops bleeding from superior and inferior branches and transverse pancreatic artery
- To avoid injury to CBD—probe passed into CBD
- Duodenotomy—closed transversely

- TV is added to control of bleeding than *H. pylori* control alone—reasons
  - Only 40–70% bleeding DU are *H. pylori* +
  - In bleeding, rapid urease test may be false negative in 18% vs 1% in nonbleeding
  - Risk of rebleeding 50%, if acid reducing surgery is not done
- Pyloroplasty most commonly done Heineke-Mikulicz

Perforated DU

- Occurs in 2–10% of DU
- Sudden onset, severe pain
- Small subset perforation may seal by itself
- But, surgery needed in almost all
  - Perforation—highest rate of mortality of all complications of PUD—15%

Treatment

- Perforation—a surgical disease
- <1 cm perforation—primary closure with omental buttressing
- Larger perforation—Graham's omental patch
- >3 cm perforation—omental/jejunal serosal patch
  - Duodenal exclusion
  - Antrectomy—Roux-y

Acid Reducing Surgery in

- *H. pylori* negative on NSAID which cannot be discontinued
- Failed medical therapy

Postop

- NGT—until bowel activity returns
- Drain—until eaten without any drain change
- Contrast study is optional
- *H. pylori* positive—triple therapy
- Simple closure of perforation in
  - NSAID induced, never been treated for PUD
  - In shock and in morbid patients
- *H. pylori* positive—in 81% DU perforation
- After *H. pylori* eradication—recurrence at 1 year—5%
- After PPI alone recurrence is 38%
- To consider acid reducing surgery if *H. pylori* status is not known

Perforation non-operative Treatment

- >24 hours duration
- Stable
- Elderly, co-morbid—high risk

- Gastrografin study shows—sealed perforation
- Conservative treatment of perforated GU not recommended because *higher rate of reperforation and complications*

Gastric Outlet Obstruction (GOO)

- Acute inflammation of duodenum
  - Functional obstruction
  - Anorexia, vomiting
  - Hypochloremic, hypokalemic, metabolic alkalosis
- In chronic DU—fibrosis—stenosis
  - Painless, large quantity vomiting
    - Dilated—atonic stomach
  - Weight loss

GOO: Treatment

- Represents 5–8% of ulcer complications
- Rule out cancer by endoscopy
- Eradication and endoscopic dilatation is mainstay: In *H. pylori* positive
- In idiopathic GOO on acid suppression treated by endoscopic dilatation
- *H. pylori* role in GOO less 33–57%

GOO—Surgical Treatment

- TV + antrectomy
- In scarred duodenum—TV+ drainage
  - Pyloroplasty—not indicated due to scarring
- Preferred method is GJ with vagotomy or lifelong PPI

Intractable Peptic Ulcer

- Failure to heal after 8-12 weeks of therapy
- On endoscopy shows ulcer >5 mm
  - Or relapsing after completion of treatment
- Rare in DU
- Eradicate *H. pylori*, eliminate NSAID use
- Rule out cancer
- Do serum gastrin estimation
- Treated with acid reducing surgery
- Recurrent ulcer—on endoscopy—ulcer >5 mm develops within 12 months after complete ulcer healing

Surgery in DU
Indications

- *H. pylori* cannot be eradicated
- Cannot stop NSAIDs
- Non-compliant acid suppression

Surgeries

- Vagotomy, antrectomy (gastrin) or both
- Truncal vagotomy reduces
  - Basal acid by 75%, stimulated acid secretion by 50%
- Vagotomy +antrectomy—reduces stimulated acid by 80%
  - Basal acid is virtually abolished
- Truncal vagotomy with drainage
  - Heineke-Mikulicz
  - Finney
  - Jaboulay—gastroduodenostomy
  - GJ
- Bile reflux is more after GJ
- Diarrhoea is more after pyloroplasty
- Dumping is same with both
- Vagus—celiac branch from posterior vagus—mediates SI motility
- Hepatic branch from anterior vagus—bile flow and GB motility

Truncal Vagotomy

- Acid secretion reduced—due to diminished cholinergic stimulation
- Cephalic phase eliminated
- BAO reduction—75%
- MAO reduction—50%
- Due to raised intraluminal pH, there is loss of negative feedback and lead to gastrin cell hyperplasia
- Loss of reflex relaxation of fundus leads to rapid emptying of liquids
- Affects distal gastric motility leads to delayed emptying of solids resulting in stasis and distension

Selective Vagotomy

- Divide vagus distal to celiac and hepatic branches
- Pyloric drainage done
- Higher recurrence than TV
- Complications—same
- Not popular

Highly Selective Vagotomy
Parietal Cell Vagotomy, Proximal Gastric Vagotomy

- Divided vagal branches to acid producing portions of body and fundus of stomach
- Preserves innervation to pylorus—so no need for drainage
- Crow's feet divided 7 cm proximal to pylorus or the area in the vicinity of antrum
- Superiorly carried 5 cm proximal to GEJ on to esophagus
- 2–3 branches to antrum and pylorus preserved
- BAO reduction 75%, MAO—50%

- 10–15% recurrence
- Lesser rates of diarrhea and dumping
- Solids emptying—normal
- Nerves for receptive relaxation are divided. so produce rapid emptying of liquids.

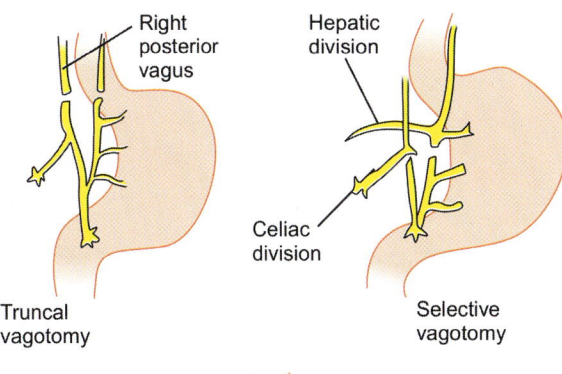

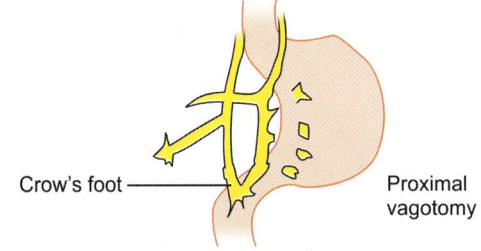

TV + Antrectomy

- Done rarely in DU more in GU
- Antrectomy = 40% distal gastrectomy
- Relative contraindications
  - Cirrhosis
    - Duodenal scarring
  - Previous surgery like CDJ
- Recurrence rate—0–2%
- But more postvagotomy syndromes—20%
- More morbidity and operation time
- Anastomosis by: GD (Billroth I), GJ (Bill II), Roux-y

DU—Other Procedures

- Hill-Baker procedure—posterior TV + anterior HSV
- Taylor procedure—posterior TV + anterior lesser curve seromyotomy
- Supradiaphragmatic truncal vagotomy
  - In failed abdominal vagotomy
  - Thoracotomy/scopy

Taylor Procedure

Posterior TV+anterior seromyotomy

- Seromyotomy starts 6 cm proximal to pylorus
- 1.5 cm away from lesser curvature
- Divides circular fibers
- Not the oblique muscle or mucosa
- Air inflated to check mucosa
- Closed with suture
- Linear staples can be used

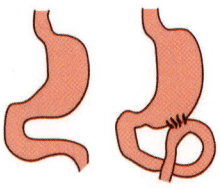

Gastrojejunostomy

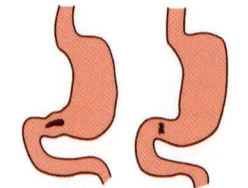

Heineke-Mikulicz pyloroplasty

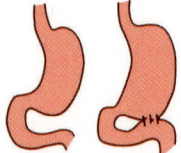

Jaboulay gastroduodenostomy

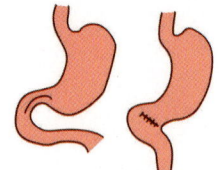

Finney gastroduodenostomy

Drainage Procedures

Gastrojejunostomy

- Retrocolic, short loop
- Avoiding long afferent limb and afferent limb obstruction
- Most common indication when duodenum is scarred/edematous which are contraindications for pyloroplasty
- Always done with vagotomy as jejunum lacks Brunner's glands like duodenum which secrete mucus to neutralise acid
- Vagotomy: Not required in malignancies as they have achlorhydria

Billroth-1

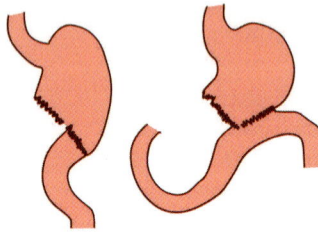

Billroth 1   Billroth 2

Billroth 1 advantages

- Normal GI continuity
- Specialised duodenal mucosa left next to stomach
- No afferent/efferent limbs
- ERCP possible in future
- Reduced cancer
- Braun anastomosis: GJ with JJ
- Finsterer-Hofmeister—partial closure of stomach stump and end to side GJ

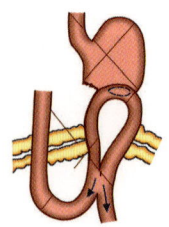 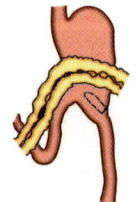 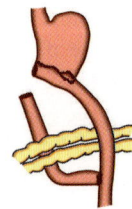

Braun Finsterer-Hofmeister Roux-en-Y

Uncut Roux

Anastomosis is done without dividing the afferent limb, only stapler is fired.

- Reduces bile reflux
- Stapler line may give way causing reflux in future

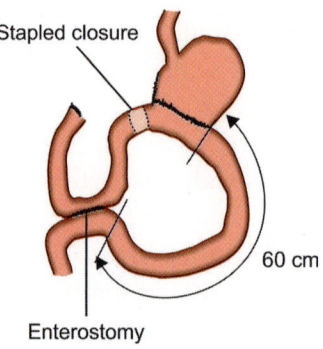

Uncut Roux-en-Y

Pyloroplasty

- In adults duodenal mucosa—adherent to muscle—so pyloromyotomy alone would not work
    - Heineke-Mikulicz
    - Finney
    - Jaboulay gastroduodenostomy anastomosis between stomach and D1 and D2
- Jaboulay causes more bile reflux
- Heineke-Mikulicz—most common drainage procedure done
- In intractable DU—choice is HSV
- Next is TV+Antrectomy

Surgery	Ulcer recurrence (%)	Risk of side effects
TV with drainage	10	Highest
TV with antrectomy	2	High
Proximal gastric vagotomy	15	Low

Giant DU

- Benign and >2 cm
- Seen in 1–2% of all DU
- Stricture formation—involve >50% of bulb circumference
- Less associated with *H. pylori*
- More with NSAIDs
- Risk of malignancy—19%

Giant DU: Treatment

- PPI, *H. pylori* eradication, stop NSAID
- More chance of complications—penetration, perforation, bleeding
- Surgery—vagotomy with duodenal excision, if possible
- Or Billroth 1 or Billroth 2 anastomosis
- Duodenal stump—leak is high
- **Nissen closure**—duodenal stump closed with pancreatic capsule
- **Bancroft closure**—stomach transected proximal to pylorus—gastric mucosa is dissected away and purse string suture of duodenum is done followed by seromuscular layer.

Gastric Ulcer

Type	Location	Acid secretion
I	Lesser curvature	Low
II	Body of stomach and duodenum	High
III	Prepyloric only	High
IV	High on lesser curve	Low
V	Diffuse ulcers due to medication	Low

Modified Johnson Classification

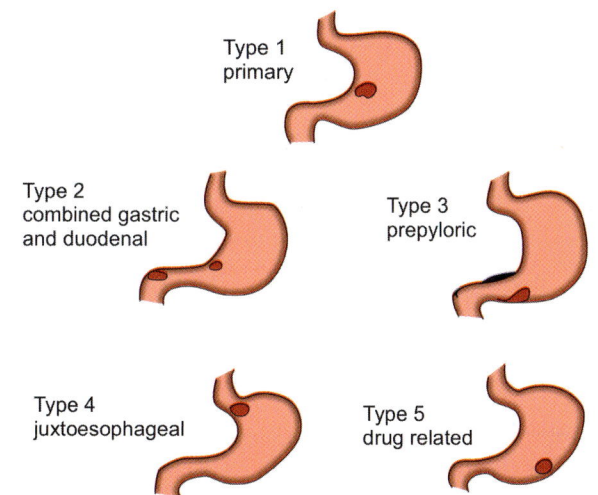

Type 1
primary

Type 2
combined gastric
and duodenal

Type 3
prepyloric

Type 4
juxtoesophageal

Type 5
drug related

Type 1

- Most common site incisura lesser curvature
- Type 1: 60% (most common)
- Not associated with hyperacidity—may be even low acid
- Most occur within 1.5 cm within fundic-antral transition
- Not associated with pyloric, duodenal mucosal abnormality

Type 2 GU

- Represents 15%
- Occurs at body of stomach and duodenum
- Associated with hyperacidity
- Large, deep, poorly defined margins

Type 3 GU

- Prepyloric
- Constitute 20%
- Associated with hyperacid secretion
- May harbor cancer

Type 4 GU

- High on lesser curve—near GEJ
- Constitute <10%
- No hyperacid secretion
- Antral mucosa may extend 1–2 cm off GEJ
- Type 4 is a subset of type 1
- Present with dysphagia and reflux

Type 5 GU

- Anywhere in stomach
- NSAID and drug induced
- Ulcers on greater curvature—<5%

Treatment

- Stop NSAIDs
  - PPI
- Surgery—TV+antrectomy—if cannot stop NSAIDs

Gastric Ulcer

- Rare before 40 years of age
- Peak incidence 55–65 years
- More common in
  - Low socioeconomic group
  - Nonwhites
- Most caused by *H. pylori* or NSAID
- Others
  - Smoking, alcohol, steroid, intra-arterial therapy
- Acid is essential—but total acid less important
- *H. pylori* related GU has normal or less acid
- Ulcer develops due to inflammatory response to bacteria (maximum concentration at junction of body and antrum)
- H2B, PPI, vagotomy—heal the ulcer

Clinical Features

- Pain—quiescence and relapse
- Benign vs malignant
- Most frequent complication—perforation

- Most common site—anterior aspect of lesser curvature
- Older patients—more perforations
- Hemorrhage in 35–40%
  - Unlikely to stop spontaneously
  - More in elderly

Malignant vs Benign Gastric Ulcer (Barium)

Benign
- Outpouching of ulcer crater beyond the gastric contour (exoluminal)
- Smooth rounded and deep ulcer crater
- Smooth gastric fold that reach margin of ulcer
- Hampton's line sign

Malignant
- Does not protrude
- Irregular and shallow ulcer crater
- Nodular and regular ulcer mound
- Nodular gastric folds that do not reach margin
- Carman meniscus sign

Haudek's Niche
- An archaic term for radiographic appearance in profile of contrast material filling the gastric ulcer in the wall of the stomach
- Obsolete these days
- Hampton's line—is a thin millimetric line seen at the neck of a GU in Barium—indicating benign—caused by a thin line of mucosa overhanging ulcer crater
- Carman meniscus sign—large GU seen on endoscopy convex in towards the lumen of stomach, rolled edges—suggestive of cancer

Treatment
- Stop NSAID
- Treat *H. pylori*

Type 1 GU
- Concern about malignancy
- Chronic ulcer—wedge excision
- Depend on location of ulcer
  - Proximity to GEJ
  - Length of lesser curve
- Distal gastrectomy: Billroth I or II
- HSV with ulcer excision
- Recurrence <5%
- Gastrectomy is not superior to wedge excision
- Do not require vagotomy

Type 2
- Treatment—similar to DU
  - Vagotomy drainage
  - HSV

Type 3
- Distal gastrectomy +TV-choice
- HSV has a poorer outcome

Type 4 GU
- Depend on
  - Distance from GEJ
  - Ulcer size
  - Level of inflammation
- Ulcer should be excised
- Or total gastrectomy—esophageal jejunostomy Roux-en-Y

Csendes Procedure
- GU 2–5 cm from GEJ
- Distal gastrectomy + Vertical resection of lesser curvature with ulcer + EEA GD or GJ-Roux

Kelling-Madlener Procedure

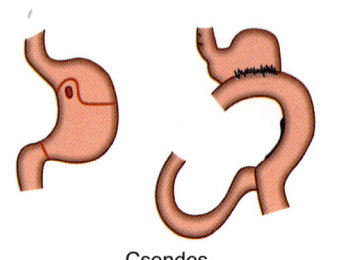 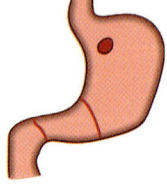

Csendes   Kelling-Madlener

- Distal gastrectomy
- After biopsy, ulcer left alone
- In ulcers <2 cm from GEJ
- Nonresective

Pauchet Procedure
- Distal gastrectomy and freehand resection of ulcer using scissors

Schoemaker Procedure
- A modification of Billroth 1
- Tube-shaped resection of high GU
- Duodenum anastomosed to greater curvature
- Nonresective procedures are not advisable—risk of cancer

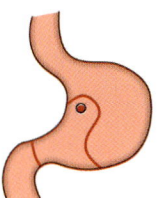 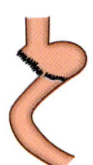

Pauchet   Schoemaker

Type 5 Treatment

- Stop NSAID
- If cannot: Excision +TV

Bleeding GU

- 70% *H. pylori* +
- Endoscopic control—biopsy for Ca and *H. pylori*
- If bleeding controlled—*H. pylori* treatment
- If not, surgery—excision of ulcer +Vagotomy/Distal gastrectomy +TV
  - For intractable ulcers not due to *H. pylori* or NSAID
- Type 2 and 3—vagotomy is added

GU Perforation

- Mortality—10–40%, more in 65 age

Type 1

Stable—distal gastrectomy with Billroth 1

- Unstable—biopsy, Graham's patch
  - *H. pylori* treatment
  - Repeat endoscopy
  - Vagotomy—no use

Type 2

- Patch closure with or without TV + pyloroplasty
  - *H. pylori* treatment
- Similar to DU
- Biopsy must
- PGV/TV with drainage—in recurrent ulcer disease, previously treated for *H. pylori*

Type 3

- Patch closure—may develop GOO
- Antrectomy with vagotomy—choice

Type 4

High—patch closure with biopsy—preferred

- Ulcer excision done whenever possible

Giant GU

- Defined as > 2 cm
- On lesser curvature
- Higher chance of malignancy—10% (6–30% depending on size)
- Penetrate to near structures
- More complications
- Medical therapy—heals 80% ulcers
- For complications/failure—gastrectomy + vagotomy in type 2 and 3
- Local excision + TV + pyloroplasty in unstable cases

2.3 GASTRITIS

- Any histologically confirmed inflammation of gastric mucosa

Autoimmune Gastritis

- Antibodies against parietal cell—atrophy of parietal cell—hypo and—achlorhydria—intrinsic factor deficiency—B_{12} malabsorption—pernicious anemia
- Antrum not affected so produce high gastrin from G cells—hypertrophy of ECL cells in body—microadenomas in the ECL cells—rarely become malignant
- These predispose to Ca stomach
- Screening is needed

H. pylori Gastritis

- Also known as type B gastritis
- Affects antrum
- Prone to PUD
- *H. pylori* produce cytotoxins—Cag A and Vac A products—gastritis—PUD—cancer
- *H. pylori* associated pangastritis is common
- But gastritis involving corpus alone—not *H. pylori* associated
- Pangastritis—most prone for cancer
- Pangastritis—intestinal metaplasia and need screening

Reflux Gastritis

- Enterogastric reflux following gastric surgery
- Seen following cholecystectomy also
- Bile chelating/prokinetics—treatment
- Surgery—for more severe cases

Erosive Gastritis

- Destroying gastric mucosal barrier
- Due to NSAID and alcohol

- NSAID—inhibition of cyclo-oxygenase 1 (COX1)—reducing cytoprotective PG
- Beneficial effects of NSAIDs are through COX2 inhibition
- COX2 inhibitors—reduce side effects
  - But have high CVS complications

Stress Gastritis

- Due to reduction of blood supply to mucosa
- Sequel of a serious disease
- Seen in cardiopulmonary bypass
- Prevention—H2B/sucralfate
- Multiple, superficial erosions—nonulcerating
- Begin in the proximal acid secreting portions of stomach—progress distally
- Occurs secondary to trauma, shock, respiratory distress—may lead to severe bleeding
- In CNS disease—Cushing's ulcer
- In thermal injury (>30%)—Curling's ulcer
- Lesions change with time
- Early lesions—within 24 hours—multiple, shallow, erosions and hemorrhage or adherent clot
- If erodes, submucosa can cause bleeding
- Microscopy—wedge-shaped hemorrhages and coagulation necrosis of mucosa
- Mostly on fundus
  Late lesions
  - When tissue reaction
  - Organised clot
  - Inflammatory exudate
- In 24–72 hours
- Features similar to GU

Pathophysiology

- Acid
- Reduced defence mechanisms
  - Reduction in blood flow, mucus and bicarbonate
- Stress produce mucosal ischemia—loss of defense mechanisms—gastritis
- Acid is necessary—but no hypersecretion is seen
- Acid block precludes stress gastritis
- Develops within 1–2 days of stress
- Pain abdomen
- Microscopic lower GI bleeding
- Flecks of blood in NGT—drop in Hb

Erosive/Stress Gastritis

- Endoscopy—'Blood under Saran Wrap' appearance—1–5 mm shallow erosions (Cling film appearance)

Prophylaxis

- Two major risk factors
  - Coagulopathy
  - Mechanical ventilation >48 hours
- Prophylactic increase in gastric pH—lead to ventilator associated pneumonia and *C. difficile*
- So only if risk factors are there—prophylaxis is started
  - Early enteral feeding
  - PPI—not H2B or sucralfate

Treatment

- Correction of coagulopathy, platelets
- Treat sepsis
- 80% bleeding stop by conservative means
- Selective infusion of vasopressin through left gastric artery
  - 0.2–0.4 IU/min—for 48–72 hours
  - Not in cardiac/liver disorders
- Angiography embolization
- Endoscopic—less effective
  - Surgery may be indicated in refractory bleeding and requiring >6 units of blood
  - **Surgery**
    - Anterior gastrotomy
    - Over sewing
    - TV+pyloroplasty
- Partial/total gastrectomy—rarely

Lymphocytic Gastritis

- Infiltration of mucosa by T cells
- Associated with *H. pylori*
- Inflammation similar to coeliac disease or lymphocytic colitis

Other gastritis
- **Eosinophilic gastritis**—allergic—steroids, cromoglycate
- **Granulomatous gastritis**—in Crohn's and TB
- **AIDS related**—infection with cryptosporidiosis
- **Phlegmonous gastritis**—a rare bacterial infection in severe intercurrent illness

Gastritis

Type A	Autoimmune
Type B	*H. pylori*
Stress	HI/burns
HIV	Cryptosporidium
Granulomatous	Crohn's, TB
Eosinophilic	Allergic
Phlegmonous	Severe sepsis

2.4 GIST

- Most common sarcomatous (mesenchymal) tumor of GIT
- Comprise—1 to 3 % of all GIT tumors
- From interstitial cell of Cajal—pacemaker
- Stomach 40–60%
- Small intestine—30%
- Colon—15%
- Esophagus—2%
- Rarely genitourinary, omentum

Intestitial Cells of Cajal (ICC)

- Santiago Ramón y Cajal—in 1893 described ICC
- Interstitial—between smooth muscle cells and nerve endings in the gut wall
- ICC have very few contractile elements—but very high mitochondria
- Arise from mesenchymal cells
- Role in the propagation of intrinsic slow wave gut peristalsis
- ICC—also found outside GIT
  - GUT, portal vein, pancreas

Pathophysiology

C-KIT mutation

- KIT contains 21 exons—mutation in GIST seen at exons 9, 11, 13, 17
- Most common site—juxtamembrane domain within exon 11—responsible for 70% GIST
- Next common—extracellular domain—in exon 9–10–20% GIST—more common in SI

Others

- Kinase I-exon 13
- Activation loop-exon 17—common in familial type

PDGFRA Mutations

- PDGFRA—alternative oncogene—activate intracellular phosphorilation

Wild Type

- Negative for c-KIT and PDGFRA
- But similar histology
- 10–15% of GISTs
  - SDH deficient—50% of wild type
  - NF1 associated
  - Others—BRAF V600E or RAS mutation ETV6-NTRK3 gene fusion
- Microscopic GIST seen in 10–25% of stomach
- Succinate dehydrogenase (SDH) deficient GIST occurs in young females
- There are no predisposing conditions for KIT and PDGFRA mutated GIST
- SDH deficient predispose to
  - Carney's triad
  - Carney-Strataki's syndrome: GIST and familial paraganglioma
  - Neurofibroma 1
- In wild type, children and in syndromes
  - More chance of LN mets
  - More multifocal and multicentric

Pathological Variants

- Spindle cells—70%
- Epitheloid cells—20%
- Myxoid stroma
- Neuroendocrine
- Signet ring type
- Marked lymphocytic infiltrate
- In 10–20% characteristic hyaline or fibrillary structures—skeinoid fibers
- All GISTs have some ability to metastasise—not truly benign
- Except small gastric GIST (<2 cm) with no high risk histology
- Gastric GISTs—less aggressive
- Low risk cases can become high risk if left untreated

Gastric GIST Clinical Features

- Age—mostly >50
- Slight, male preponderance
- Most develop *de novo*
- Familial syndromes
  - Paraganglioma syndrome (Carney's syndrome/triad)—
  - Neurofibromatosis-1
  - von Hippel-Lindau

Carney's Triad

Paraganglioma, GIST, pulmonary chondroma

- Most females <30
- Mostly gastric GISTs
- Lack c-KIT or PGDFRA mutation
- Indolent course

Other Clinical Features

- Most common symptom—bleeding
  - Most common—melena
- Many are asymptomatic—discovered incidentally
- OGD—smooth, round, submucosal lesion
- Occasionally central ulceration
- EUS-FNAC—diagnostic sensitivity—82%
  - Specificity—100%
- CT for staging

Histopathology

- Smooth muscles and neuroendocrine cells

> **EUS—high risk features**
> - Irregular border
> - Cystic spaces
> - Ulceration
> - Echogenic foci
> - Internal heterogeneity

- PET CT
  - Useful in preop staging
  - Assessing response to treatment
  - **Ring-shaped uptake** on preop PET—an independent adverse prognostic factor for postop recurrence
- GISTs grow out from organ—not submucosally

GIST-IHC

- C-KIT proto-oncogene CD 117—overexpression in 95%
- CD 34 in 60–70%
- DOG 1 (discovered on GIST)—overall sensitivity 95%
- PDGFRA—in 15%

Gastric GIST

- Very small <2 cm
- Mini 1–2 cm
- Micro <1 cm
- In micro GIST EUS is done and can be observed
- In mini lesions do EUS with or without CT and may be observed
- Surgery is considered if high risk

Modified Fletcher (Joensuu Modification)

Joensuu Modification of NIH Consensus Classification for selecting patients with GIST for adjuvant therapy			
Risk category	Size of tumor (cm)	Mitotic figures/ 50 HPFs	Tumor site
Very low risk	<2.0	≤5	Any site
Low risk	2.1–5.0	≤5	Any site
Intermediate risk	2.1–5.0	>5	Gastric
	<5.0	6–10	Any site
	5.1–10.0	≤5	Stomach
High risk	Any size	Any number	Tumor rupture
	>10 cm	Any number	Any site
	Any	>10	Any site
	>5	>5	Any site
	2.1–5	>5	Non-gastric
	5–10	≤5	Non-gastric

Treatment

- Mainstay—surgery
  - >2 cm size—resected
- < 2 cm with **high risk features** on endoscopy/EUS should be resected
  - Heterogeneity
  - Irregular borders
  - Ulceration
- Others followed-up—endoscopy/EUS 6–12 monthly
- Wide excision (1–2 cm), enucleation, gastrectomy
- No specific margins for resection—achieve R0 resection
- LN dissection—not required—LN mets rare
- Avoid pseudocapsule violation
- >10 cm—consider neoadjuvant
- **R1 resection—no worse prognosis than R0**
- **R1 resection—further treatment individualised**
- GIST ruptured during surgery—considered metastatic
- Lap surgery—**Privette classification**

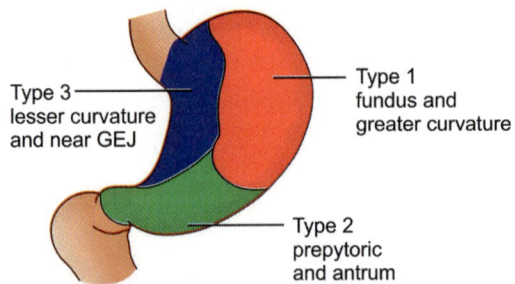

Type 3 lesser curvature and near GEJ

Type 1 fundus and greater curvature

Type 2 prepytoric and antrum

- Microscopic positive resection margin—resurgery to achieve R0—not indicated
- No survival advantage—but should be macroscopically negative

Postop

- Recurrence/metastasis—40–50%
- Most common hematogenous metastasis—liver, peritoneum
- One-third can have local recurrence
- Long-term follow-up is warranted
- Long-term disease-free survival—50%

Follow-up

- Spiral CT: 3–6 months
- Clinical evaluation every 6 months—for 2 years
- Annually for years 3 to 5

Benign vs Malignant

- Tumor size >10 cm
- Mitoses >5/50 HPF
- Tumor site

Adjuvant Therapy

- Tyrosine kinase inhibitor—preventing phosphorylation—Imatinib
- Imatinib was originally used for
  - In mets, unresectable and high risk groups
  - Minimum 3 years
  - 400 mg daily

Imatinib

- Side effects:
  - Most common—periorbital and peripheral edema, diarrhea, fatigue
  - Hypertension, GI bleeding—rare

Sunitinib

- In GISTs refractory or intolerant to imatinib
- Inhibits CD117, PDGFRA, BRAF and VEGFR

Regorafenib

- Tyrosine kinase inhibitor
- Effective against KIT
- In failed cases with imatinib and sunitinib

Neoadjuvant followed by Surgery

In metastatic, locally advanced, recurrent

- Imatinib for 4–12 months—PET/CT, then surgery after 4–12 months of therapy, continue imatinib for 1 to 2 years postop
- 70–80% show some response—makes it operable
- Drug related tumor necrosis, hemorrhage, perforation—in <5%
- Complete response in <2%
- No response in 10%, should proceed to sunitinib or clinical trials

- Surgery is not indicated, they are not curative and cause more morbidity

Metastatic

- Treatment of choice—imatinib
- Should be continued unless toxicity
- Surgery—limited role
- Only in isolated with limited morbidity and organ preserving
- Optimal timing 4 months

Radiotherapy

- Mainly in bone metastasis
- Intra-abdominal metastasis—not clear

Pediatric GIST

- Extremely rare
- Different genetics
- More of epitheloid than spindle cell morphology
- More in females
- Most common site—stomach—85%
- Most common presentation—GI bleed: Anemia
- Higher rate of metastasis, but favourable outcome
- Nearly all express CD117
- But only <15% harbor c-KIT or PGDFR mutation
- So less response to imatinib
- There is role for IGF1R
- Wild type is the predominant type

Small Bowel GIST

- More common in jejunum and ileum
- More in males
- Malignant—>5 cm
- Grow from muscularis propria
- Most common indication for surgery—bleeding and obstruction
- Most useful indicator of survival and risk for metastasis—size, mitotic index, invasion to lamina propria

Treatment

- Complete resection
- Capsule rupture—100% recurrence
- Capsule rupture—should receive adjuvant therapy
- Lymphadenectomy—not indicated
- Radiology—unresectability—infiltration of CA, SMA, PV
- <2 cm—surgery only, no further treatment
- Imatinib—blocks unregulated mutant c-KIT tyrosine kinase
- High risk patient should receive 3 years of imatinib

- Not recommended for low risk patients after R0
- Deletions affecting exon 11, codon 557/558 of c-KIT gene and D842VPGDFR alfa—have high risk for recurrence
- In D842VPGDFR—imatinib not indicated—resistant to this agent
- In mets and unresectable—imatinib 400 mg once daily
- In exon 9 mutation increasing to 400 mg twice—reduces chance of recurrence—dose dependent
- Desatinib—tyrosine kinase inhibitor of c-KIT, PDGFR
  - Effective in imatinib and sunitinib refractory GIST
  - Also in D842VPDGFR mutation

Others

- Regorafenib—second generation tyrosine kinase inhibitor
- Effective in advanced GIST and resistant GIST
- Nilotinib
- Sorafenib
- Imatinib with Doxorubicin—effective in wild type

> **Hereditary GIST**
> - <5% GIST—familial
> - NF mutation
> - Carney's triad
> - Familial GIST syndrome (c-KIT, PDGFRA mutation)
> - Carney-Stratakis
> - If suspected—genetic tests done in family
> - Treatment similar to pediatric GIST

2.5 GI LYMPHOMA

- Involvement of stomach or intestine either as a sole site of involvement or as clinically dominant site (>75%) volume.

> **Dawson's criteria**
> - No peripheral lymphadenopathy
> - No mediastinal lymphadenopathy
> - Peripheral smear/BM—normal
> - Liver and spleen not involved
> - Predominance of GI involvement

Non-Hodgkin Lymphoma

- 30% extranodal
- Among extra nodal site, GI tract is the most common site.

Within GI Tract

- Stomach 60%
- Small intestine 18%
- Colorectal 15%
- NHL mainly in LN
- 20–30%—extra nodal
- GIT comprises 50% of extra nodal lymphomas
- Represent 8–10% of all GI neoplasms
- Stomach—most common site of GI lymphomas
- Accounts for <15% gastric malignancies
- Gastric lymphoma—2% of all lymphomas
  - B symptoms are rare
  - Present with vague symptoms
  - >50% present with anemia—frank bleeding rare

Cells of Origin

- B—cell 90%
  DLBCL 50–60%
  MALT 25–30%

Others

- Follicular—more common in duodenum
- Mantle cell—in ileum
- Burkitt lymphoma—associated with EBV
- **T Cell: 5%**
  - Enteropathy associated T cell lymphoma
  - Most often—jejunum
  - In refractory celiac disease

Among Bowel

- B cell lymphoma mainly affect ileum
- T cell lymphoma jejunum

Primary GI Lymphoma

- Low grade
  - MALT
  - FL
  - MCL
- High grade
  - DLBCL
  - BL
  - PTLD
- **Risk factors**
  - *H. pylori*
  - Immunosuppression
  - Celiac disease
  - IBD
  - HIV, EBV

DLBCL

- Most common histologically
- 50% of gastric lymphoma
- May have mixed MALT lymphoma

MALT Lymphoma

- 30% of PGIL
- Stomach most common
- *H. pylori* positive or negative

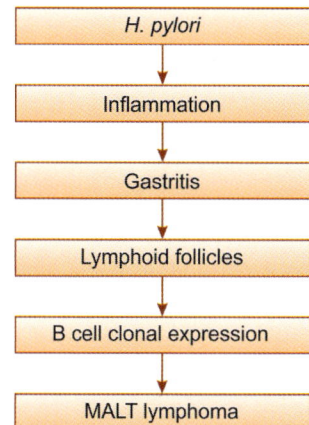

Gastric Lymphoma

- Common in 6–7th decade
- Second most common cancer of stomach
- M:F = 2:1
- Most common location—*Antrum or distal body*—but from any part
- Gastric lymphoma—if stomach is exclusive or predominant part

Types of Lymphoma Stomach

- Most common—diffuse large B cell (55%)
- Next common—MALT lymphoma (40%)
- Burkitt—3% (3–15)
- Mantle cell—1% (<10)
- Follicular—1% (<10)

MALT Lymphoma

- No native lymphoid tissue in stomach mucosa
- MALT—chronic inflammation—lymphoma
- *H. pylori* infection—strong association
- Mostly antrum and distal body
- Develops from B cells—clonal expansion
- Other sites
  - Thyroid
  - Parotid
  - Subconjunctiva

Diffuse Large B Cell Type

- Generally primary lesions
- May occur from progression of CLL, small lymphocytic lymphoma, MALT lymphoma

- Risk factors—immunodeficiency
  - *H. pylori*

Burkitt Lymphoma

- Associated with Epstein-Barr virus
- Aggressive
- Affects younger
- Found in cardia or body of stomach
- Increased cell turnover—attracts macrophages—'starry sky' appearance

Gastric Lymphoma

Clinical Features

- Most common symptom—abdominal pain
- 'B symptoms'—in 10–12%

Evaluation

- They are submucosal lesion
- So endoscopy and biopsy may be nondiagnostic
- EUS—most accurate for local staging
- Staging investigations
  - CT chest, abdomen
  - Bone marrow
  - Laryngoscopy—Waldeyer's ring
    □ LN biopsy
- *H. pylori* evaluation

PET CT

- Standard for staging
- Treatment response assessment
- Follow-up
- False positive results in
  - GI lymphoid tissue, IBD, Crohn's, TB
- **MR enteroclysis**
- **Capsule enteroscopy**
- **CBC**
- **Metabolic profile**
- **LDH**
- **Serum protein electrophoresis**

Disease site	% incidence	Risk factors	Path subtype
Esophagus	<1%	EBV, HIV	Majority DLBCL
Gastric	60–75%	*H. Pylori, C. jejuni,* HTLV, EBV	DLBCL, MALT FL, Burkitt
Small intestine	20–30%, distal ileum most common	Celiac diseases, IBD, HIV, EBV	DLBCL, MALT, Burkitt FL, MCL
Colon	5–10%	Celiac disease, EBV, UV	Burkitt, DLBCL, MALT

- **Clinical evaluation**
  - History and examination
  - Performance status
  - B symptoms
  - Nutritional evaluation
  - CBC, LDH, uric acid, Hep B, HIV.
- **Diagnosis**
  - Endoscopy
  - EUS
  - Biopsy

Other Studies

- FISH, IHC, PCR
- Cytogenetics/karyotyping
- Flow cytometry
- Gene expression profiling

Work Up

- Surgical pathology
- IHC
- CD79a, CD3, CD5, etc. in DLCBL
- CD20, CD22 CD79a, CYCN D1 in MALT lymphoma

Cytogenetics

- 4 contributory translocations—three of them affect NF-kB pathway
- Most common—t(11; 18) (q21; q21)—associated with disease unresponsive to *H. pylori* eradication and aggressive disease
- Others t(1;14) (p22; q32), t(14; 18) (q32; q21), t(3; 14) (p14; q32)

- **Metastatic Workup**
  - CECT abdomen and chest, pelvis
  - PET—CT-DLBCL
  - BM biopsy
  - Laparoscopy
- **Others**
  - Pregnancy test
  - Multigated acquisition scan—MUGA for cardiac status assessment
  - ECHO

Staging Systems

- **Ann Arbor staging**
- Mushoff modifications to Ann Arbor for extranodal lymphoma

Mushoff modifications	
Stage	
I or IE	Single lymphatic organ/ extranodal site
II1	Regional node involved
II2	Distant node involved
III	LNs on both sides of diaphragm
IV	Disseminated disease, bone marrow, liver, etc. involved

- **Lugano staging for gastrointestinal lymphoma**

Lugano staging for GI lymphoma	
Stage	
I	Confined to GIT (single primary/noncontiguous lesions)
I1	Limited to mucosa
I2	Infiltrates submucosa, muscularis propria, subserosa or penetrates serosa
II	Abdominal lymph nodes
II1	Local (paragastric) LNs
II2	Distant LNs
IIE	Infiltrates adjacent organs/tissues by direct infiltration
IV	Extranodal LNs. Noncontinuous involvement of separate site GIT (stomach, rectum). Noncontinuous involvement of other organs or tissues. Bone marrow uninvolved
A	Absence of systemic symptoms
B	Presence of systemic symptoms (fever, night sweats, weight loss >10% BW)
X	Lesion >10 cm longest diameter

- In Lugano—no stage III. Any supradiaphragmatic disease—stage IV
- Paris TNM staging
- **Treatment of gastrointestinal lymphoma**

MALT Lymphoma Stage I1, I2, II1, *H. pylori* Positive

- *H. pylori* eradication
- 70–100% resolve
- Endoscopy at 3 months for *H. pylori* and tumor remission

After 3 Months Reassessed

- If *H. pylori* negative, tumor free—observation
- If *H. pylori* persists—second line antibiotics
- *H. pylori* negative, tumor persists—may observe with 3 monthly endoscopy
- Progressive disease consider—RT and antibiotics
- *H. pylori* regimens
  Second line *H. pylori* treatment
  - Bismuth quadraple therapy
  - Levofloxacin, Amoxycillin, PPI
  - Levo, Amoxy, PPI, Bismuth
  - High dose regimen

H. pylori positive and t (11;18) positive
- Antibiotic + ISRT (involvement site RT)
- Rituximab if ISRT contraindicated
- Rituximab is the monoclonal antibody against CD20 B cell antigen

MALT Lymphoma

H. pylori Negative 1E, 2E

- Antibiotics with Clarithromycin
- ISRT or Rituximab
- Endoscopy 3 monthly

Stage 4: MALT Lymphoma

Induction chemoimmuno therapy (R CHOP)

or

Rituximab + RT

MALT Lymphoma SI and Colon

- Stages 1 and 2: ISRT + Rituximab and surgery
- Stage 4: RCHOP

Other drugs used in MALT lymphoma
- Chlorambucil
- Bendamustil
- Purine analogues
- **MALT-Chemo (CHOP or RCHOP), RT, surgery indications**
  - Transmural extension
  - LN involvement

- Transformation to large cell phenotype t (11;18)
- Nuclear BCL10 expression
- *H. pylori* negative

DLBCL: Treatment

- *Stage 1 and 2: RCHOP*
- *ISRT for bulky disease (>7.5 cm)*
- *Non-bulky—3 cycles RCHOP + ISRT or 6 cycles RCHOP with no RT*

RCHOP—first line
- Second line—EPOCH R
- Etoposide Prednisolone Vincristine Cyclophosphamide Doxorubin Rituximab
- **Stages 3 and 4**—high dose therapy
  - Clinical trial
  - Autologus stem cell rescue

Evolving Therapy

- Targeted
- Tumor cell signalling pathway
- Surface antigen
- Ibrutinib
- Idelasilib
- Venetoclax
- Next generation CD20 monoclonal antibody Obinutuzumab
- AntiCD 19 CART therapy (chimeric antigenic receptor T cell)

> **Chemotherapy in GI lymphoma**
> - DLBCL—CHOP
> - MALT—*H. pylori* eradication
> - MCL, FL—RCHOP
> - Burkitt-CHOP—Prednisolone replaced with methotrexate

Follow up—DLBCL

- Clinical, labs 3–6 monthly for 5 years—then as indicated
- CT scan 6 monthly for 2 years
- In relapse, recurrence or progression—second line chemo, clinical trial, ISRT or palliation
- **Role of surgery**
  - Very limited mainly biopsy

Gastric lymphoma—stages 1 and 2

- Chemotherapy alone
- Surgery + chemotherapy

S.I and colon: Role of surgery
- Same as stomach
- Surgery for complications

Complications
- Intestinal obstruction
- Bleeding
- Perforation
- During surgery it is not necessary to achieve microscopically negative margins, though it is desirable

Prognosis
- MALT—best prognosis—irrespective of location
- Gastric lymphoma better than SI
- B cell lymphoma better than T cell
- Depends on grade and stage

International Prognostic Index

Risk factors	Ann Arbor stage III to IV (advanced disease)
	>1 extranodal site
	Age greater than 60
	High LDH
	Performance status ≥2 (ECOG)
Risk assessement	
Low risk	0 to 1 risk factor
Low intermediate risk	2 risk factors
High intermediate risk	3 risk factors
High risk	4 to 5 risk factors

2.6 CARCINOMA STOMACH

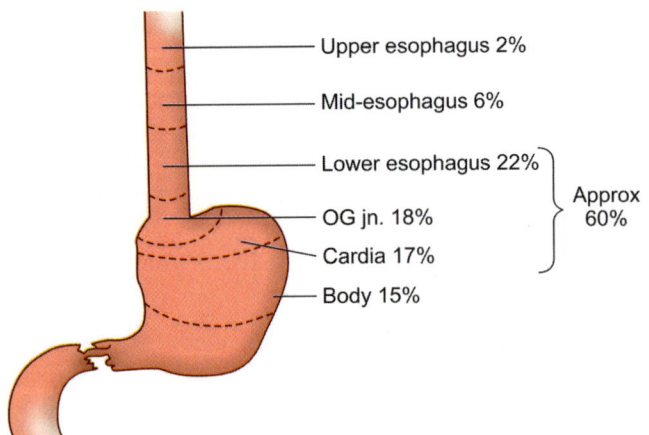

Lymph Nodes
- First echelon—1–6
- Second echelon along named arteries 7–12
- Third echelon 13–16

- Pathophysiology of sister Mary Joseph nodule—hepatoduodenal LN—falciform ligament—periumbilical deposits
- No normal lymphoid tissue seen in gastric mucosa
- But most common site of GI lymphoma
- More males
- 6–7th decade
- Highest rate in Japan and Korea

Risk Factors
- *H. pylori*
  - Relative risk between 3.6 and 17
  - Primary mechanism—chronic inflammation
  - Infection—gastritis—primarily in body-ventral gastric atrophy
  - Intestinal metaplasia—dysplasia—intestinal type ca stomach
  - GEJ tumors—not related
- *H. pylori*—**Molecular alterations**
  - Overexpression of cyclooxygenase 2 and cyclin D2
  - p53 mutations
  - Microsatellite instability
  - Decreased p27 expressions
  - Altered transcription factors CDX1, CDX2
  - Individuals with high levels of interleukin 1—high risk
  - Presence of **Cytoxan associated gene A(CagA)**—has high chance of Ca

Dietary Factors
- Salted/smoked food—contains high levels of nitrates—converted to N-nitroso compounds by bacteria in the stomach
- N-nitroso compounds found in tobacco smoke
- Fresh fruits—contain vitamin C—remove N-nitroso compounds and oxygen free radicals

H. pylori and diet
- Synergism
- *H. pylori* increasing carcinogen production
- Inhibition of removal
- Promote growth of bacteria that produce N-nitroso compounds
- Inhibit secretion of vitamin C
- Refrigeration—reduced the rate of ca

Hereditary Risk Factors
- **Hereditary diffuse gastric cancer**
  - Mutation to cell-cell adhesion molecule—E-cadherin
  - 80% lifetime incidence of ca
  - Prophylactic total gastrectomy—indicated

- **FAP**
  - Fundic gland polyps seen in 85%
  - 40% of these having dysplasia
  - >50% contain somatic adenomatous polyposis coli mutation—risk of cancer
  - Gastric polyps and duodenal polyps—warrant surveillance
- **Li-Fraumeni syndrome**
  - Autosomal dominant
  - Mutation of p53 tumor suppressor gene
  - Risk of ca stomach
- **Lynch syndrome**
  - Microsatellite instability
  - Increased risk of ca stomach and ovary
  - Account for 2–3% of ca colon

Genetics

- Activation of oncogenes
- Inactivation of tumor suppressor
- Reduction of cellular adhesion
- Reactivation of telomerase
- Microsatellite instability
- C-met proto-oncogene—receptor for hepatocyte growth factor—overexpressed
- K-sam, c-erbB2 oncogenes
- Inactivation of TSG p53, p16—in diffuse and intestinal type
- Adenomatous polyposis coli gene—in intestinal type
- Microsatellite instability
  - In 20–30% intestinal type
- Reduction in E-cadherin in 50% of diffuse type

Molecular Subtypes

- Mesenchymal like type—worst prognosis
  - Early age, more recurrence
  - Lauren—diffuse type
- **Microsatellite unstable**
  - Best over all prognosis
  - Least recurrence, intestinal type
  - Immunotherapy—most useful
- **TP53 active**
- **TP53 inactive:** HER2 target therapy most effective

Other Risk Factors

- **Pernicious anemia**
  - Autoimmune—destruction of parietal and chief cells—mucosal atrophy—antral and intestinal metaplasia
  - Relative risk for Ca stomach—2.1–5.6 in population
- **Polyps**
  - Adenomatous polyps—risk
  - Risk 10–20 %—increases with size
  - <2 cm pedunculated, no foci of invasive ca—endoscopic removal sufficient
    - >2 cm, sessile, invasive cancer—surgery indicated

- **Fundic gland polyps**
  - Result from glandular hyperplasia and decreased luminal flow
  - Strong association with PPI
  - Dysplasia rare
  - Excision, cessation of treatment with PPI, or regular surveillance—NOT indicated
- **PPI**
  - Block acid—hypergastrinemia—which reverses after stoppage
  - Low acid—more *H. pylori*—colonise body—corpus gastritis—one-third of them—atrophic gastritis—increased ca risk
  - Atrophic gastritis reverses on *H. pylori* eradication

Protective and risk factors for adenocarcinoma stomach
Protective
Antioxidants
Vit A, C
Selenium, zinc, iron
Citrus fruits
Raw vegetables
Green tea
Genetic risk factors
Pernicious anemia
Family history
HNPCC
Peutz-Jeghers syndrome
FAP
Type A blood
Li-Fraumeni
Acquired risk factors
H. pylori
EBV
Previous stomach surgery
Coal workers
Rubber workers
Well water
Smoked/cured food
Smoking
High salt/nitrate diet
Radiation exposure
Precursors
Adenoma
Intestinal metaplasia
Atrophic gastritis
Ménétrier disease
Dysplasia

Pathogenesis

- Gastric cancer stem cells situated at the isthmus of gastric glands
- Most common type—tubular adenocarcinoma—followed by papillary and mucinous
- Signet ring cell type—10%

Pathology

- Borrmann classification—in 1926

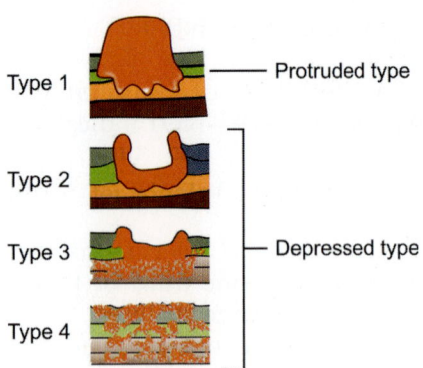

Type 1 — Protruded type

Type 2 ⎤
            ⎬ Depressed type
Type 3 ⎦

Type 4

Borrmann's classification

- Based on macroscopic appearance
- 5 types—fungating or polypoid
  - With elevated edges
  - Ulcerated and infiltrative
  - Diffusely infiltrative
  - Cannot be classified in any

Lauren 1965—Intestinal, Diffuse

Intestinal

- More well differentiated—form glands
  - From a precancerous lesion—atrophic gastritis or int. metaplasia
  - More in men
  - Incidence increases with age
  - Metastasis by hematogenous route to distant sites
  - Dominant where ca stomach is epidemic— environmental—*H. pylori*
  - More microsatellite instability
  - APC gene mutations, p 53 and p16 inactivation.

Diffuse

- Tiny clusters of signet ring cells
  - Poorly differentiated
  - Lack glands
  - Spreads submucosally, less inflammatory infiltrate
  - Early metastasis—transmural and lymphatic
  - Not associated with—chronic gastritis
  - More common in women and younger age
  - Association with blood group A and familial
  - More chance of intraperitoneal metastasis and it is a less favourable sign
- E. cadherin, p53 and p16 inactivation
- **Linitis plastica—involvement of entire stomach— diffuse type—constitute <10% of all gastric adeno-carcinoma**

Spread

- Into duodenum—rare—0.5–1% through muscular layer and subserosal lymphatics
- Into esophagus—via submucosal lymphatics

Lymphatics

- Extensive submucosal plexus

Diagnosis

- **Tumor Markers**
  - CEA, CA19–9, CA 72–4, CA 50—combined evaluation—elevation correlate stage of disease

Endoscopy

- 6–8 biopsies
- Single biopsy—yields 70%
- seven biopsy—98%
- <2 cm—resect EMR or ESD
- EUS
  - Stomach is filled with water
  - 5 layers
  - Mucosa and submucosa (T1)—first 3 layers
  - Muscularis propria—4th layer (T2)
  - Serosa—5th layer (T4a)
  - Accuracy—T stage—85%
    - N stage—80%
- **CECT**
  - CECT chest, abdominal and pelvis—IV and oral contrast—mandatory
  - Primary method for intra-abdominal metastasis
  - Overall detection—85%
  - Peritoneal metastasis—51%
  - For T and N stages—less accurate than EUS
  - Main role to detect metastasis
- **PET**
  - Limited use—only 50% of ca stomach are—PET avid
  - Role in detecting response to neoadjuvant treatment
  - NCCN recommends PET in routine staging in without metastasis in CT
  - Signet ring type—PET nonavid due to decreased expression of glucose transporter GLUT1
- **Laparoscopy**
  - Staging—accuracy— >95%
  - Integral part of work up
  - Can avoid unnecessary laparotomy in 9–60%
  - CT nondetectable metastasis—<5 mm
  - Indicated in >cT3 and suspicious nodes in the absence of distant metastais in CT/PET
  - 200 ml saline instilled all quadrants—shake patient aspirate at least 50 ml and do cytology if malignant cells seen on cytology—M1 disease
  - Lap US and extended laparoscopy—an option
- In metastatic disease
  - HER-2 neu testing

- Distal extension of tumor into duodenum will not affect T3 staging
- Tumor deposits in subserosal fat adjacent to gastric cancer, without evidence of LN tissue—considered LN mets
- Tumor deposit—discrete tumor nodules within lymph drainage area of primary carcinoma without identifiable LN tissue, vascular or neural structure. Shape, contour and size not considered

Japanese Gastric Cancer Association Staging System

Tumor Stage	
T1	Tumor invasion of mucosa and/or muscularis mucosa or submucosa
T2	Tumor invasion of muscularis propria or subserosa
T3	Tumor penetration of serosa
T4	Tumor invasion of adjacent structures
TX	Unknown
Nodal Stage	
N0	No evidence of lymph node metastasis
N1	Metastasis to group 1 lymph nodes but no metastasis to group 2-3 lymph nodes
N2	Metastasis to group 2 lymph node but no metastasis to group 3 lymph nodes
N3	Metastasis to group 3 lymph nodes
NX	Unknown
Hepatic Metastasis Stage (H)	
H0	No Liver metastasis
H1	Liver metastasis
HX	Unknown
Peritoneal Metastasis Stage (P)	
P0	No peritoneal metastasis
P1	Peritoneal metastasis
PX	Unknown
Peritoneal Stage Cytology (CY)	
CY0	Benign/indeterminate cells on peritoneal cytology
CY1	Cancer cells on peritoneal cytology
CYX	Peritoneal cytology was not performed
Other Distant Metastasis(M)	
M0	No other distant metastasis (although peritoneal, liver, or cytological metastases may be present)
M1	Distant metastases other than peritoneal, liver or cytological metastasis
MX	Unknown

Stage Grouping	N0	N1	N2	N3
T1	IA	IB	II	
T2	IB	II	IIIA	
T3	II	IIIA	IIIB	IV
T4	IIIA	IIIB		
H1, P1, CY1, M1				

Early Gastric Cancer

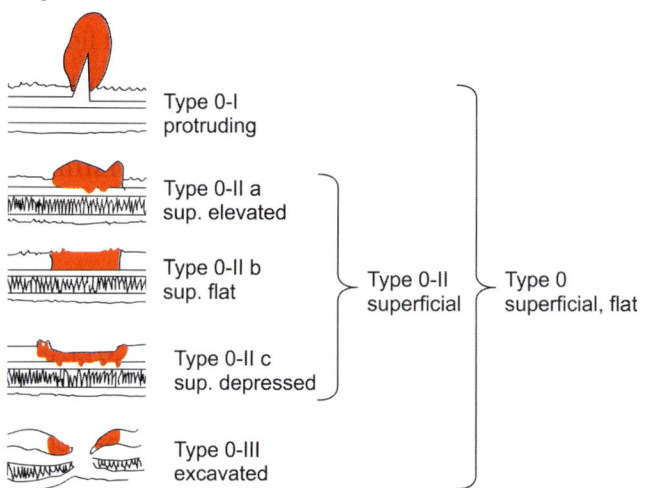

Type 0-I protruding

Type 0-II a sup. elevated

Type 0-II b sup. flat

Type 0-II c sup. depressed

Type 0-III excavated

Type 0-II superficial

Type 0 superficial, flat

- Type I > twice the thickness of mucosa
- Type II < twice the thickness
- **Endoscopic resection**
  - Absolute indication—possibility of LN mets <1%, therapeutic effect equal to surgery
  - Expanded indication—as an investigational treatment, LN mets <1%, possible same result as surgery
  - Relative indication—surgery the treatment—when not possible—endoscopic which may be an option
- **EMR**
  - For early ca
  - Major disadvantage—incomplete resection and unrecognized LN metastasis

Guidelines

- Limited to mucosa T1a
- No L–V invasion
- Size <2 cm
- No ulceration: UL0
- Well or mod differentiated
- Any of these positive—need formal surgery

EMR—ESD

- **Extended criteria**
  - All intramucosal lesions without ulceration
  - Differentiated mucosal tumor <3 cm regardless of ulceration
  - Limited submucosal tumor (SM1) without ulceration and <3 cm
- **Absolute indication for ESD**
  - Differentiated adenocarcinoma
  - Not ulcerated UL0
  - T1a
  - Differentiated adenocarcinoma with ulceration (UL1), depth T1a, diameter <3 cm
- After EMR/ESD
  - Differentiated type—papillary, tubular types
  - Undifferentiated—poorly differentiated adeno-carcinoma, signet ring types, mucinous type

Surgery

- Margins-intestinal—5 cm
  - Diffuse 8–10 cm
- T1 lesions—proximal margin 2 cm
- T2 and more with expansive growth pattern (Borrmann type 1 and 2)—at least 3 cm
- With infiltrative growth (Borrmann type 3 and 4)—5 cm margin
- Infiltrating esophagus—5 cm margin

Gastrectomy

- Standard gastrectomy—performed curative intent. Resection of at least two-thirds of stomach with D2 LN dissection
- Nonstandard gastrectomy—anything less than the earlier criteria
- Modified surgery—the extend of gastric resection and/or LN dissection reduced
- Extended surgery—gastrectomy with adjacent organ resection or LN dissection >D2

Noncurative Surgery: Palliative or Reduction

- **Palliative surgery**—in bleeding or GOO—either palliative gastrectomy or GJ—to relieve symptoms
- **Reduction surgery**—No tumor related complications but with liver, peritoneal mets—to reduce tumor load—to prolong/delay onset of symptoms
- **Total gastrectomy**—total resection of stomach including cardia and pylorus
- **Distal gastrectomy**—stomach resection including pylorus, cardia preserved. Two-thirds—standard
- **Pylorus preserving gastrectomy (PPG)**—preserving upper third of stomach and pylorus along with a portion of antrum
- **Proximal gastrectomy**—resection including cardia, preserving pylorus
- **Segmental gastrectomy**—circumferential resection of stomach—preserving cardia and pylorus
- **Local resection**—noncircumferential resection
- **Nonresectional**—bypass, gastrostomy, Jejunostomy

Gastric Remnant Surgery

- Completion gastrectomy—total resection of cardia and pylorus remnant
- Subtotal resection—distal resection of remnant preserving cardia

In Gastrectomy

- If we cannot obtain proximal margin—total gastrectomy is done
- If pancreaticosplenectomy done due to infiltration—total gastrectomy is preferred even if we can get proximal margin and irrespective of site of primary lesion
- Tumor on greater curvature with LN 4sb—splenectomy done

Lymphadenectomy

- Minimum nodes removed—15
- D2 resection
- Spleen preserving
- **LN dissection**
  - D2 LN dissection in tumors >cT2 and cN+
  - D1 or D1+ dissection is acceptable for cT1N0 tumors
  - Since tumor invasion and LN involvement—unreliable—D2 resection done whenever possible

D1 LN Dissection May be Done in

- cT1a—that do not meet criteria for EMR/ESD
- cT1bN0—which are differentiated type and <1.5 cm
- D1 + LN dissection in—for cT1N0 other than above
- D2 LN dissection is indicated in potentially curable cT2-T4 and cT1N + tumors
  - Spleen and distal pancreas are preserved. In greater curvature tumors, spleen may be removed

D2 + LN dissection: Beyond D2—non-standard Gastrectomy

- Dissection of No. 10 LN in greater curvature tumor
- Level 14V—in distal tumor with metastasis to No. 6 LN (D2 + 14V)
- Level 13 in cancer invading duodenum (D2 + No. 13)—No. 13 for stomach is M1—but for duodenum it is regional
- Level 16—after NACT for cancer with extensive LN involvement (D2 + No. 16)

D1 vs D2

- **MRC trial**—found no recurrence free survival or survival advantage
- **Dutch D1 D2 trial**—lower recurrence rate and better DFS, but no difference in overall survival

- Japanese trial showed improved survival with D2
- Spleen preservation—improved survival—only removed when involved

Total gastrectomy	
D0	Less than D1
D1	1–7
D1+	D1 + 8a, 9, 11p
D2	D1 + 8a, 9, 11p, 11d, 12a

For tumors invading esophagus: 110 added to D1+ and 19, 20, 110, and 111 to D2

Proximal gastrectomy	
D0	Less than D1
D1	1, 2, 3a, 4sa, 4sb, 7
D1+	D1 + 8a, 9, 11p

Distal gastrectomy	
D0	Less than D1
D1	1, 3, 4sb, 4d, 5, 6, 7
D1+	D1 + 8a, 9
D2	D1 + 8a, 9, 11p, 12a

- **Current guidelines node station 10 dissection is D2+**

Current Guidelines

- Vagal preservation
- In PPG—hepatic branch should be preserved—to preserve pyloric function

Omentectomy

- Removal of greater omentum part of standard gastrectomy for T3 or deeper tumors
- For T1 and T2—omentum >3 cm away from gastroepiploic artery preserved

Bursectomy

Removal greater omentum + anterior leaf of transverse mesocolon and pancreatic capsule

- No survival advantage

Reconstruction

TOTAL GASTRECTOMY

- Roux-en-Y esophagojejunostomy
- Jejunal interposition
- Double tract method

DISTAL GASTRECTOMY

- Billroth 1 gastroduodenostomy
- Billroth 2 gastrojejunostomy

- Roux-en-Y gastrojejunostomy
- Jejunal interposition

PYLORUS PRESERVING GASTRECTOMY

- Gastro-gastrostomy

PROXIMAL GASTRECTOMY

- Esophagogastrostomy
- Jejunal interposition
- Double tract method

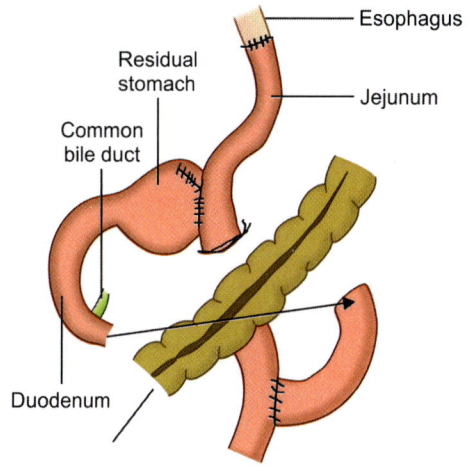

- Double tract anastomosis
  - Technically simple
  - Preserved passage of food through duodenum
  - No duodenal stump—and blow out
  - Endoscopic access to duodenum

Adjuvant/Neoadjuvant Therapy

- **South West Oncology Group SWOG0116**
  - Gastrectomy alone vs postop 5FU and RT
  - Showed better OS, and RFS
- **CLASSIC trial**—D2 alone or with postop eight 3-week cycles on capecitabine and oxaliplatin
  - Significant improvement in OS and DFS
- **ARTIST trial**—D2 + Chemo with capecitabine and cisplatin with or without RT
  - Improved DFS in LN + group
- **MAGIC trial**—in stage 2 or higher
  - Three 3-week cycles of ECF—surgery—3 cycles ECF vs surgery alone
  - 5-year OS, distant mets, local recurrence—improved in chemo group
- **ACCORD trial**—perioperative chemotherapy (CF) vs surgery alone
- **FLOT4 trial**—ECF/ECX vs FLOT

- **INT116 trial**—surgery alone vs adjuvant 5-FU based chemo
- **CRITICS trial**—pre and postoperative chemotherapy ECC/EOC
- **ACTS GC trial**—surgery alone vs adjuvant S1 (12 months)
- **GOIRC trial**—surgery alone vs adjuvant PELF
- **Macdonald protocol**
  - 5-FU based adjuvant chemo RT

Chemotherapy for Adenocarcinoma

- ECX
  - Epirubicin
  - Cisplatin
  - Capecitabine
- EOX
  - Epirubicin
  - Oxaliplatin
  - Capecitabine
- ECF
  - Epirubicin
  - Cisplatin
  - 5-FU
- FLOT
  - Doxetaxil
  - Oxeplatin
  - 5-FU
  - Folic acid

Treatment in Nutshell

- **Stage I (EGC):**
  - EMR/ESD
  - Limited resection
  - Gastrotomy full thickness excision
  - D1 gastrectomy
- **EGJ tumors**
  - Siewert 1—as esophageal cancer
  - Siewert 2—no consensus—individualized
  - Transabdominal vs THE vs transthoracic
  - Siewert 3—as Ca stomach
- **Intraperitoneal chemotherapy**
  - HIPEC-hyperthermic
  - Normothermic intraop intraperitoneal CT-(NIIC)
  - Early postop intraperitoneal CT-(EPIC) normo-thermic
  - Delayed postop intraperitoneal CT—normothermic
- **Palliative**
  - Chemotherapy
  - In morbid—single or 2 agents preferred
  - Epidermal growth factor receptor inhibitor—cetuximab—shows early good results—in phase 3 trial stage
  - HER2 antagonist—trastuzumab
  - 6–35% ca stomach—HER2 positive
  - ToGA trial—better median survival

- **Metastatic disease**
  - HER2 neupositive in 12–23%: Trastuzumab
  - More in intestinal type, mod differentiated
  - In MSI-H and dMMR: Pembrolizumab
- MMR is assessed by IHC
- MSI by PCR
  - In PDL-1 (programmed death ligand) expression pembrolizumab can be given
  - Emerging marker
    - EBV
- **Target therapy**
  - Trastuzumab—monoclonal antibody
  - Cetuximab—monoclonal antibody
  - Vascular endothelial GF—MCA: Bevacizumab
  - Tyrosine kinase inhibitors: Sunitinib, apatinib
  - Inhibition of mammalian target of
  - Rapamycin—everolimus
- Ramucirumab: VEGFR-2 antibody
- Pembrolizumab: PD-1 antibody

Locally Advanced

- **Role of multiorgan resection**
  - In T4—if can achieve R0 resection, there is survival benefit
  - Only palliative resection—survival similar to chemo group only
  - In unresectable tumors on surgery—with no symptoms warranting resection—palliative resection is avoided
  - CT scan predictive value for T4 disease—50% only
- **Carcinoma stomach with GOO**
  - Predicted short survival (metastasis)
  - Endoscopic dilatation
  - Stenting
  - Chemo RT
  - Predicted long survival
  - GJ or palliative gastrectomy
- **Outcomes**
  - Overall 5-year survival—25%
  - Following curative resection 5-year—24–57%
  - In early—80%
  - >63% present with locally advanced or mets
- **Recurrence**
  - Recurrence—40–80%
  - Most occur in first 3 years
  - Locoregional—38–45%
  - Most common site gastric remnant at anastomosis, gastric bed, regional LN
  - Peritoneal—54%
  - Isolated distant metastasis—uncommon

Prophylactic Gastrectomy

- 1–3% gastric cancers are hereditary
- Most common hereditary diffuse gastric cancer
- Autosomal dominant
- Diffuse signet ring type
- Germline mutation of CDH1 (E-cadherin)
- Hereditary diffuse gastric cancer
  - In women
  - Average age of diagnosis—37
  - Women—with CDH1 mutation—high risk for lobular carcinoma breast
- Lynch syndrome
  - Risk 1 to 13%—second most common extracolonic malignancy after endometrium
- Juvenile polyposis syndrome
  - When UGI is involved, lifetime risk of gastric cancer—21%
- Peutz-Jeghers syndrome—risk of GC—29%
- FAP—1–2% risk
- In hereditary diffuse gastric cancer, once mutation is diagnosed, prophylactic gastrectomy is done between age 18 and 40.
- Other hereditary GC syndromes

Syndrome	Genes	Inheritance
Ataxia-telangiectasia	ATM	Autosomal recessive
Bloom syndrome	BLM/RECQL3	Autosomal recessive
Hereditary breast ovarian cancer syndrome	BRCA1, BRCA2	Autosomal dominant
Cowden syndrome	PTEN	Autosomal dominant
Li-Fraumeni syndrome	TP53	Autosomal dominant
Xeroderma pigmentosum	7 genes	Autosomal recessive

> **Pearls**
> - Localised cancer—Tis, T1a
> - Locoregional—T1b-T4a, M0
> - Metastatic—T4b, M1
> - Tis,T1a—EMR
> - T1b—primary surgery possible
> - >T2—periop chemo

2.7 MISCELLANEOUS

Hypertrophic Gastritis (Menetrier's Disease)

- Hypoproteinemic hypertrophic gastropathy
- Rare acquired premalignant disease
- Massive gastric folds at fundus and body
- Cobblestone or cribriform appearance
- Histology
- Foveolar hyperplasia—expansion of surface mucosal cells
- **Absence of parietal cells**

Causes

- Unknown
- Cytomegalovirus—in children
- *H. pylori*—in adults
- Increased transforming growth factor-alfa seen in gastric mucosa

Clinical Features

- Pain abdomen
- Weight loss
- Anorexia
- Peripheral edema

DD

- Carcinoma, lymphoma

Investigation

- Chromium labelled albumin test indicative of GI protein loss
- 24 pH test—achlor/hypochlorhydria

Treatment

- **Medical**—inconsistent results
  - Anticholinergic
  - Acid suppression
  - Octreotide
  - anti *H. pylori*
- **Total gastrectomy**
  - Massive protein loss with failed med treatment
  - Dysplasia, carcinoma
- **Protein loss from stomach**
- **Excessive mucus secretion**
- **Achlor/hypochlorhydria**

> - Gross hypertrophy of gastric mucosal folds
> - Mucus production
> - Hypochlorhydria
> - Premalignant
> - Present with anemia and hypoproteinemia
> - Due to overexpression of TGF-alfa—bind to EGF receptor
> - Only treatment—gastrectomy

Mallory-Weiss Tear

- Associated with forceful vomiting, retching, coughing, straining: Against unrelaxed glottis
- Disruption of gastric mucosa *on lesser curvature at GE junction*
- Account for 15% GI bleeding
- Rarely massive bleeding
- Overall mortality 3–4%—especially in PHT

Treatment

- Endoscopic—choice
  - Laser, clips, thermal
- Angiography—embolisation
- Surgery—gastrostomy—oversewing

Dieulafoy's Lesion

- Account for 0.3–7% of nonvariceal bleed
- Bleeding from a 1–3 mm artery coursing in submucosa
- Pulsation of this artery—erosion of the overlying mucosa—artery exposed to gastric contents—erosion—bleeding
- Mucosal defect 3–5 mm—surrounded by normal mucosa
- 6–10 cm from GEJ—commonly fundus near cardia
- Men, 5th decade
- Commonest presentation—sudden onset, painless, recurrent hemetemesis with hypotension
- Diagnosis by OGD—identifies lesion in 80%
- May need repeated scopy
- Endoscopic treatment—choice
- Angiogram: Ectatic vessel in the left gastric artery branch—embolisation
- Surgery—wedge resection: Endoscopic tattooing to identify lesion

Gastric Volvulus

- Along stomach's longitudinal axis—organoaxial—two-thirds of cases
- Along vertical axis—mesenterico axial—one-third of cases

Organoaxial

- Associated with diaphragmatic defect
- Acute—obstruction both ends
- Associated with diaphragm defects in adults following trauma, paraesophageal hernia
- Children—foramen of Bochdalek hernia/eventeration
- Upside down stomach
- Obstruction at cardia and pyloroduodenal ends
- Along longitudinal axis

Mesenterico Axial

- Recurrent
- Partial <180 degree rotation
- Not associated with diaphragmatic defect

- Stomach folds itself on transverse axis
- Pyloroduodenal obstruction

Clinical Features

- Pain abdomen, hemetemesis
- **Borchardt's triad:**
  - Severe upper abdominal pain
  - Retching with little vomitus
  - Inability to pass RT
- **Diagnosis**
  - X-ray chest—gas filled viscus in the chest/upper abdomen
  - Confirmed by Barium study or endoscopy

Treatment

- Surgical emergency
- Laparotomy—stomach reduced and uncoiled—diaphragmatic defect repaired—fundoplication in PEH
- Strangulation (5–28%)—part resected
- Spontaneous without diaphragmatic defect—detorsion—stomach fixed by gastropexy or tube gastrostomy
  - Untwisting and gastropexy to anterior abdominal wall.
  - Gastrectomy—if stomach gangrenous.
  - Treat hiatus hernia or eventration.
  - Tanner's gastropexy

Bezoars

- Phytobezoar—vegetable fibers most common
- Trichobezoar—hair
- Pharmacobezoar—medicines or vitamins with its coating
- Lactobezoar—undigested milk—in infants
- Collection of nondigestable material

Phytobezoar

- Seen in previous gastric surgery
- Diabetics
- Impaired gastric emptying
- Following bariatric surgery

Rapunzel Syndrome

- Gastric trichobezoar
- Tail-like extension to duodenum or small intestine
- May cause jaundice or pancreatitis

Management

- Present with early satiety, pain, abdominal mass
- **Diagnosis**—barium/endoscopy

- **Treatment**
  - Papain (Adolph's meat tenderiser)
  - 1 tsp in 150–200 ml water—several times
  - Contain sodium so it can cause hypernatremia
- Followed by endoscopic fragmentation
- Also cellulase
- In case of failure, surgery is indicated

Trichobezoar

- In women with long hair
- Trichophagy
- GOO, abdomen mass, ulceration, SI obstruction
- Form cast of stomach
- Small bezoars treated by enzymatic/endoscopic
- Majority need surgery
- Inspect small intestine
- Psychiatric management

Gastric Antral Vascular Ectasia (GAVE)

- Also known as—watermelon stomach—because of appearance
- Seen in elderly
- Occult blood loss—anemia
- Associated with systemic sclerosis, PHT
- Endoscopy—linear red streaks along gastric rugal folds in the antrum—watermelon appearance
- Also have angiomata
- **Treatment**—endoscopic—argon laser plasma, heater probe, rubber band
- TIPS—not very effective in PHT
- Refractory—distal gastrectomy

Glomus Tumor

- Gastric glomus tumor—most common site antrum
- Pain abdomen, bleeding
- DD: GIST, paraganglioma, carcinoid
- **Treatment**—excision/gastrectomy

Heterotopic Pancreas

- Rare
- >70% near antrum
- Mostly incidental—rarely pain, bleeding
- **Endoscopy**—conical with central umbilication—'Volcano' sign
- Submucosal lesion
- EUS-FNAC can diagnose
- May contain malignancy—so excised

2.8 POSTGASTRECTOMY SYNDROME

- Gastric reservoir dysfunction
  - Dumping syndrome
  - Metabolic aberrations

- Vagal denervation
  - Diarrhea
  - Gastric stasis
  - Gall stones
- Aberrations in reconstruction
  - Bile reflux gastritis
  - Afferent/efferent loop obstructions

- **Dumping**
  - GI and CVS symptom complex
  - 25% of patients following PUD surgery get
  - Very low after HSV
  - Approx 1% only permanently disabled

Early Dumping

- 20–30 minutes after eating
- Seen more in gastrectomy with Bill II
- Less with Bill I or vagotomy with drainage
- More of GI symptoms than CVS
- Nausea, vomiting, crampy pain. fullness, explosive diarrhoea

CVS

Palpitation, diaphoresis, tachycardia, flushing blurred vision

Pathophysiology

- Rapid passage of high osmolar fluid into SI—due to bypass, stomach unable to deliver isoosmolar fluid slowly—rapid shift of fluid from ECF into lumen—autonomic response
- Also cause release of humoral agents—serotonin, bradykinin-like substances, neurotensin, enteroglucagon, renin-angiotensin-aldosterone, peptide YY

Diagnosis

- Scintigraphic gastric emptying study
  - 50% of isotope labelled solid meal has emptied in 1 hour

Late Dumping

- Larger amount of carbohydrate in SI—absorbed—intestinal hormones glucagon like peptide-1(GLP-1)—induce insulin release—overcompensation produce profound hypoglycemia and release of catecholamines
- Diaphoresis, tremulousness, tachycardia, lightheadedness
- Similar to insulin shock
- Rarer than early dumping
- Develops in >70% after bariatric surgery

Treatment

- Dietary measures
- Avoid food with larger amount of sugar

- Frequent small feeds
- More of lipids and protein
- Separated liquids and solids in meal
- Octreotide
- Alfa-glucosidase inhibitor: Acarbose—in late dumping
- Octreotide in dumping—will not control diarrhea and may form gall stones

Early vs late dumping		
	Early	*Late*
Incidence	5–10%	5%
Relation to meals	Immediate	2nd hour after meal
Durations of attack	30–40 min	30–40 min
Aggravated	More food	Exercise
Precipitating	Carbohydrate rich/wet food	As early
Relief	Lying down	Food
Symptoms	Fullness, sweating, light headedness, tachycardia, diarrhoea	Tremor, faintness, prostration

Surgical Treatment

- Majority respond to conservative methods
- <1% surgery required
- If primary procedure involved no gastric resection—only pyloric dysfunction—reconstruction of pylorus
- Previously resected with Billroth 2 reconstruction, convert it into Billroth 1 anastomosis
- Interposition of iso or anti-peristaltic loop of jejunum—slows down peristalsis
- Roux-en-Y GJ—choice
- Electrical and mechanical activity in Roux—travel towards stomach—aborad—so slows the gastric emptying
  - Most durable

Metabolic Disturbances

- Most common—anemia
- Iron deficiency—more common
  - >30% following gastrectomy
  - Reduced intake/absorption
  - c/c blood loss
  - Iron supplements—corrects
- Iron needs acidic environment for absorption
- Vit B_{12} bioavailability is facilitated by acidic environment
- So even in partial gastrectomy with acid reduction—deficiency of B_{12} can occur

- Total gastrectomy—lifelong cyanocobalamine—inj every 3–4 months
- Megaloblastic anemia occur in vit B_{12} deficiency
  - Subtotal/total gastrectomy
  - Should receive lifelong B_{12}
- Osteoporosis/osteomalacia
  - Bone disease develops 4–5 years after surgery
- Supplement calcium 1–2 g, vit D 500–5000 U/day
- Can get fat malabsorption
- In Bill II/Roux—by passing duodenum supplementation of fat soluble vitamins is indicated

Postvagotomy Diarrhea

- Mechanisms
  - Bile acid malabsorption
  - Infection—due to lack of acid
  - Rapid gastric emptying
- 5–10% following vagotomy—clinically significant diarrhea
- 1%—sustained problem

Treatment

- Usually gets corrected by itself
- Cholestyramine—bile salt binding
- Antibiotics
- If incapacitating diarrhea 1 year after surgery and failed medical management remedial surgery may be indicated
- Octreotide—not useful
- For postvagotomy diarrhea
  - Interposition of 10 cm reversed jejunum

Afferent Loop Syndrome

- Partial obstruction to afferent loop—accumulation of pancreatic biliary secretions—distension—crampy pain—forcible emptying into stomach—bilious vomiting—relief of symptoms
- In obstruction—bacterial growth—bind with B_{12}—anemia
- Can perforate
- Due to long afferent limb
- Endoscopy—failure to visualise afferent loop
- Radionuclide scan of the biliary tree—look for excretion (HIDA)

Treatment

Surgical

- Billroth 2 convert to Billroth 1
- Enteroenterostomy
- Convert to Roux-en-Y

Efferent Loop Obstruction

- Rare—causes intestinal obstruction
- Due to adhesions or retroanastomotic herniation of SI in right to left direction
    - 50% occur within first month
- Pain and bilious vomiting
- Diagnosed by Barium—failure to enter efferent limb
- Surgery—repair retroanastomotic hernia and close that space
- JJ can solve this problem

Alkaline Reflux Gastritis

- Reflux of bile—gastritis—bilious vomiting
- HIDA scan—demonstrate
- Endoscopy—beefy red, friable gastric mucosa with erosions
- More common in gastrectomy with Billroth 2

Treatment
Medical

- PPI, anticholinergics, cholestyramine

Surgical

- Conversion to Roux-en-Y—40–45 cm
    - Interposition of isoperistaltic jejunal loop between gastric remnant and duodenum (Henley loop)
- In Billroth 2—do a Braun JJ
- Braun GJ-JJ
- Uncut Roux anastomosis
- Interposition of 40 isoperistaltic jejunum between stomach and duodenum—alkaline gastritis
    - Henley loop

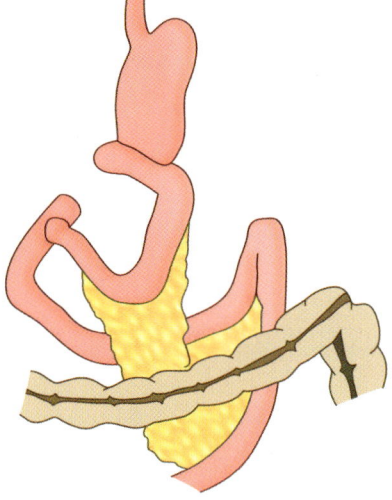

Gastric Atony

- More common after TV, SV—not HSV
- Confirmed by scintigraphy
- Endoscopy

DD

DM, electrolyte imbalance, drug toxicity, neuromuscular

Treatment

- Functional GOO
- Metochlopromide—dopamine antagonist and cholinergic agonist
- Erythromycin—motilin agonist
- Domperidone
- Gastrostomy/jejunostomy feed
- TPN
- Intractable cases gastrectomy—delayed for at least 3 months

Gall Stones

- Due to division of hepatic branch of vagus—dysmotility—stones
- Prophylactic cholecystectomy—not indicated
- But can be done when further intervention is difficult—gastric bypass for morbid obesity
- GB is abnormal with sludge

Roux Syndrome

- Difficulty in gastric emptying
- Vomiting
- Dilated stomach and Roux limbs—no mechanical obstruction
- CT/GI series—show delayed gastric emptying
- Cause—abnormal propulsive force towards stomach
- More common in large gastric remnant or vagotomy

Treatment

- Motility drugs
- Surgery
- Convert to 95% gastrectomy
    - Resect Roux limb—construct another Roux
- Billroth 2 with Braun JJ
- Interposition of jejunal limb between stomach and duodenum

Jejunogastric Intussusception

- Most commonly in simple GJ
- Efferent limb gets intussuscepted into stomach
- Also in Billroth 2
- Pain, bloody vomiting, tender mass

- Surgical emergency
- Resection of the loop
- Fixing the afferent and efferent limbs to other structures like colon, stomach
  - Convert Billroth 2 to Billroth 1

Gastrojejunal Colic Fistula

- Anastomotic ulcer penetrates transverse colon
- Severe diarrhea follows every meal
- Foul breath—may vomit feces
- Weight loss—DD cancer
- Major factor contamination of jejunum with colonic bacteria
- Endoscopy—may not show fistula in 50%
- Barium—not useful
- When GJ-colic fistula develops, patient complaints relief of pain
  - Diarrhoea is due to enteritis.

- *Investigation of choice is CT with oral contrast/ Barium enema*
- NO role to drug therapy
- Surgery is the treatment of choice—triple resection of the involved gastric, jejunal and colonic segments with anastomosis is the choice

Small Stomach Syndrome

- Early satiety follows all PUD surgery
- Also in HSV—due to loss of receptive relaxation
- Gets better with time—no need for surgery

Malignant Transformation

- Gastrectomy or vagotomy + drainage independent risk factors
- Risk 4 times than control population
- Lag phase at least 10 years
- HSV—not associated with increased incidence of cancer in the long term

Bariatric Surgery

The surgical treatment of morbid obesity is known as bariatric surgery.

Two unique aspects of the field of bariatric surgery.

- This surgery involves the alteration of metabolic processes by changes in appetite, energy regulation, satiety, and metabolism, and weight loss.
- Long-term follow-up is required to really know the effect of these operations on a patient's overall health.

Morbid obesity (severe obesity) is defined as

- Body mass index of 40 kg/m^2—this definition is more accepted internationally
- 100 pounds above ideal body weight.
- Twice ideal body weight

Pathophysiology and Associated Medical Problems

- Genetic and environmental factors
- Familial predisposition
- The genetic abnormality of leptin deficiency leads to severe childhood obesity.

Specific Genes That Are Associated with Obesity

- FTO gene (fat mass and obesity related)—role in controlling feeding behaviour and energy expenditure.
- MC4R deficiency gene (melanocortin 4 receptor)—associated with obesity, increased fat mass, and insulin resistance
- β_2-adrenergic receptor obesity genes—role in regulation of lipolysis and thermogenesis
- Environmental component—easily available, cheap, high-density, calorie-rich foods and physical inactivity
- Another theory—bacteria within the gut, known as the microbiome, play a role in the metabolism and immune system.

Ghrelin

- Orexigenic gut hormone
- Also known as the hunger hormone
- Secreted by P/D1 cells of the gastric fundus
- Stimulates release of various neuropeptides, such as neuropeptide Y and growth hormone, from the hypothalamus increasing appetite state.

- Increased levels develop in individuals after low-calorie diets, thus suggesting that one possible mechanism for the failure of most diets after 6 months is the increase in the appetite hormone ghrelin.

Morbid obesity is a metabolic disease associated with numerous medical problems
- Most common—arthritis and degenerative joint disease
- Sleep apnoea.
- Asthma
- Hypertension in more than 30%
- Diabetes in more than 20%
- Gastroesophageal reflux in 20% to 30% of patients

The metabolic syndrome includes type 2 diabetes mellitus caused by insulin resistance, dyslipidaemia, and hypertension.
- The syndrome is characterized by impaired hepatic uptake of insulin,
- Systemic hyperinsulinemia, and
- Tissue resistance to insulin.

Medical Therapy

- Short-term success

Medical Vs Surgical Trials

- **SOS** study, most common cause of death in surgery patient—cancer
- **Adam trial,** compared RYGB with no surgery group, mortality decreased by 40% after surgery
- **O'Brien RCT**, comparison in obese adolescents between LAGB and diet control
- **Schauer study** with 150 obese patients also showed surgery as superior to medical.

Pharmacological Therapy

- **Phentermine:** Decreases appetite, increases resting energy expenditure
- **Orlistat:** Inhibits pancreatic lipase
- **Phentermine topiramate combination:** Induces 5% body weight loss in 80%

- **Lorcaserin:** Less side effects, showed 5% weight loss after 1 year of treatment
  - But weight regained after 12 to 18 months after medication is stopped

Indications for Bariatric Surgery

- BMI >40 kg/m^2 with or without other medical problems
- BMI >35 kg/m^2 with comorbidities which may improve after surgically induced weight loss—diabetes, hypertension, hyperlipidemia, Pickwickian syndrome, NAFLD, GERD
- BMI: 30 to 35 kg/m^2 with diabetes or metabolic syndromes

Bariatric Surgery in Adolescents

- BMI >40
- Has followed 6 months of weight reducing attempts
- Shows skeletal maturity
- Psychologically stable

Contraindications for Bariatric Surgery

- No absolute contraindications (SAGES)
- Should be avoided in (European guidelines)
  - Psychologically unstable
    - □ Substance abuse
    - □ Serious medical disease
    - □ Secondary type 2 diabetes
  - Antibody positive diabetes, presence of islet cell antibody
  - Cirrhosis, PHT
    - □ Active cancer
    - □ Prader-Willi syndrome
    - □ Pregnancy
- Pregnancy should be avoided 12 to 18 months after bariatric surgery

Mechanism of Action of Bariatric Surgery

Classified as

1. **Restrictive:** LAGB and LSG: Decrease in appetite and early induction of satiety
2. **Malabsorptive:** BPD and DS: Brain gut interaction enteroencephalic endocrine axis affected, ghrelin levels suppressed
   - Increase insulin sensitivity of liver and muscle
   - Also, many metabolic effects
   - Weight independent effects on glucose metabolism is due to the incretin stimulation due to the bypass of duodenum. Incretins are peptides affecting synthesis and release of insulin, and are synthesised in small and large intestines. Bypass of duodenum in RYGB causes stimulation of incretin secreting cells and increased GLP-1 secretion and thereby improving glucose metabolism
   - Alteration in gut microbiome due to bypass

3. **Hybrid procedures: RYGB**
   - RYGB has effect on beta cell function that can result in remission of DM

Preoperative Evaluation and Selection

- Eligibility
- Selection based on currently accepted NIH and AHA/ACC/TOS guidelines

General Bariatric Preoperative Evaluation and Preparation

- Counseling and educating
- Preop antibiotic (first generation cephalosporin)
- DVT prophylaxis
- If there is any associated hernia, repair usually done after weight loss
- If associated gall stone, cholecystectomy can be considered (incidence of gall stone or sludge after gastric bypass is 30%)

Operative Procedures

Restrictive

1. Vertical banded gastroplasty:

- Now not done due to poor long-term weight loss and late stenosis.
- Lesser curvature was used to make restrictive pouch, as this part was resistant to dilation with pressure

2. Laparoscopic adjustable gastric banding

2 bands approved: LAP band and Realize band.
Pars flaccida technique is used—the proximal area of gastrohepatic ligament (pars flaccida) is where the band is placed. This is 2–3 cm below GE junction. Port is placed below costal margin and saline is injected to adjust the band pressure

- Band is initially placed without adding saline to distend it, saline is added in 1–1.5 mL increments to produce desired weight loss of 1 to 2 kg/week.
- Nutritional deficiency will be low
- Potential problem is esophageal dilatation from chronic obstruction secondary to band slippage
- Resolve type 2 DM in 50% and improve in 83%, hypertension may be resolved in 40% and remission in 70%

Advised in Patients

- Who wish for moderate weight loss
- Who had successful control of weight with diet control
- Physically active

Relative Contraindications

- BMI >50, morbidity, poor diet control

Absolute Contraindications

- Previous anti-reflux surgery
- Large hiatal hernia
- Esophageal motility disorders

Band is adjusted so that patient can eat and drink optimally.

Complications

- Stenosis
- Perforation
- Prolapse of stomach. Stomach below the band herniates into the lumen of the band—produce symptoms of GERD and obstruction. Treated by releasing the fluid in the band—if not relieved—swallow studies done—may need surgery to release the buckle and pressure
- Slippage—band slips down onto stomach leads to obstruction
- Leak is very rare unlike other surgeries
- Band slippage in pars flaccida approach—4% (diagnosed by a plain X-ray with band in horizontal position 10 o' clock to 4 o' clock position is diagnostic), can result in obstruction, strangulation, stenosis and esophageal dilatation.
- Erosion of band (seen in 1 to 3%)
- Port access problems: Leakage (11%) or kinking of access tubing can occur
- Port site infection

3. Laparoscopic sleeve gastrectomy

- Involve resection of greater curvature of stomach and creating small stomach based on lesser curvature with its blood supply
- Removes about 80% of stomach
- Simple procedure, nomal absorption, and no internal herniation
- While making gastric tube, orally placed bougie is used of size 32–50 F—most common 36 F
- Average size of stomach that remains is about 150 ml
- Oversewing the staple lines has no clear benefits
- Can place omentum at the suture site
- GERD is a problem postoperatively
- Due to high morbidity after DS in BMI >60, performed in two stage, with sleeve gastrectomy alone in first stage, reducing BMI to 45
- Very low serious complication
- Improvement in comorbidities similar to that of RYGB

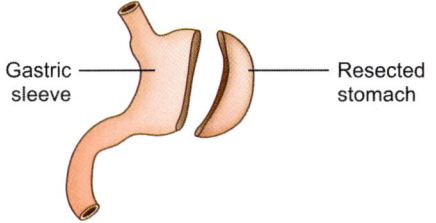

Gastric sleeve — Resected stomach

Advantages

- Good control of diabetes
- Decrease Ghrelin levels
- Decrease in gastric emptying time and increase in incretins like glucagon like peptide (GLP1) due to early presentation of food to ileum.

Complications: Most common—leak along gastric staple line and bleeding (1%). Most common site of leak proximal third of stomach near GE junction. CT or gastrografin study done. Early leaks are managed by surgery. Late leaks are managed conservatively and surgery only if peritonitis and sepsis develop

- Mortality .07–.11
- VTE, infection, reoperation
- Malabsorption is less
- Leak more common

Stricture—most common site near incisura angularis

Largely Restrictive, Moderately Malabsorptive
Roux-en-Y Gastric bypass

- Most commonly performed bariatric surgery and is the gold standard
- Causes weight loss and improves DM, but sustained long-term weight loss appears essential for its effect on DM
- Resolves symptom of pseudotumor cerebri and cure venous stasis ulcers
- Immediate resolution of symptoms of GERD in 90%

Indications

- BMI >40
- BMI >35 with other morbidities of obesity
- Failure of trial dieting
- Patients with GERD and diabetes and obesity—have best results in patients with GERD and type 1 DM

Absolute Contraindications

- Drug abuse
- Morbid medical conditions
- Psychiatric disabilities
- Age <15 and >70—relative contraindications

Technique

- Length of roux limb is according to patient: BMI 40, roux limb 80 to 120 cm
- In patients with BMI >50, roux limb 150 cm
- Stomach is divided in the proximal part, from lesser curvature up to angle of His, avoiding fundus from the newly created gastric pouch
- Most common long-term adverse effect—weight gain
- Others—marginal ulcers, obstruction

Complications

- Lap approach has less complication, but more early bowel obstruction due to internal hernia
- Anastomotic leak 2%
- Pulmonary embolism 1%, 30% of cause of death
- Nausea, vomiting, dehydration and Wernicke encephalopathy, if there is prolong vomiting
- Stenosis of GJ (2–14%), more with circular staplers, manifest at 4 to 6 weeks, treat with endoscopic balloon dilatation (not in marginal ulcer)
- Marginal ulcer (2–10%), incidence can be decreased by preoperative treatment of *H. pylori*
- Iron and B12 (15–20%) deficiency

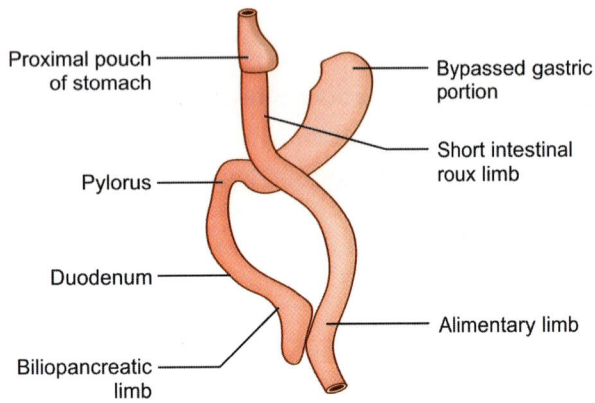

Largely Malabsorptive

1. Biliopancreatic Diversion

Reconstructed GI tract with short common channel of 50 cm distal ileum for fat absorption, proximal stomach anastomosed to distal ileum.

Procedure includes—distal gastrectomy, with 400 ml gastric pouch, division of small bowel 250 cm proximal to ileocecal junction. Roux-en-Y gastro-enterostomy is done and biliopancreatic limb is anastomosed to small intestine creating a 50 cm common limb.

Produce weight loss. But also nutritional deficiencies, so, not popular, indicated only in super obese individuals who have failed with other methods.

- Excess weight loss in patients noted (70%), so preferred in super obese

- More side effects
- Highly effective in treating comorbid conditions
- Vitamin supplements needed monthly

Complications

- Mortality 1.1%
- Leak 1.8%
- Reoperation in 4%
- Malnutrition is more (12%), manifest within months. vitamin D deficiency and vitamin A deficiency
- Marginal ulcers
- Bloating in 30%
- Bone pain
- Due to complication and dangers of surgery, it is the least preferred surgery

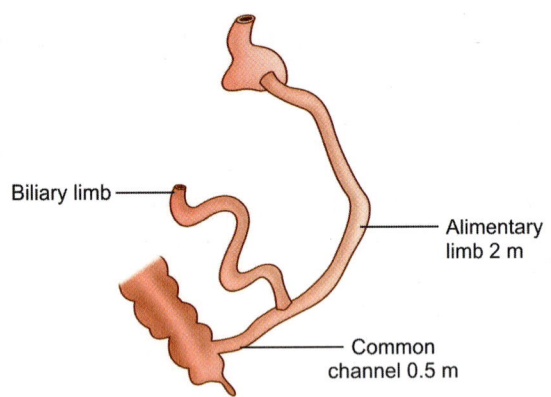

2. Duodenal Switch

Sleeve gastrectomy of greater curvature, duodenum divided 2 cm beyond pylorus, distal connection like BPD 100 cm proximal to IC valve, proximal anastomosis between bowel 250 cm from ileocecal valve and first portion of duodenum

- Cholecystectomy is also done
- Not very popular procedure

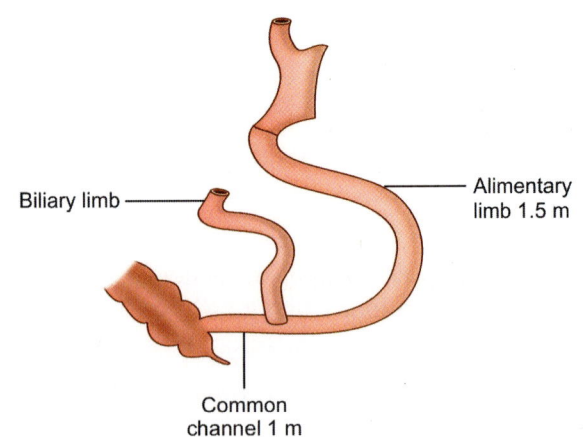

Postoperative Care and Follow-up

- Most dreaded complication is a leak from GI tract
- DVT prophylaxis, early ambulation within 4 to 6 hours, LMWH, (pulmonary embolism is a major cause of death)
- A goal of 1–2 lb/week weight loss
- After RYGB, visit within 2 weeks to assess wound healing, to start solid diet, subsequent visit at 3, 6, 12 months and annually, to monitor weight loss and nutrition assessment (vit A, D, B$_{12}$)
- After BPD and DS, patient seen within 2 weeks to be certain that diarrhea is not prolific and there is no dehydration
- Follow-up to assess fat soluble vitamin, LFT and metabolic stability

Results

- Beneficial in diabetes and obesity

Other Procedures

One Anastomosis Gastric Bypass (Omega Loop Gastric Bypass) Mini Gastric Bypass

- Proximal gastric pouch is created on entire lesser curvature
- GJ is done using jejunal loop 200 cm distal to ligament of Treitz in antecolic manner

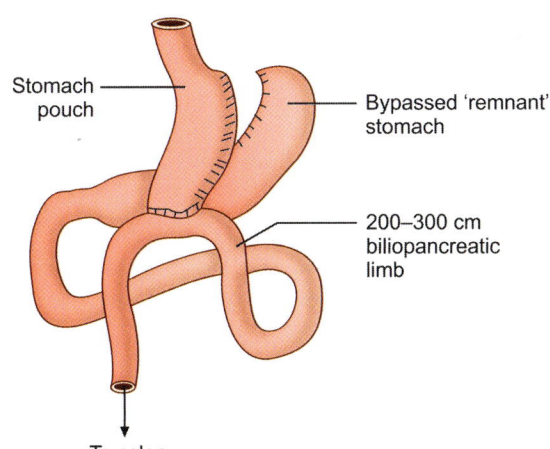

Stomach pouch
Bypassed 'remnant' stomach
200–300 cm biliopancreatic limb
To colon

Single Anastomosis Duodenal Switch

- Single duodeno-ileal anastomosis 200 cm proximal to ileocecal valve is done

Endoscopic Procedures

Intragastric Balloons

- Obera balloon—single balloon
- Reshape balloon—double balloon

- Both work on the same principle—create a space occupying object inside stomach

Endoscopic Sleeve Gastrectomy

- Performed using overstitch device
- Creates limited size gastric lumen by performing sutured gastroplasty
- Trans oral gastroplasty system (TOGA). A stapled pouch is made along lesser curvature and creates gastroplasty as a 8 cm long tube from GE junction

Malabsorptive Procedures

- Endobarrier GI liner. 60 cm polymer implant sleeve
- Duodenal jejunal sleeve placed endoscopically into duodenum or GE junction. Food passes quickly to jejunum through the sleeve. Avoids mixing of chyme with proximal jejunum

Neurohormonal Modulatory Procedures

- Implantable gastric devices are used to manipulate neurohormonal signals to induce satiety

Primary Obesity Surgery Endoluminal (POSE)

- Endoscopic restrictive procedure. Reduces the size of stomach by endoscopic suturing

Bariatric Surgery and its Effect of Weight Loss and Glycemic Control

Foregut theory of bariatric surgery

- On exclusion of duodenum from alimentary pathway, can eliminate the physiologic influence of duodenal gut hormones and the enzymes like glucagon, CCK, and biliopancreatic enzymes
- **Hindgut theory**
  - Rapid transit of food to distal bowel induces secretion of distal gut hormones called incretins like glucagon like peptide (GLP1) and peptide YY which cause early release of insulin
- **Gut microbiome**
  - Change in the composition of gut microbiome occurs after bariatric surgery which may contribute to weight loss and glycemic improvements
- **Bile acids**
  - Stimulate secretion of GLP1 and increase energy expenditure in brown adipose tissue. They also inhibit gluconeogenesis, increase glycogenesis, enhances insulin sensitivity. Plasma bile acids are elevated after RYGB

Liver

4.1 ANATOMY

History

- Anatomy of blood vessels of liver—Francis Glisson
- First documented partial hepatectomy—Berta
- Digital compression of hilar vessels to control bleeding—J Hogarth Pringle
- Segmental nature of liver—Couinaud, Goldsmith, Woodburne
- First documented anatomic liver resection—Lortat Jacob

Anatomy

- Weight—1.2 to 1.6 kg
- Areas without peritoneal covering
  - GB fossa
  - Porta hepatis
  - On either side of inferior vena cava
  - Bare area—portion on right of IVC

Ligaments

- Coronary ligaments are peritoneal reflections of diaphragm.
- R&L triangular ligament—lateral margin on either sides of coronary ligaments.
- Falciform ligament—arises from centre of coronary ligament and connects diaphragm, anterior abdominal wall and umbilicus.
- Ligament teres—obliterated umbilical vein, runs along inferior edge of falciform from umbilicus to umbilical fissure (contains left portal pedicle)
- Ligamentum venosum—obliterated sinus venosum, on posterior surface of liver running from left portal vein towards left hepatic vein and IVC
- Division of R&L triangular ligament helps in mobilization of liver
- Division of superior leaflets of falciform ligament. Exposes suprahepatic IVC and that of left triangular ligament exposes IVC.

Liver Ligaments

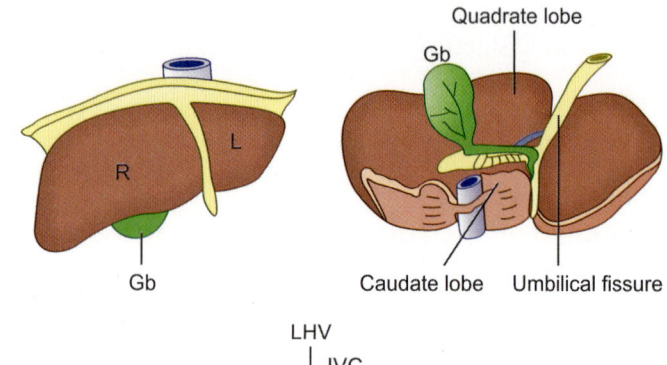
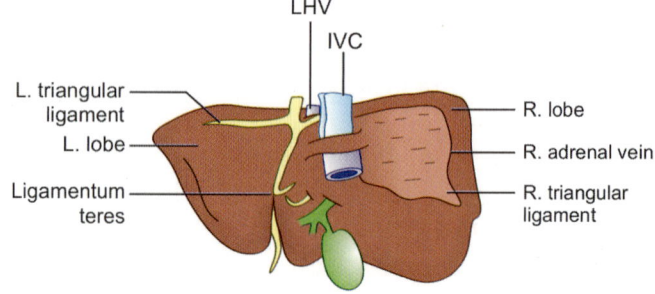

Functional Anatomy

- 8 segments, each with separate pedicle.
- These 8 segments are divided into four sectors separated by scissure containing 3 main hepatic veins
- Main scissura (aka Cantlie's line)—contains middle hepatic vein, runs anteriorly from GB fossa to the left of IVC, divides liver into left and right lobes
- Right liver comprises 2/3rd of total liver volume
- Right liver is divided into anterior (segment 5&8) and posterior (6&7) by right scissura which contain right hepatic vein.
- Umbilical fissure on posterior surface of left liver contains left portal pedicle.
- Each segment has a portal pedicle (PV, HA and BD)
- Scissura containing portal pedicles—called hepatic scissura
- Segment IV is divided into superior IVa and inferior IVb

- IV b is also drained by umbilical vein
- Left portal scissura divides left lobe into anterior (3&4) and posterior (2) and contain left hepatic vein.
- Right portal triad has a short extrahepatic course (1 to 1.5 cm) as compared to left portal triad (3–4 cm)
- Connective tissue of left portal triad forms hilar plate.

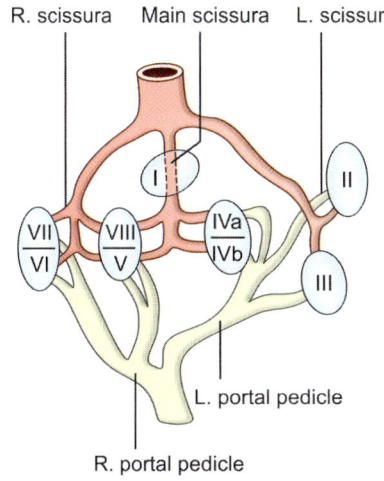

- **Caudate lobe:**
  – Dorsal portion of liver
  – Relations—superiorly—left and middle hepatic vein, posteriorly IVC, anteriorly portal triad
  – Derives arterial, venous and biliary drainage from both right and left pedicles
  – Right portion mainly from right pedicle and left from left pedicle
  – Hepatic venous drainage of caudate is unique as it drains directly to IVC
  – Constitutes 1–2% of total liver volume.
  – 3 subsegments—caudate process, paracaval caudate, Spiegel's lobe

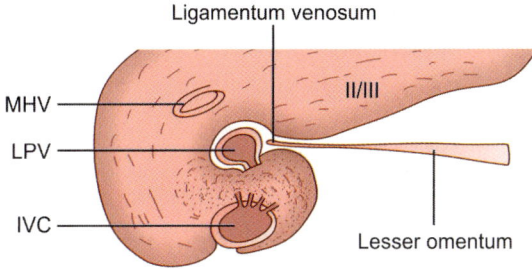

- Main bulk of caudate lobe is to the left of IVC
- Gastrohepatic omentum separates caudate lobe from segments II and III and it is attached to ligamentum venosum.

- Left portion of caudate lobe passes to the right between LPV and IVC—the caudate process—fuses with right lobe of liver
- Caudate lobe's—right lobe is variable
- Portion of liver between right part of caudate lobe and segment VIII is called segment IX—not much significance
- Posterior edge of caudate lobe—fibrous attaches to crura of diaphragm—extends posteriorly behind IVC—links to fibrous tissue called vena caval ligament which protrudes from segment VII
- In 50%—this may be replaced by hepatic tissue, thus caudate lobe may encase IVC
- Anteriorly abuts segment 4 and on right merges with segments 6 and 7
- Portion of caudate lobe on right side—segment IX also called paracaval caudate

Blood Supply
- Inflow—from right and left PV and LHA and right sectorial artery
- Venous drainage directly into IVC—only segment to do so

Hepatic Veins
- RHV is largest—short course of 1–2 cm
- Left and MHV may join together
- Umbilical vein—runs beneath falciform ligament—empties into terminal portion of LHV
- Accessory RHV—present in 15%
- Fibrous tissue extension from IVC to caudate lobe—ligament of vena cava
- Systemic drainage of the entire splanchnic circulation
- Normal pressure 1 to 2 mmHg
- Pressure gradient between PV and IVC is 5 mmHg
- HV blood may be two-thirds saturated with oxygen

Riedel's Lobe
- Anomalous development of liver where a tongue of liver tissue extending from inferior part of right liver.

Structures of Hilum
- Hepatic artery, bile duct, portal vein within the lesser omentum (hepatoduodenal ligament) + nerves and lymphatic enters the porta hepatis.

Note

For patients with tumor related cholestasis or marked underlying disease, a 40% liver remnant is necessary to avoid cholestasis, fluid retention and liver failure.

Portal Vein

- Supplies 75% of hepatic inflow, length 5.8 to 8 cm, diameter ~1 cm

- Forms by the union of SMV and splenic vein behind neck of pancreas

- Divides into left and right branch at hilum of liver

- Right portal vein has short extrahepatic course, enters substance of liver and divides into anterior and posterior sectoral branches.

- Left portal vein runs along base of segment 4 into umbilical fissure

- Portal vein lies posterior to hepatic artery and bile duct

- 90 degree turn at base of umbilical fissure to become umbilical portion before entering liver parenchyma

- Parasympathetic innervation—vagus

- Sympathetic innervation—greater splanchnic and celiac ganglia

- PV is valveless

- PV pressure 6 to 10 mmHg

- Due to large volume—may supply 30–70% of oxygen

- If PV flow is reduced, increase oxygen extraction from HA occurs, not by increasing flow

Hepatic Artery

- 25% blood flow, 30–50% oxygenation

- In hilum, hepatic artery lies anterior to portal vein and to the left of bile duct

- Left hepatic artery supplies segments 2, 3, 4

- Right hepatic artery runs posteriorly to common hepatic duct and enters Calot's triangle and gives off cystic artery.

- Anatomy of hepatic artery is highly variable

- Liver constitutes 2.5% of total body weight

- Receives 25% of cardiac output

- Total blood flow—800 to 1200 ml/minute equivalent to 100 ml/min/100 g of liver

- Liver blood volume 25 to 25 ml/100 g of liver (10–15% of blood volume)

- Sinusoids hold 60% of blood remaining in PV, HV and HA

- Liver is a good reservoir of blood

- Accessory vessel—aberrant origin of a branch that is in addition to normal branching pattern.

- Replaced vessel—aberrant origin of branch that substitute for lack of normal branch

- Accessory or replaced right hepatic artery arise from SMA—incidence 11–21%

- Replaced or accessory left hepatic artery arise from left gastric artery 12–15%

- Accessory cystic artery can arise from proper hepatic or gastroduodenal artery

- If common HA is ligated—vascularity is derived from inferior phrenic artery and GDA

- If proper HA is ligated, vascularity is through inferior phrenic artery only

- If RHA or LHA ligated—intrahepatic translobar anastomosis maintains vascularity

Common Bile Duct

Please refer to Chapter 5: Gall Bladder and Biliary System

Variation in anatomy of cystic artery
- MC arises from right hepatic artery (57%) and posterior to bile duct
- Double cystic artery, 2nd branch arises from proper hepatic artery

Nerve Supply

- Sympathetic fibres—T7–T10
- Parasympathetic—vagus

Microscopic Anatomy

- Functional unit of liver—acinus/lobule
- Structure of lobule—each consists of a central terminal hepatic venule surrounded by 4–6 terminal portal triad that forms a polygonal unit.
- Between terminal portal triad and venules 3 zones are there

  - **Zone 1**—periportal rich in oxygen and nutrients

  - **Zone 2**—intermediate zone

  - **Zone 3**—perivenular zone poor in nutrients

- Hence, centrilobular necrosis seen in hypotension, occurs in zone 3.

- Blood flow occurs from zones 1–2–3 in that order.

- Sinusoids (which are endothelial lined) in the hepatic lobule is the functional unit.

- Space between basal surface of hepatocyte and the sinusoid lining cells—*space of Disse*

- Diameter of sinusoids—7 to 15 micrometer.

- Peripherally the portal tracts (branches of HA, PV and BD) are grouped in *space of Mall*

- A classic lobule has endocrine function—blood flows towards centrilobular vein

- B-portal lobule has exocrine function—flow of bile is from classic lobule to bile duct. Area drained by each bile duct is triangular.

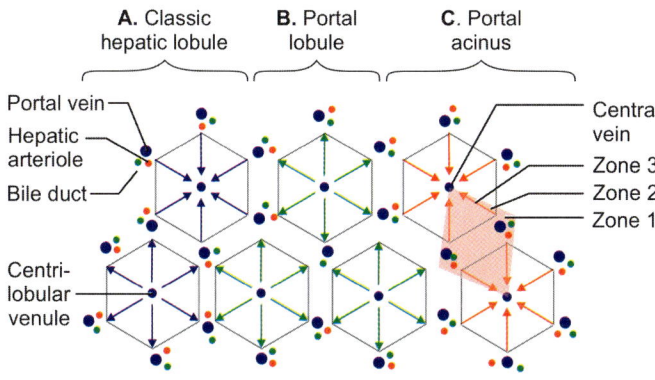

- C—Liver acinus (portal acinus) concept by Rappaport zones I, II and III. Distance from sinusoids determines delivery of oxygen and nutrient contents

- Sinusoidal endothelial cells are separated from hepatocytes by space of Disse—extracellular space to which hepatocytes projects microvilli

- Kupffer cells—found in sinusoidal endothelial lining, derived from macrophage monocyte system, they are phagocytes, class 2 antigens are exposed on Kupffer cells.

- Stellate/Ito cells found in space of Disse, have high retinoid content, functions are vitamin A storage and extracellular collagen synthesis and matrix proteins, plays role in fibrosis and cirrhosis

Blood Flow Regulation

- Liver cannot control PV flow

- Main regulation is on HA flow—regulated by adenosine—a vasodilator

- Adenosine secreted into space of Mall—causes—dilatation of HA—can buffer 25–60% decreased portal flow

Measurement of Liver Blood Flow

Doppler US—most common first line method

Small for Size Syndrome

- In living donor liver transplant—small remnant—pressure of full portal flow—leads to decreased arterial flow due to buffer system—can develop ischemia

- Also due to splenic artery (steal) syndrome—in patients with hypersplenism—arterial flow is shifted to splenic artery—reduces HA flow

- Can be reduced by prophylactic splenic artery ligation/embolisation

- More due to PHT than blood siphoning

Functions of Liver

- Energy—storage, metabolism and distribution, 2 major sources—glucose and acetoacetate

- Bile formation—1500 ml/day

Concentration of Hepatic Bile

- Sodium—132–165 mEq/L

- K—4.2–5.6 mEq/L

- Calcium—1.2–4.8 mEq/L

  □ Mg—1.4–3 mEq/L

  □ Chloride—96–126 mEq/L

  □ Osmolality—300 mOsm/kg

  □ HCO$_3$—17–55 mEq/L

  □ Protein—300–3000 mEq/L

  □ Cholesterol—60–320 mEq/L

  □ Phospholipid—25–810 mEq/L

Enterohepatic Circulation

- Primary bile salts—cholic acid and chenodeoxycholic acid

- Secondary bile salts—deoxycholic and lithocholic acid
- Bile acids are reabsorbed actively in ileum and passively in jejunum
- Bile salts help in absorption of fats, fat soluble vitamins and drugs

Bilirubin Metabolism

- Product of heme metabolism. Early phase of metabolism yields 20% (~3 days) of bilirubin, whereas late phase yields 80% (~120 days)
- Circulating bilirubin is bound to albumin which protects tissue from harmful effects
- This complex enters hepatic sinusoidal and get dissociated in space of Disse
- Free bilirubin is taken up by hepatocyte and it gets conjugated with glucuronic acid
- Secreted actively into bile—reach GIT—gets deconjugated by intestinal bacteria into urobilinogens—further oxidized and reabsorbed into enterohepatic circulation.

Carbohydrate Metabolism

- Stores and breakdown of glycogen
- Contains 65 gm/kg of liver weight
- Gluconeogenesis and Cori cycle

Protein Metabolism

- Synthesis, storage and catabolism of protein occur in liver
- Synthesis of acute phase reactants
  - Albumin, alpha-1 antitrypsin, ceruloplasmin
- IL1, IL6, TNF

Coagulation

- Synthesis of vitamin K dependent coagulation factors 2, 7, 9, 10, protein C, protein S

Metabolism of Drugs and Toxins

- By phase 1&2 reactions
- Phase 1—oxidation, reduction, hydrolysis
- Phase 2—mainly conjugation

Maintenance of Core Body Temperature

- pH balance

Removal of Gut Endotoxin and Foreign Body

Liver imaging
- USG—standard first line
- **CT—Gold standard**
  - Early arterial phase of contrast detects small liver cancers
  - Inflammatory lesions exhibit rim enhancement
  - Hemangioma shows characteristic late venous enhancement
- MRCP for—biliary tract
- ERCP—imaging and removal of stones
- PTC—biliary tract imaging when ERCP is failed
- Laparoscopic USG—to detect superficial peritoneal metastasis and superficial liver metastasis
- **Intraoperative USG**—gold standard for detecting liver lesions

Tumor staging, vascular structures, guidance of resection.

Volumetric Assessment

- CT or MRI used
- FLR volume = FLR/TLV
- Remanent liver volume is calculated by subtracting the tumor volume from TLV
- Total estimated liver volume (TELV) = −794 + 1267 × BSA (body surface area)
- FLR/TELV is standardized FLR (sFLR)

Specific Diagnostic Tests In Liver Disease

- Aminopyrine breath test—useful in prognosis of CLD (tests hepatic function)
- Lidocaine breath test—same as above, monoethylglycine xylidide (MEGX) is a metabolite of lidocaine, easy to estimate—metabolised primarily in liver
- Galactide elimination test—measures hepatic function
- Indocyanine green dye—only test shown to have prognostic ability in cirrhotic patients undergoing liver resection
  - Exclusively cleared by liver and excreted unchanged in bile
- GGT not very specific, 5' nucleotidase increased level suggests hepatic disease
- Measurement of specific clotting factors 5 and 7, used in evaluation of function in transplantation population
- Quantitative tests—Child-Pugh score is used for cirrhotic

Nuclear Imaging Techniques

- Tc 99 labelled galactosyl serum albumin scintigraphy
  - Uptake is reduced on hepatocytes in diseases
  - Can assess total and localised liver function
- Tc 99 labelled IDA scintigraphy
  - Tc 99 Mebrofenin—a derivative of IDA
  - **MRI with contrast**
- Gadolinium ethoxybenzyl dimeglumine (Gd-EOB-DTPA)—has 50% hepatobiliary excretion
- Provides liver function and details about focal lesions

Transient Elastography

US transient elastography to assess extent of fibrosis

4.2 PORTAL HYPERTENSION

- Portal hypertension when portal pressure is >5 mm Hg
- HVPG >12 mm Hg leads to PHT
- Collateral circulation begins when pressure >8–10 mmHg

Collaterals

- Esophagogastric junction—between coronary and short gastric vein to azygos vein
- Caput medusae—recanalized umbilical vein from left portal vein to esophageal venous system, superior and inferior epigastric vein
- Retroperitoneal collateral vessels—hemorrhoidal venous plexus
- Posterior abdominal vein—colic and omental vein with retroperitoneal veins
- Bare area of liver—hepatic venules and right branch of portal vein with phrenic and intercostal vein

Prehepatic Portal Hypertension

- MC: Portal vein thrombosis
- ~50% portal hypertension in children is due to portal vein thrombosis.
- Isolated portal vein thrombosis (left portal hypertension) is secondary to pancreatic inflammation/neoplasm, here left gastroepiploic vessel becomes major collateral and gastric varices develop instead of GE varices.
- Massive splenomegaly (Banti syndrome)

Intrahepatic Portal hypertension

- Intrahepatic presinusoidal—most common schistosomiasis NASH, sarcoidosis, vinyl chloride

- Intrahepatic sinusoidal—alcoholic cirrhosis, PBC, Wilson's disease, metastasis

Posthepatic Postsinusoidal

- Budd-Chiari syndrome
- Splanchnic AV fistula
- CCF
- Restrictive cardiomyopathy

Budd-Chiari Syndrome

- Congestive hepatopathy characterized by the obstruction of hepatic venous flow
- Thrombotic or non-thrombotic along the venous outflow system
- Primary—endoluminal obstruction
- Secondary—veins are compressed or invaded by neighboring lesions
- Primary myeloproliferative lesion—accounts for approx. 35–50% cases
- Caudate lobe hypertrophy seen in 50%
- USG—spiderweb hepatic veins
- MRI—hepatic vein thrombosis
- Liver biopsy—congestion, hepatocyte loss, centrilobular fibrosis
- Rx—percutaneous angioplasty, TIPSS, thrombolytic shunt

Variceal Hemorrhage

General measures
- Resuscitation, avoid hypervolemia, vit K, platelet transfusion (for thrombocytopenia due to hypersplenism), antibiotics

Endoscopic band ligation or sclerotherapy ~85% bleeding can be controlled (gold standard)
- Sclerosants—enthanolamide oleate, STS, polidocanol

Balloon Tamponade with Sengstaken Blakemore Tube

- Gastric balloon filled ~300 ml air
- Esophageal balloon filled ~40 ml air
- Balloons are temporarily deflated after 12 hours to avoid pressure necrosis
- Side effects—pressure necrosis and aspiration

Medical Management of PHT

- Factors influencing progression of size of varices
  - Decompensated cirrhosis
  - Red wale markings on endoscopy
  - HVPG >10 mm Hg, if >12 very high risk

Varices—diagnosis
Lab Markers
- Platelet count decreased
- PT increased
- Serum albumin low
- Child score
- Inflammatory markers
- Very low clinical utility
- Transient elastometry
  - Normal pressure—8 kPa
  - 13–18 kPa suggestive of cirrhosis
  - Not useful for screening
- Ultra thin endoscopy and capsule endoscopy
- Limited vision and no therapeutic option

Pharmacotherapy
- Octreotide or somatostatin is as efficient as endoscopic treatment—reduce splanchnic pressure
- Usually endoscopy + octreotide is standard treatment
- In severe cases vasopressin is used, terlipressin has longer half life and fewer side effects—generalised vasoconstriction
- But due to side effects—nitroglycerin should be simultaneously infused to achieve BP control

Prevention of Variceal Bleeding
- All medium and large-sized varices—should be treated
- Small varices with decompensated liver—treated

Primary prophylactic therapy for esophageal varices: Prevention of initial bleeding	
Variceal grade	*Recommended therapy*
No varices	No treatment
Small, CTP class A and no red wale markings	No treatment
Small, CTP class B or C or red wale markings	β-blocker
Medium/large, CTP class A and no red wale markings	β-blocker preferred, endoscopic variceal ligation if patient can't take β-blocker
Medium/large, CTP class B or C or red wale markings	

Secondary Prophylaxis
- Risk of recurrent bleeding—70%
- All who have bled—should be treated to prevent further bleeding

- Sclerotherapy has no role
- Carvedilol—non-selective beta blocker

Gastric Varices Classification
- Continuous with esophageal varices in the lesser curvature—GOV1
- Continuous into fundus—GOV2
- Isolated varices in gastric fundus—IGV1
- Isolated in other than fundus—IGV2
- Prophylaxis by endoscopic ligation is not useful
- Most used—beta blocker/cyanoacrylate injection

Pharmacotherapy
- Propranolol—diminish portal inflow
  - Reduce cardiac output
  - Beta-1 blockage on cardiac and beta-2 receptors in splanchnic vessels—unopposed alfa-1 action—vasoconstriction—decrease in portal flow and pressure
- Serotonin antagonists

TIPSS (Transjugular Intrahepatic Portosystemic Stent Shunts)
- Main treatment of variceal bleeding not responding to above managements
- Shunts are inserted under local anesthesia and fluoroscopic and ultrasound guidance, via internal jugular vein and superior vena cava, a guidewire is inserted into hepatic vein and through liver parenchyma into a branch of portal vein
- The track through the parenchyma is then dilated with a balloon catheter, and then a stent is inserted which connects portal and systemic circulation.
- Side effects—main complication—haemorrhage due to rupture of liver capsule
  - Stent occlusion due to variceal recurrence
  - Postshunt encephalopathy—due to portal blood bypassing detoxification ~40%
  - Long-term—stenosis of stent ~50%
- Contraindications—portal vein occlusion
- Use of PTFE covered stents reduces stent-related complication

Surgical Approaches
Indications
- Failed endoscopic/TIPSS
- Haemorrhage from gastric vessels

- Portal hypertension gastropathy
- Failure of long-term endoscopic treatment
- With grade A Child-Pugh in whom initial bleeding has been controlled with sclerotherapy
  - High mortality ~25%

Options

- **Portocaval shunt (nonselective shunt)** done in emergency when there is active severe variceal bleed. It rapidly and effectively decompresses the portal circulation
- **Selective shunt** (distal splenorenal shunt) more complex operation done in patient whom bleeding is temporarily controlled with tamponade/ sclerotherapy
  - Advantage—preserve blood flow to liver while decompressing the left-sided portal circulation, incidence of postsystemic encephalopathy is less

Prophylactic shunting and TIPS in patients who have not bleed, as prophylaxis, have no documented benefits and also sclerotherapy

Prevention of Recurrent Variceal Hemorrhage

- Pharmacotherapy
  - Beta blocker
  - Long-acting nitrates
- Endoscopic therapy
  - Variceal ligation is more effective and has less side effects than sclerotherapy
  - Incidence of rebleed after variceal ligation ~50% within first year
- TIPSS
- Surgical intervention

Bleeding Gastric Varices

- 20% with cirrhosis have
  - Greater risk and mortality
- EVO—(endoscopic variceal obturation) with N-butyl-cyanoacrylate—better than variceal ligation
- If this is not available—TIPS
- In recurrent bleeding—TIPS preferred

Surgical Therapy
Devascularisation

- 10–15% require surgery
- Maintain liver circulation—less encephalopathy and hepatic dysfunction
- Done in
  - Patients not candidates for LT

- Hypersplenism
- Absence of suitable veins for shunt
- Contraindicated in Child C
- Can also be used as a bridge to LT—do not alter vascular anatomy
- Two components
  - Devascularisation of OG junction
  - Splenectomy

Hassab Procedure (1957)

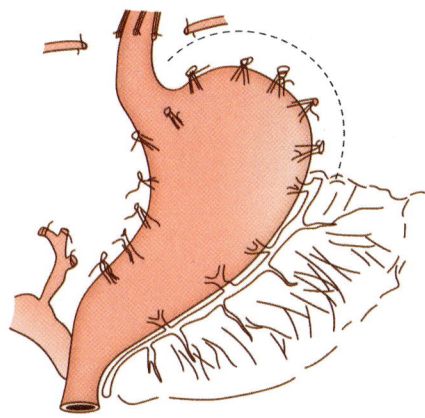

- Transabdominal
- Devascularization of lower 7–10 cm of esophagus and proximal stomach
- Vagotomy is done
- Ligation of left gastric artery and vein
- Splenectomy after ligating SA and SGA
- No transection of esophagus and pyloroplasty
- Splenectomy and devascularization prevent extramural connections.
- For intramural connections—sclerotherapy be added

Sugiura and Futagawa Procedure (1967)

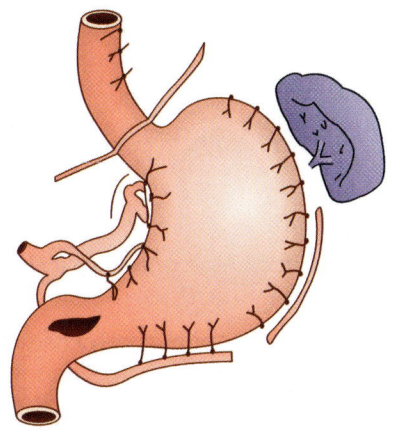

- Originally transthoracic and transabdominal through separate incisions
- Thoracic—extensive devascularization up to inferior pulmonary vein and esophageal transection
- Abdominally—splenectomy, devascularization of abdominal esophagus and cardia, 7 cm of lesser curvature, selective vagotomy and pyloroplasty

Modified Sugiura

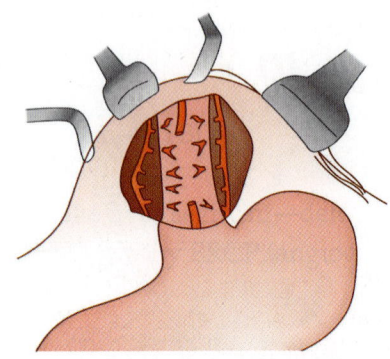

- Only abdominal approach
- EG devascularisation preserving coronary vein and the longitudinal periesophageal collateral veins
- Esophageal transection using staplers

Peracchia Modification

- Included splenectomy, devascularization of gastric corpus, fundus and distal esophagus, resection—anastomosis of distal esophagus using circular stapler, selective vagotomy with pyloromyoplasty and antireflux cardioplasty

Ginsberg

- Through left thoracoabdominal incision. Proximal vagotomy, no pyloroplasty, circular stapler anastomosis
- Loose fundal wrap is also done

Sugiura—has better results in controlling varices

TIPS

- Nonselective side to side portacaval shunt only one involving suprahepatic IVC
- Complications—encephalopathy, shunt stenosis, bleeding
- PTFE—covered stents—better result

- Stenosis—dilated with balloon or re-stented
- Effective in acute variceal bleeding
- Most frequent use—to prevent recurrent bleeding
- Most rebleeding after TIPS due to—stent stenosis or thrombosis
- Primary patency—40–70% in 1 year
- Assisted primary patency—with revision of stenotic stents—79–88%
- Secondary patency—after thrombectomy or revision—95–100% at 1 year

Shunt Surgery

- Not recommended for prophylactic surgery
- In acute bleeding—portacaval shunt—if ascites are present, side to side shunt
- Main role in preventing rebleed

Partial—preserve hepatic portal perfusion and minimise risk of liver failure and encephalopathy and preventing bleeding

Nonselective Shunts

- Completely divert portal flow

Types
- End to side portacaval shunt (ECK shunt)
- Side to side portacaval shunt (most effective)
- Large diameter interposition shunt
  - Portacaval
  - Mesocaval
    □ Mesorenal
- Conventional splenorenal shunt

Indications

- When TIPSS fails
- Patient with both variceal bleed and intractable ascites
- May accelerate hepatic failure
- Higher postshunt encephalopathy (splenorenal shunt has lesser incidence)
- Splenorenal shunt—after splenectomy splenic vein is anastomosed with renal vein
  - Risk of shunt thrombosis
  - Hypersplenism is eliminated
- For mesocaval shunt—IJV may be used
- Meso-rex shunt
  - In extrahepatic PV occlusion without cirrhosis
  - Use autologous left IJV

- SMV to left PV
- Restores blood flow to liver and relieves PHT
- In Budd-Chiari—side to side portacaval shunt
- In mesocaval shunt using left IJV—proximal end of IJV is anastomosed to SMV

Selective Shunts

- **Distal splenorenal shunt**
- Anastomosis of distal splenic vein to renal vein along with the disruption of the collateral vessels (coronary and gastroepiploic vessels) that connects left gastric vein.
- Contraindications—medically intractable ascites
  - Prior splenectomy
  - Splenic vein diameter <7 mm, as chance of thrombosis

Disadvantages—DSRS

- Technically demanding procedure
- Loss of portal blood flow due to collateralization of high pressure mesenteric system to low pressure shunts—more common in alcoholic, if coronary vein ligation is omitted, gradual diversion can occur through pancreatic siphon, can be prevented by complete pancreaticosplenic disconnection

Advantages

Preserve portal flow

Less incidence of PSE

Less rebleeding

Less incidence of thrombosis as compared to TIPSS

Partial Shunts

- Objective—effective decompression of varices
- Prevention of hepatic portal perfusion
- Maintenance of some residual portal hypertension
- A small diameter interposition portacaval shunt using PTFE graft combined with ligation of coronary vein and other collaterals
- Ideal diameter of prosthetic graft ~10 mm
- Liver transplantation

If LT is being Considered

- In acute bleeding
  - Endoscopic control/pharmacologic—TIPS
  - If shunt surgery is done—distal splenorenal or mesocaval shunts preferred—away from porta
  - More appropriately—TIPS

NEOPLASMS OF LIVER

4.3 BENIGN LIVER TUMORS

Adenoma

- Benign proliferation of hepatocytes
- Young, female, 20–40 years
- Associated with OCP/anabolic steroids
- Female: Male—11:1
- Usually single, multiple in 12–30% (in females)
- Multiple adenoma are not associated with OCP or steroids
  - Seen in type 1 glycogen storage disease
- Normal architecture of liver is absent in the lesion (**nonfunctioning**)
- Consists of normal hepatocytes
- Can present with spontaneous bleeding—more in if size >5 cm
- Risk of malignant transformation 4–10%—more in males
- Well delineated—sometimes capsulated
- Contains hepatocytes arranged in trabecular pattern with intracellular fat and glycogen

Adenoma: Subtypes

- Beta catenin mutated adenoma—increased risk to malignancy
- HNF1A (hepatocyte nuclear factor) mutated adenoma—steatosic
- Inflammatory/telangiectasia adenoma
- Not otherwise specified adenoma

Factors

- Estrogen
- Androgen
- Obesity
- Syndromes associated—
  - Fanconi
  - McCune-Albright
  - Type 3 diabetes in young
  - NASH

Clinical Features

- Most are asymptomatic
- Most common symptom—upper abdominal pain—due to hemorrhage or local compression, severe intraperitoneal rupture may occur

Diagnosis

- USG
- CECT—heterogenous lesion with peripheral enhancement with centripetal progression

- MRI—well-demarcated heterogenous mass containing fat and hemorrhage
- CEUS—can differentiate vascular lesions from FNH
- Biopsy to differentiate FNH from adenoma

Complication

- Rupture (30–50%),
- Malignant transformation to HCC (10%)—most common in beta catenin mutated type and if size >5 cm—both of this are indication of surgery
- HCC in HCA—well differentiated with normal AFP
  - No satellite nodules
  - Better prognosis—usually diagnosed after resection
- Pregnancy with adenoma >5 cm—need close follow-up
- Risk for malignant transformation
  - Male sex
  - Androgen use
  - Beta catenin mutated adenoma type
  - Tumor >5 cm
- **Treatment—HCA**
  - In males—should be resected regardless of size
  - In females—tumor < 5 cm—cessation of hormonal treatment—annual MRI follow-up
  - In females—tumor >5 cm after cessation of hormones—surgery
    - □ Preop biopsy—not required
- Only indication for biopsy—in a steatotic lesion—to confirm HNF1A-type—then conservative treatment
- Only tumors >5 cm resected
- If all are <5 cm—observe—most remain stable or disappear
- In bleeding—transarterial embolization—choice
  - Tumor also may regress—so no need to resect later
  - If tumor persists—later resection
  - RFA
- LT rarely indicated in multiple unresectable HCA
  - Intrahepatic venous shunt
  - Glycogen storage disorder

Focal Nodular Hyperplasia

- Second most benign tumour of liver
- 10 times more common than adenoma
- Most common in middle aged women
- There is focal overgrowth of functioning liver tissue supported by fibrous stroma
- FNH contains both hepatocytes and Kupffer cells
- No malignant potential
- Some regard FNH as congenital vascular malformation

Pathology

- Steatosis cholestatic degeneration with Mallory bodies seen
- IHC—with glutamine synthetase—positive focal hepatocellular areas around hepatic veins—map-like pattern
- Hyperplastic reaction due to increased arterial blood flow
- Central stellate scarring with spoke wheel pattern of vascular branching
- CECT—strong hypervascularity in arterial phase with nonenhancing scar and isodense in portal and delayed mode
  - Lack of capsule
- MRI—100% specific
  - Hypointense T1
  - Hyperintense T2
- Combination of CEUS and MRI—yield highest
- DD—fibrolamellar HCC

Special Tests

- MRI with gadoxetic acid contrast or supra-paramagnetic iron oxide dye

Treatment—no treatment required

- If symptomatic—resection, RFA, HA embolization

Hemangioma

- Most common benign tumor—70% of all benign lesions
- F:M—3:1
- Mean age 45
- Due to congenital vascular malformation
- Usually single and <5 cm
- Incidence equal in both lobes
- Giant hemangioma >5 cm (10 cm)

Clinical Features

- Most common asymptomatic, incidentally found, rarely rupture
- Have estrogen receptors—accelerated growth seen in high estrogen states

Kasabach-Merritt Syndrome
Coagulopathy—consists of intravascular coagulation, clotting and fibrinolysis—thrombocytopenia—reversible after removal of hemangioma

Imaging

- CE US–typical peripheral nodular enhancement pattern
  - Isoechoic on late phase
  - Sulphurhexafluoride microbubble or perflurobutane is used as contract agents
- CECT—low attenuation on noncontrast CT
  - Peripheral and globular enhancement followed by central enhancement on CECT
  - Delayed contrast enhancement
- MRI:
  - Hypointense on T1
  - Hyperintense on T2—'light bulb' pattern

Indication for surgery

- Significant increase in size
- Rupture
- Development of Kasabach-Merritt syndrome
- No treatment for asymptomatic—irrespective of size
- Surgery—resection choice
  - Enucleation with arterial inflow control—for peripheral lesions
  - HA ligation, RT, RFA
- Hemangioma in children: ~12% of all liver tumors in children
- Large hemangioma can cause CCF secondary to AV shunting
- Rx embolization
- No malignant potential
- Capillary hemangioma resolve spontaneously

Other Benign Solid Tumor

Macro Degenerative Nodule/Adenomatous Hyperplasia

- Bile stained bulging
- Nodule associated with cirrhosis
- Has malignant potential

Nodular Regenerative Hyperplasia

- Usually <2 cm
- Associated with
  - Lymphoproliferative disorders
  - Collagen vascular disorders
  - Chemotherapy/steroid

- Not associated with cirrhosis, no malignant risk

Mesenchymal Hamartoma

Large cystic mass in right liver, painless abdominal distension

Angiomyolipoma

- Comes under perivascular epithelial cell tumors (PEComas)
- More common in kidneys
- 3 components—smooth muscle, vascular, fat
- MRI—choice—arterial enhancement without washout in delayed phase
- Liver biopsy mandatory—HMB-45 is the stain used.
- <5 cm lesions—observed
- >5 cm—resection

Biliary Hamartoma

- von Meyenburg complex
- Multiple <5 mm nodules—scattered all over liver—confused with metastasis
- Constitute abnormal development of small intrahepatic bile duct—composed of bile ductules and fibrosis
- Confused with caroli but they do not communicate with bile duct
- MRI-T2—hyperintense
- No treatment is needed

Bile Duct Adenoma (Benign Cholangioma)

- <5 mm, subcapsular
- Proliferation of non-cystic biliary structures within dense fibrous stroma
- BRAFV600E mutations seen in >50%—unlike BD hamartoma
- No treatment recommended

Leiomyoma—associated with HIV and organ transplantation

Heterotopic Tissue

Most common—**liver splenosis** due to autotransplantation of splenic tissue after traumatic rupture

- Asymptomatic—most common on left lobe
- Hypervascular—DD HCC/metastasis
- Diagnosis—TC 99 heat denatured RBC scan
  - Biopsy

- Hepatic endometriosis
  - Usually >5 cm—diagnosis difficult
- Others
  - Pancreas, adrenal

Peliosis

- Multiple, small blood filled pools in liver
- Size vary from mm to cm without lobular systemization
- Results from focal rupture of sinusoids
- Associations
  - Chemotherapy with oxaliplatin in CRC secondaries
  - Androgenic steroids
  - TB
  - Hodgkin's
- MRI—hypervascular lesions
- Treatment—withdrawing the cause which produce regression of tumor

4.4 CYSTIC NEOPLASMS

Simple Cyst

- Serous fluid, does not communicate with biliary tree
- No septations, single (50%), may be as large as 20 cm
- Most common complication—intracystic bleeding
- Treatment—follow-up
  - Sclerotherapy
  - Surgery—fenestration or unroofing of the extrahepatic portion of the cyst

Two Types

1. With ovarian stroma—MCN-L
2. Communicating with bile duct—IPMN-B

MCN-L

- Most common cystic neoplasm
- Biliary in origin—most common location—liver
- Solitary, large
- Most common in segment IV
- Lobulated, contain mucin—bile very unusual
- No communication to bile duct
  - Epithelium—stain for CEA and CA 19–9
  - Stroma—express ER and PR and inhibin-alfa
  - Hyalinized pseudocapsule
- Origin—ectopic ovarian cells—migrated to liver
- Cells covering the gonads—get detached and get attached to peritoneal surface

Clinical Features

- Exclusively in women, 4–5 decades
- Mass—slow growing and may present as large tumors
- Jaundice—due to migration of mucus to bile duct or compression
- Tumor rupture
- DD—simple cysts, cystic mets from ovary, colon, hemangioma

Diagnosis

- USG—anechoic mass with septations
- CECT—multiloculated
- MRI—fluid containing multiloculated cyst
- CEUS
- US and MRI better than CT
- Differentiation with simple cyst
  - MCN is single
  - May show upstream bile duct dilatation
  - ALP may show rise in MCN

Complications

- Cystadenocarcinoma
- Fistulation to bile duct
- Treatment
- Excision—hepatectomy/enucleation
  - Partial excision can cause recurrence

MCN without Ovarian Stroma

- Multilocular
- Seen in both sexes
- CA 19–9 and CEA raised
- Similar to MCN-L

Cystadenoma

- Large cystic mass 10–20 cm
- Contains mucinous fluids
- Most common in female >40 cm
- USG—cystic structure with varying wall thickness, septation, nodularity and fluid-filled locules
- CECT—enhancement of cystic wall with septa
- Differential diagnosis—hydatid cyst
- Malignant transformation very rare—cystadenoma carcinoma
- Rx—complete excision

Cystadenocarcinoma

- Most commonly in liver than bile duct
- More in females
- Present with mass, pain, jaundice
- Solitary
- Diagnosis—difficult
- CT/MRI—multiseptate, calcification
- CA19–9, CEA—elevated
- Cyst fluid study
- Cytology not helpful

Treatment

- Formal resection is preferred rather than enucleation
- Tumor with ovarian stroma—have better prognosis

IPMN-B

- Exclusively in intrahepatic bile duct or left or right bd
- Do not have ovarian stroma
- Duct ectatic type—dilated ducts
- Cystic type—large cystic mass
- Lining epithelia—pancreaticobiliary type, intestinal, gastric, or oncocytic
- Columnar type—resembles intestinal type
- Cuboidal resembles—pb and oncocytic—more commonly associated with cancer
- Epithelium positive for CK-7 and CK-20

Clinical Features

- Both genders—6th decade
- Pain, mass
- Communicate with bd—CT/MRI may not show because of very narrow communication
- ERCP or intraoperative cholangiogram more reliable
- Can cause migration of mucus—mucobilia and obstruction
- Dysplasia leads to cancer

Treatment

- Formal hepatectomy
- Prognosis better

Polycystic Liver Disease

- Associated with: ADPKD (autosomal dominant polycystic kidney disease)
- Multiple cystic lesions
- Hepatic functions are preserved
- Incidence increases with age, 0% in <20 years to ~80% by 60 years
- Usually asymptomatic

Treatment

If symptomatic—percutaneous aspiration with or without sclerotherapy, cyst fenestration, hepatic resection, or liver transplantation

4.5 HEPATOCELLULAR CARCINOMA

- Most common primary liver cancer

Etiology

- Chronic HBV infection accounts >50%
- HCV infection
- Obesity
- NASH
- DM
- Smoking/alcohol (act as a cocarcinogen, not an active carcinogen)
- In male 2–8 times more common
- Aflatoxin
  - Aspergillus grow on peanuts, grains; aflatoxin B1
- **Other chemicals**
  - Nitrites, hydrocarbons, solvents,
  - Pesticides, vinyl chloride
  - Thorotrast
- **Metabolic**
  - Hereditary hemochromatosis (phlebotomy can deplete iron but does not prevent development of HCC)
  - Alfa-1 antitrypsin deficiency
  - Wilson's disease
  - Tyrosemia
- **Hormonal**
  - OCP
  - Anabolic steroids
- >80% of HCC occur in South East Asia and Tropical Africa
- **Infective**
  - HBV—insertional mutagenesis into hepatocytes
  - Persistent carrier state with HBsAg + state
  - High titer of hepatitis B surface antigen and core antibody (HCcab) are frequently found in HCC patients.
  - In HCV chronic infection and cirrhosis cause HCC
  - It is a RNA virus so do not incorporate into host genome
- HCC—screening
  - In liver cirrhosis—USG 6 monthly
  - AFP is not recommended
  - USG—in cirrhotic nodule <1 cm—60% of them will be benign

Clinical Features

- Common in men, 50–60 years
- RUQ pain

- Weight loss
- Palpable mass
- Anorexia, lethargy
- Omnious prognostic sign—ascites and upper abdominal mass
- Hepatic decompensation especially in cirrhosis
  - Ascites, jaundice, liver failure

Rare Presentation

- Rupture—shock
- Hepatic vein occlusion—Budd-Chiari
- Obstructive jaundice
- Hemobilia
- FUO
- Erythrocytosis
- Incidental

Paraneoplastic Syndrome—<1%

- Hypoglycemia
- Erythrocytosis
- Hypercalcemia
- Most common—hypercholestrolemia

Diagnostic Investigations

- Verification of diagnosis
- Extent of disease (whether isolated to liver, whether resectable)
- Estimation of functional liver reserve

Initial Workup

- Ultrasound abdomen
- Hepatitis panel
- Assessment of comorbidity
- Metastatic workup—CT chest mandatory
- Bone scan only, if needed
- Triple phase CT/MRI

Radiology

- **USG**
  - Screening and early detection
- **CT/MRI**
  - Peritoneal, lymph nodes metastasis
  - Vascular, biliary involvement
  - Thrombus/tumor in PV, HV
- Indocyanine green clearance—for providing functional assessment
- **Triple phase CT**
  - Non-contrast, arterial phase, portal phase
  - Number, distribution of tumor, vascular invasion, nodal or peritoneal disease, tumor thrombus
  - Typical feature is arterially enhancing mass with washout of material in delayed phase

- MRI
  - With gadolinium or iron oxide as contrast
  - Characterization of small lesions <1 cm difficult—because they are isointense
- AFP
  - >20 ng/nl in 75%
- Triple phase CT/MRI
  - Typical—arterially enhancing lesion with wash out of contrast in late phases, combined with AFP > 200 is confirmatory
- In case of atypical features—biopsy indicated
- Liver mass consistent with HCC on CT/MRI with elevated AFP in a cirrhotic or hepatitis infection patient—diagnosis is confirmed
  - No need of biopsy
- Biopsy not done in potentially operable tumors
- FNAC can result in rupture, bleeding, spillage

Biopsy Indications

- Suspicious but imaging inconclusive
- No high risk factors
- Non-malignant nodules confusing with HCC
- In patients with elevated CEA or CA 19–9 to rule out intrahepatic cholangiocarcinoma
- Complications of biopsy—rupture, bleeding, spillage

Diagnosis

- Nodule >2 cm with hypervascular on CT on single dynamic study with portal venous washout and AFP >200 ng/ml—biopsy not required
- Nodule 1–2 cm on two confirmatory studies with CT—treated as HCC
- Nodule 1–2 cm—without cirrhosis and with risk factors for HCC—biopsy required
- Risk of postoperative liver failure and death should be assessed before resection
- Assess—degree of cirrhosis, presence of portal hypertension, functional liver reserve, regenerative potential response
- Clinical assessment—Child-Pugh status

Child-Pugh scoring system			
		Points	
Parameter	1	2	3
Albumin (g/dl)	>3.5	2.8–3.5	<2.8
Bilirubin (mg/dl)	<2	2–3	>3
Ascites	Absent	Slight	Moderate
Encephalopathy	None	1–2	3–4
PT (INR)	<1.7	1.8–2.3	>2.3
Score	A	B	C
Points	5–6	7–9	10–15

- Mainly metastasis to lung, bone, peritoneum
- Assess liver for multiple lesions—CECT/MRI
- CT chest
- Bone scans—only if suggestive signs/symptoms
- Laparoscopy

HCC—Work up

- LFT
- PHT—very important
  - Measured by hepatovenous wedge pressure
  - Characterized by splenomegaly thrombocytopenia and varices
- Liver function assessment
- LFT, PT/INR, PLC, CBC, RFT
- Measure of pretransplant mortality

> **MELD score**
>
> Model for end stage liver disease scoring system
> $= 0.957 \times \log (\text{creatinine mg/dl})$
> $+ 0.378 \times \log (\text{bilirubin mg/dl})$
> $+ 1.120 \times \log (\text{INR})$
> $+ 0.643$

- To prioritize the allocation of transplants

Functional Liver Reserve

- Indicate postop liver function
- CT: Direct measurement
- Future remnant/total liver volume—tumour volume should be 25% without cirrhosis and 30–40% in CLD
- Indocyanin blue clearance test
- ICG retention rate of 14% at 15 minutes is the cutoff for resection
- Aminopyrine breath test
- Hepatic venous wedge pressure

> **Serum biomarkers**
> - **AFP**
> - **DCP (Des-gamma carboxyprothrombin)**
> - **AFP L3**
> - **Neurotensin**
> - **PIVKA 2**
> - **Vit B$_{12}$ binding globulin**

Alpha-fetoprotein

- Helpful in diagnosis
- >400 ng/ml is diagnostic
- May be elevated or normal
- Low sensitivity and specificity

- Also elevated in chronic active hepatitis, colorectal metastasis, intrahepatic cholangiocarcinoma, germ cell tumors
- Only as adjunctive test
- Useful in monitoring treated patients for recurrence
- AFP, a protein, produced by fetal hepatocytes and tumor cells
- Not produced by healthy, mature hepatocytes
- Normal range 10–20 ng/ml
- Normal value varies in various ethnic groups
- With liver mass, value >200 ng/ml—highly predictive of HCC
- An absolute value of >400 ng/ml is diagnostic irrespective of ethnicity and liver disease
- >1000 ng/ml—predictor of vascular invasion
- Value >1000—a contraindication for LT

HCC—Staging Systems

- **Okuda**

> **Okuda staging**
> Factors representing advanced disease
> - Tumor size >50% of liver
> - Ascites
> - Albumin <3 g/dl
> - Bilirubin >3 mg/dl
>
> | | |
> |---|---|
> | Stage I | no factors |
> | Stage II | 1–2 factors |
> | Stage III | 3–4 factors |

- **TNM**
- **Cancer of the liver Italian program**

Cancer of the liver Italian program score		
Clinical parameters	*Cutoff values*	*Points*
Child-Pugh class	A	0
	B	1
	C	2
Tumor morphology	Uninodular, <50% extension	0
	Multinodular, <50% extension	1
	Massive/extension >50%	2
AFP level	<400 ng/dl	0
	>400 ng/dl	1
Portal vein thrombosis	No	0
	Yes	1
Range 0–6; 4–6: advanced disease, 0–3: long-term survival potential +		

- **Chinese University Prognostic Index**
- **Barcelona clinic liver cancer (BCLC) system**

Barcelona clinic liver cancer staging classification

Stage	PST	Tumor status		Liver function
Stage A: Early HCC				
A1	0	Single	I	No PHT and normal bilirubin
A2	0	Single	I	PHT and normal bilirubin
A3	0	Single	I	PHT and abnormal bilirubin
A4	0	3 tumors <3 cm	I–II	Child-Pugh A–B
B: Intermediate HCC	0	Large multinodular	I–II	Child-Pugh A–B
C: Advanced HCC	1–2	Vascular invasion/ extrahepatic spread	I–II	Child-Pugh A–B
D: End stage HCC	3–4	Any	III	Child-Pugh C
PST: Performance status test				

Treatment schedule for HCC cirrhotic patients according to BCLC

Stage	Treatment intervention	1st/2nd choice
Stage A: Early HCC		
A1	Radical	Surgical resection
A2		Surgical resection –OLT/ percutaneous
A3		OLT/percutaneous
A4		OLT/percutaneous
B: Intermediate HCC	Palliative	Transarterial embolization Chemoembolization
C: Advanced HCC	Palliative	New agents
D: End-stage HCC	Symptomatic	Supportive treatment

- BLCL staging—considers—liver function, tumor burden and presence of cancer related symptoms

HCC: Pathology
- **Infiltrative type**
  - Infiltrates vessels
- **Small tumors <5 cm**
- **Multifocal**
  - PV–metastasis
  - Multiple primary and metastasis
- **Hanging type**
  - Connected to liver by a thin stalk
  - Large size—but easy to resect

- **Pushing type**
  - Well demarcated
  - Fibrous capsule
  - Displaces vascular structures
  - Microscopically—trabecular, solid, tubular types

Fibrolamellar Type
- In younger
  - No H/O cirrhosis
  - Well demarcated
  - Well encapsulated
  - Central fibrotic area
- Does not produce AFP
- Elevated neurotensin
- Better prognosis
- Better resectability and no cirrhosis
- Surgery is mainstay
- Long-term survival 50–75%
- Chimeric protein containing catalytic domain of protein kinase A is detectable in this, so believed to have role in pathogenesis, so targeted therapy can be developed

Comparison of standard HCC and fibrolamellar HCC

Parameter	HCC	Fibrolamellar HCC
Male: female ratio	2:1–8:1	1:1
Mean age	56	26
Cirrhosis	80–90%	5%
AFP+	85%	5%
Hep B+	65%	5%
Tumor	Invasive	Well circumscribed
Resectability	<25%	50–75%

Clear Cell HCC
- Resemble renal cell neoplasm
- Has better prognosis

Pleomorphic or Giant Cell HCC
- Contains pleomorphic large multinucleate giant cell arising in hepatocyte

Sarcomatoid Variant or Carcinosarcoma
- Sarcomatous differentiation
- Do not produce AFP
- Higher incidence of metastasis

Childhood HCC
- Associated with viral hepatitis, metabolic liver disease
- Treatment complete resection, liver transplant

Intrahepatic Cholangiocarcinoma
- 10% of all cholangiocarcinoma
- It is the second most primary liver neoplasm

- Clinical features similar to HCC
- Jaundice is rare
- AFP is normal but CEA and CA 19-9 can be raised
- Biopsy shows adenocarcinoma
- CT/MRI—focal hepatic mass associated with peripheral biliary dilatation
- Treatment—complete resection, resectability~60%

Hepatoblastoma

- Most common primary hepatic tumor of children
- Median age—18 months, rare after 3 years
- Associated with FAP
- Clinical features—may be asymptomatic, mild anemia with thrombocytopenia
- AFP elevated in 90%
- Treatment—initial chemo followed by resection
- 50% of patients with pulmonary metastasis can be cured with hepatic tumor resection with chemotherapy or resection of pulmonary metastasis

Angiosarcoma

- It is a primary hepatic sarcoma
- Associated with vinyl chloride or thorotrast exposure
- Typically appears as multiple hepatic masses
- Poor prognosis

Treatment

- HCC is a therapeutic challenge
- **3 factors**
  - Usually associated with cirrhosis
  - Late presentation
  - Resistance to cytotoxic drugs

Four Types of Patients

- Potentially resectable or transplantable, operable by performance status or comorbidity
- Unresectable
- Inoperable by performance with local disease
- Metastatic disease

Surgery

- Resections can be
  - Segmental
  - Multiple segments
  - Hemi/partial hepatectomy
- Central hepatectomy—segments IV, V, VIII
- **Negative prognostic factors**
  - Tumor size
  - Cirrhosis
  - Infiltrative growth
  - Vascular invasion
  - Intrahepatic metastasis
  - Multifocal

- LN metastasis
- Margin <1 cm

Liver Resections

Segments	Couinaud	Goldsmith and Woodburne	Brisbane
5, 6, 7, 8	Right hepatectomy	Right hepatic lobectomy	Right hepatectomy
4, 5, 6, 7, 8	Right lobectomy	Right hepatic lobectomy	Right trisectionectomy or extended right hepatectomy
2, 3, 4	Left hepatectomy	Left hepatic lobectomy	Left hepatectomy
2, 3	Left lobectomy	Left lateral segmentectomy	Left lateral segmentectomy bisectionectomy
2, 3, 4, 5, 8	Extended left hepatectomy	Extended left lobectomy	Left trisectionectomy extended left hepatectomy
5, 8			Right anterior sectionectomy
6, 7			Right posterior sectionectomy
4			Left medial sectionectomy or resection of segment 4

Pre-op Portal Vein Embolization

- When sFLR (standardised) is low
- In post-chemo sFLR should be 30%
  - In cirrhosis—40%
  - Normal liver—20%
- Absolute contraindications
  - Established PHT
  - Extensive thrombus on ipsilateral PV

Approaches

- Transileocolic venous
  - Under general anesthesia—laparotomy, this approach is not in favor
- Transhepatic contralateral—through FLR
- Transhepatic ipsilateral
- Mainly done for extended right hepatectomy
- RPV is embolized. Segment IV, PV also should be embolized—otherwise it also hypertrophies which is undesirable in extended right hepatectomy
- Left portal vein embolisation is rarely indicated, as the FLR will be adequate without this for left hepatectomy

Sequential PVE

- First HA branches chemoembolised—followed 2 weeks later—PVE
  - Treats the disease—if resection becomes not possible due to lack of hypertrophy
  - Eliminates arteriovenous shunts
  - If PV embolised alone—more blood drawn from HA called arterialization
- Degree of hypertrophy 5% and
- sFLR volume >20% predicts good response

Associating Liver Partition and PV Ligation for Staged (ALPPS) Hepatectomy

- Two surgical techniques—right portal vein ligation
  - *In situ* splitting of liver

Indications

- In CRC metastasis bilobar, HCC
- When extreme volume gain is needed
- When minimal hypertrophy is needed—PVE better having lesser morbidity
- In the first stage—FLR can be cleared of tumor
- Can be done in failed PVE
- Undivided PV at hilum—absolute anatomic contraindication

Stage 1

- Tumor bearing lobe PV ligation, preserving ipsilateral artery and parenchymal transection

Stage 2

- Performed in 7–14 days later
- HA and BD ligated and corresponding HV taken down—remove specimen

In ALPPS

- Divides all PV connections
- Trauma of division release cytokines and regeneration
- HA maintains vascularity
- Most common complication—bile leak

Different types of ALPPS

ALPPS—complete transection of liver parenchyma

Partial(p) ALPPS—incomplete transection of liver (>50% divided)

ALTPS (associating liver tourniquet and portal ligation for staged hepatectomy)—partial transection and occlusion by tourniquet

RALPP (radiofrequency assisted liver partition with PV ligation)—complete transection, RF-induced necrosis

Hybrid ALPPS—PV embolization and complete transection of liver, used when RPV is compromised by tumor

- Can enhance tumor proliferation also

Liver Transplantation

- Live donor
- Orthotopic

Non-surgical

Percutaneous ethanol injection/acetic acid

- Causes dehydration
- Coagulative necrosis
- Vascular thrombus
- <2 cm single ablation sufficient
- Can be done if tumor is subcapsular, near heart or near GB (usually contraindications)

Thermal Ablative Techniques

- Cryotherapy
  - Laparotomy/laparoscopy/percutaneous
  - Freeze and thaw tumor causes necrosis
  - Can have heat sink effect
  - Monitored by ice ball formation by USG

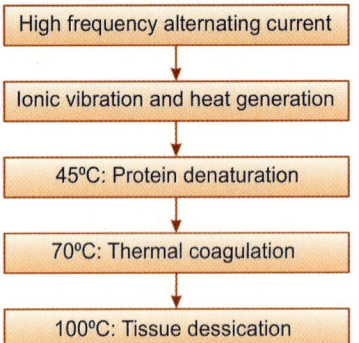

RFA

- Uses high frequent ac 300–500 kHz—friction—heat by Joule effect
- Temp >60 degree—cell death
- Does not ablate well near blood vessels—convective cooling (heat sink effect) if more than 3 mm
- Spherical ablation zone
  - If temp >100 deg C causes charring which can increase impedance

Percutaneous

- USG/CT used to guide
- Large lesions—ablation starts at posterior aspect—probe withdrawn at 2 cm increments
- Not ideal near surface—can injure—introduce artificial ascites/CO_2

Lap/open

- Can assess the tumor
- Pringle maneuver to reduce heat sink effect

- Can be combined with resection
- RFA is an alternative to small HCC compared to resection
- Used in secondaries
- A bridge to LT

Microwave Ablation

- Achieves heat destruction through passive and active heating
- Reaches operating frequency 2450 MHz
- Heating needs dipolar molecules—like water
- Microwave electromagnetic transmission in water molecules causes vigorous movement generating friction heat—also due to ionic polarization
- Microwave produce nonionizing radiation for heating—homogenous heating—makes it superior
- They cause passive heating (transmission of heat by conduction). So cause larger ablation zones
- Current sinking means due to proximity of vessels, diversion of current this is more with RFA
- So both heat sink and current sink—less with MWA
- Even charring or water vapor generation have less effect on MWA—as energy is uniform through the electromagnetic field
- Done via percutaneous, lap/open
- Ablation success—no tumor on imaging within 4 weeks
- Local recurrence—evidence of viable tumor after 4 weeks within 1 cm from prior ablation
- Nonlocal hepatic recurrence > 1 cm away

Irreversible Electroporation

- Nonthermal—uses multiple short pulses (70–90 micro secs), high voltage (2250–3000 volt) electrical energy—electroporation of cell membranes—destruction of tumor
- Affects only target tissues—vital structures not affected
- Need deep paralysis/general anesthesia
- Electrical field 2500 V/cm^2—nano pores created—unsealable—cell death by disruption of cellular homeostasis
- Well-defined area of destruction
- 8–10 weeks required for the efficacy

- Bile ducts and vessels—have high collagen content and lack the cell membrane—so not damaged
- It would not disrupt smooth muscle
- Indications—<4 cm size, <5 mm from a vital structure
- Ideal spacing of probes—1.5 to 2.3 cm
- <1.5 cm—ineffective, reversible electroporation or thermal damage
- >2.3 cm—ineffective
- Ablation success—no tumor on CT/MRI after 3 months

Tumor Location, Size and Options

- RFA—if <3 cm tumor, non-perivascular
- MWA—intermediate size 3–5 cm or in perivascular
- Proximity to vital structures, vessels—non-thermal like IRE, PEI
- PEI only for small HCC

Cryo Ablation

- Subzero temp—tissue destruction—normal and tumor
- Gradient of temperature in the ice ball from –170°C at tip of probe to 0° at the periphery
- Liquid nitrogen system
- New method argon-helium system

Cooling Rates

- Maximal cell death achieved at slow and rapid cooling rates
- In slow cooling (<1°C/min)—ice formed more in extracellular compartment—fluid shift from IC space—dehydration
- In intermediate cooling (cooling rate 1–10°C/min)—also freezes the intracellular space—stops further dehydration and ionic influx—survival can be achieved which is a limitation, greatest cell survival—seen with intermediate cooling rates
- In rapid cooling (cooling rate ~50°C/minute). Due to mechanical action of ice crystallisation and expansion
- Normal hepatocytes die at temp –15 to –20°C
- Tumors need temp –40°C
- Ice ball should be extended 1 cm beyond tumor
- Thawing process—further destroys cells
- If >40% liver affected—contraindication for cryo

Important notes			
	Cryo	*RFA*	*MWA*
Sites avoided	Liver surface	Adjacent to GB, porta, bowel	Adjacent to GB, porta, bowel
Ideal size	<5 cm	<3 cm	<3 cm
Bleeding	1.6%	2.6%	3.5%

- Cryo shock—DIC—lung and renal failure
- Local recurrence maximum with cryo and least with MWA, among these three.

Transarterial Therapy

- 90–100% blood supply to liver tumors from HA
- Hepatocarcinogenesis—multistep arterialization
- Encapsulated HCC—almost exclusively supplied by HA
- Extracapsular infiltration edge and well-differentiated HCC supplied both by PV and HA
- Metastasis:
  - <200 micro m—exclusively by sinusoidal blood
  - As size grows—progressive arterialization—metastasis always have some PV supply—may be resistant to TACE
- Lipiodol emulsion in 4:1 ratio—accumulates in tumor and stays in tumor—due to absence of Kupffer cell in tumor so cause slow release
- When lipiodol is given, tumoral spaces may be overfilled. So additional volume may flow back to PV through arteriovenous communications which allow dual embolization
- Gelatin sponge, polyvinyl alcohol, blood clots or cyanoacrylate used for embolization
- If there is prominent AV shunt—embolization of shunt is done first

Lipiodol

- Poppy seed oil contains iodine 38% by weight
- Normal hepatocytes remove lipiodol in 7 days
- HCC retains it for weeks
- Has some embolic effect
- It is radiopaque

Transarterial Therapy

- Indicated in child A or B
  - In Barcelona—intermediate
- Can be used as primary role or as bridge for LT or as neoadjuvant
- In metastasis—benefit the hypervascular ones—(NET metastasis, GIST metastasis, uveal melanoma)

- Drugs used—doxorubicin, mitomicin C, cisplatin, epirubicin
- Contraindications
  - No absolute contraindication
  - Child B and C
  - Both lobes, extensive
  - Major PV involvement
- Relative contraindications
  - GI bleeding, severe ascites, extrahepatic spread, encephalopathy

Technique

- Overnight fasting—hydrate—access though common femoral artery
- Visualize the visceral arteries and PV
- Selective cannulation of tumor vessels—lipiodol 15 ml/doxorubicin 20–75 mg—inject and then embolize—embolize AV shunts before injection
- Continue hydration and analgesics—LFT repeated 2–4 weeks later
- CT/MRI every 2–3 months—TACE can be repeated when there is progression—more chance of complications

Post-embolization Syndrome

- Pain—due to ischemia, edema, capsule distension
- Fever—tumor necrosis
- Others:
  - Inadvertent injection into cystic artery—GB inflammation—perforation
  - Accessary LGA from HA—gastric ulcer
  - Skin necrosis—due to extrahepatic collaterals—in internal mammary artery, intercostal
  - Supraumbilical discoloration due to lipiodol—due to falciform artery, this artery should be embolized
- TACE to inferior phrenic artery can cause pulmonary complications

Newer

- Bland embolization without chemo
- Drug eluting beads (DEB)—doxo/irinotecan
- Combination of TACE with RFA/microwave/alcohol
- DEB/TACE

TARE

Yttrium—90 microspheres
Pure betaemitter
Half life 64.2 hours
Decays into stable zirconium—90

- Tissue penetration 2.5 to 11 mm
- Pretreatment coiling of non-target vessels—like inferior esophageal, left inferior phrenic

artery, retroduodenal artery, supraduodenal artery

- Pretreatment—angiogram
  - Tc 99 macroaggregated albumin (Tc99MAA) scan—for evaluation for peritumoral vessels
- Radiation segmentectomy—infusing the spheres at segmental level
- Extended shelf life microspheres are used in large multifocal lesions
- Radiation lobectomy—infusion at lobar level inducing fibrosis and compensatory hypertrophy of other lobe

Other Radionucleotides

- I131 with lipiodol
  - Thyroid is medically blocked
- Rhenium—188-with iodised oil
- Phosphorus—32 glass microspheres—emit beta particles
  - Half life 14.28 days
- Milican/holmium—166 microspheres
  - Ho166 is beta and gamma emitter
  - Highly paramagnetic—so acts as a negative contrast in MRI
  - Radio-opaque on CT

TARE

- In HCC—as a bridge to LT
- As neoadjuvant
- In inoperable cases
  - In secondaries
- Unresectable, age >18
- With good systemic functions
  - Contraindications
- If scheduled for any other liver procedures
- If expected RT dose to lung >30 Gy in single or >50 Gy cumulative

External Beam RT

- Limited role

Systemic Chemotherapy

- Ineffective
- Drugs used 5FU, cisplatin, doxorubicin, etoposide, tamoxifen

Systemic Immunotherapy

- Sorafenib (Anti-serine threonine kinases)

Hormonal therapy

Combination therapy

BRIDGE THERAPY

- In patients waiting for LT
- To delay tumor progression
- RFA, TACE, TARE, DEB/TACE, sorafenib may be used

Liver Transplantation in HCC

- Recurrence of HCC after resection
  - 40–50% in 3 years
  - Up to 70% in 5 years

Milan Criteria

- Single lesion <5 cm, up to 3 lesions of 3 cm or less in size, none >3 cm
- >stage 2—higher chance of recurrence

4.6 METASTATIC TUMORS OF LIVER

- Most common malignant liver tumors
  - Common site from GIT through portal system
  - Colorectal—most important

Others

- Upper GI—stomach, pancreas, biliary
- GU—renal, prostate
- Neuroendocrine, breast, eye
- Ovary, endometrium, cervix
- Melanoma, sarcoma

Colorectal Metastases

- Most of them unresectable
- 10–20% of them potentially resectable
- ~30% have liver metastasis at time of presentation
- 20% will develop liver disease after colorectal malignancies have been resected
- FLR of ~25% is considered sufficient

Clinical Features

Symptoms of Primary

- Pain
- Ascites
- Jaundice
- Weight loss
- Palpable mass

Colorectal Metastases

Evaluation

Of primary
  - LFT
  - ALP, GGT, LDH
  - Serial CEA (with mass)
  - Imaging
  - CECT with portal venous phase
  - CECT chest
  - MRI
  - PET-CT
  - Laparoscopy

Poor Prognostic Factors After Resection

- Extra hepatic metastasis
- LN+ with primary tumor
- Synchronous tumor (shorter disease free interval)—within <1 year
- Larger number of lesions
- Bilobar tumor
- CEA >200 ng/ml
- Largest tumor >5 cm
- Involved margins

5 Worst prognostic factors
- Size >5 cm
- Disease free interval <1 year
- CEA >200 ng/ml
- More than one tumor
- LN + primary

- **Pulmonary metastasis is not a contraindication for liver resection**

Evaluation before Resection

- Medical resectability—morbidities
- Oncologic
- Technical—negative margin, FLR
  - **CT**—pre-contrast, arterial, PV, delayed—quadruple phase
- Most important—pre-contrast and delayed or venous—most metastasis are not well vascularized
- Arterial phase distinguishes from benign hemangiomas and define vascular anatomy

MRI

- Most useful in intermediate hepatic lesions
- Can detect very small lesions, subcapsular with hepatocyte specific contrast vs CT
- In macrovascular steatosis—MRI is better than CT

PET

Role in CRC

- In selection for metastasectomy
- Evaluation of recurrence, in elevated CEA—better than CT
- RT planning
- Assessment of response
- Discovery of incidental lesions

Treatment

- Resection with 1 cm margin
- Adjuvant chemo (FOLFOX4, FOLFIRI)
- Preop and postop chemo
- Neoadjuvant chemo

- HAI (hepatic arterial infusion)
- Cryoablation, RFA, microwave
- Bevacizumab (anti-endothelial GF)
- Cetuximab (anti-EGF)
- Panitumumab (EGFR-humanised)
- EGFR inhibitors are effective only if they do not have mutation of KRAS gene

Preop Chemo

- Useful in downstaging unresectable disease—FOLFOX, FOLFIRI
- Resectable metastasis—chemotherapy debatable value

Toxicity

- Oxaliplatin—sinusoidal dilatation, regenerative nodular hyperplasia
  - Fragile hemorrhagic—'blue liver'—difficult to transect
- Irinotecan
  - Hepatic steatosis
  - Toxicity rise if >6 cycles used

Preop Chemo—Disappeared Liver Mets

- Place fiducial marker prior to chemotherapy
- MRI and intraop palpation/US if still not located, resection based on vascular landmarks or observation and later interventions

Perioperative Management

- Laparoscopic assessment
- Assess peritoneum, celiac nodes
- IOUS—to assess the resection line and postresection assessment of bile ducts

Synchronous Metastasis

- Worse prognosis

Methods

- Start systemic chemotherapy—if colon lesion is not obstructing or simultaneous resection
- Resection of primary first—chemo—later liver resection
- Liver first approach—in complex liver disease, liver secondaries are operated first and allow liver regeneration, then resect primary later.
- In simultaneous resection—more infective complications

Multifocal/Bilateral Liver Metastasis

Options are:
- PV embolization
- Staged resection
- ALPPS

Postop

- Cure rate—20%
- Most common sites of failure—liver and lung
- Recurrence in liver—60%
- 5-year survival—70%
- 10-year survival—<1%

Neuroendocrine Metastases

- Gastrinomas
- Glucagonoma
- Somatostatinomas
- Nonfunctional
- Less commonly
  Insulinomas
  – Carcinoid
- Slow growing tumors with long-term survival
- Secrete peptides with hormonal effects
- Goal of treatment is improvement of quality of life than survival

Treatment

- Somatostatin analogues
- HAI
- Thermoablative procedures—RFA, cryo, microwave
- Lap RFA
- Surgery is done with minimum morbidity
  – NET metastasis is intensely hypervascular

Intra-arterial Therapy

- TAC
- TACE
- TARE

Resection

- Should debulk >90% of tumor
- Recurrence rate—60 to 80% at 5 years

Liver Transplantation May be Considered in

(Currently not recommended as a primary treatment)
- NET of GIT origin
- Resection of primary before OLT
- Absence of high grade tumor and metastasis
- Low Ki 67 index
- Age <60

Systemic Therapy

- Somatostatin analogues—mediated through receptors 2 and 5
- Chemotherapy with streptozocin, 5FU, doxorubicin
- Target therapy—sunitinib, everolimus

Prognosis

- 5 years 50–75% after complete resection

Breast, Melanoma, Sarcoma, Stomach

- Secondaries from stomach are less easy to detect with CT, as they may be having same density as liver, and may have same IV contrast enhancement as normal liver, MRI may pickup more secondaries than CT.
- Melanoma—most from cutaneous lesions
- Uveal melanoma have exclusive metastasis to liver, without other sites
- Dismal prognosis

Isolated Hepatic Perfusion in metastais

- In inoperble, multiple metastasis
- With good function
  – Melphelan is used
- Venovenous shunt by left femoral vein and right IJV to maintain circulation
- Hepatic circuit inflow by GDA, outflow by percutaneously through right femoral vein to IVC
- Liver is isolated by cross clamping at porta and suprahepatic IVC

4.7 LIVER ABSCESS
Pyogenic Liver Abscess

- Ochsner and DeBakey described
- More common in 50–60 years of age
- Male: Female—1.5:1
- Comorbid conditions associated with pyogenic abscess—cirrhosis, diabetes, chronic renal failure, h/o malignant disease

Pathogenesis

- When an inoculum of bacteria enters and exceeds ability of liver to clear

Routes

- Biliary tree—biliary obstruction, stones and cholangitis, malignancy, Caroli disease, ascariasis, biliary tract surgery
  – Hilar CCA—most common
- Portal vein—ascending portal vein infection (pyelophlebitis), untreated appendicitis, diverticulitis, pancreatitis, IBD, PID, perforated viscus, omphalitis in newborn
  – This cause has reduced
- Hepatic artery—any systemic infection (endocarditis, pneumonia, osteomyelitis) microabscess in sepsis
- Direct extension—suppurative cholecystitis, subphrenic abscess, perinephric abscess, bowel perforation
- Trauma—hematoma gets infected
- Cryptogenic—undiagnosed abdominal disease, resolved abdominal disease, diabetes, malignant disease
- Local treatment of liver tumors—RFA
- Bilioenteric anastomosis
- Most common pathology—biliary
  – Benign conditions more common in Asia

- Most common in right liver 75%

  Due to laminar flow
  - Left 20%
  - Caudate 5%
  - 50% are solitary
  - 1 mm to 3 mm thickness
  - 4 cm diameter, single or multiloculated

Microbiology

- *E. coli* and Klebsiella most common organism
- Klebsiella serotype K1 most common in Asians than K2
- *E. coli*—most common pathogen in the West
- Klebsiella is frequently associated in gas forming abscess
- Enterococci and Viridans streptococci generally found in polymicrobial abscess
- Staphalococcus most common
  - If only single organism cause abscess
  - Hematogenous route
- Less common causes Pseudomonas, Proteus, Enterobacter, Citrobacter, Serratia, Fusobacterium, Clostridium
- Abscess cultures get more positive than blood
- Pus culture negative in 20%
- Cryptogenic abscess—more negative blood culture
- Biliary source abscess—more positive blood and pus culture

Clinical Features

- Fever with chills, jaundice, RUQ pain
- Tenderness on palpation (10%)
- Cough and dyspnoea if diaphragm is involved
- Peritonitis due to rupture
- Single lesions more on right lobe
- A rare complication specific to Klebsiella hepatic abscess is endogenous. Endophthalmitis (3%), meningitis, cellulitis, lung abscess
  - Infection with *K. pneumoniae* genotype K1 and immunosuppression are the reasons
- Single lesions are usually cryptogenic
- Multiple are usually biliary in origin
- Most common locations are right lobe, then left lobe, then bilateral
- PLA <2 cm is called microabscess

- Diffuse miliary nature—more with staphylococcal because hematogenous
- Cluster pattern—in enteric organism in cholangitis in biliary obstruction—clusters may coalesce

Diagnosis

- LFT deranged
- ALP raised, ALT elevated, jaundice
- Chest X-ray is abnormal in 50%—subdiaphragmatic disease, elevated right hemidiaphragm, right pleural effusion, atelectasis
- Abdominal X-ray—air fluid levels, portal venous gas
- USG—round or oval area that is hypoechogenic than the surrounding liver
  - Thick pus may be confused with parenchyma—Doppler—distinguish solid areas
  - Sensitivity 80–95%
- CECT—sensitivity 95–100%
  - Arterial phase—parenchyma surrounding abscess show segmental enhancement—as a result of altered portal microcirculation in infected tissue
- **Target like sign**—single or multiloculated mass with a central hypodense region and peripheral contrast enhancement during portal phase
- **MRI**—distinguishing the cause of many hepatic masses and evaluating the biliary tree
  - Not preferred—takes long time.
- **Nuclear medicine**
  - Indium—111 leucocyte scintigraphy with prior Tc 99 sulfur colloid scan

Treatment

- Antibiotics—cryptogenic—ampi/genta/metronidazole
  - Biliary-imipaenam/vancomicin
- IV antibiotics—for 2 weeks—clinical improvements—afebrile and when start oral intake—switch to oral antibiotics for 2 more weeks
- Biliary source—drainage through ERCP/PTC

Percutaneous—CT Guided

- If <5 cm aspiration alone
- If biliary communication is there—PCD (PCD—Percutaneous catheter drainage PNA—Percutaneous needle aspiration)

- May cause bacteremia so avoid excessive contrast distension and saline irrigation
- Bile leak through drain, if prolonged do ERCP
- Laparotomy considered, if failure of percutaneous method
- Liver resection is occasionally required

Surgical Treatment
- Not first line
- In—rupture, bleeding, failed percutaneous methods
- Large multiloculated with thick pus
- In liver atrophy and multiple abscesses—resection may be considered

Postop
- Cavity may persist on imaging
- If patient is asymptomatic and lesion is stable, no treatment is needed
- Recurrence more common with biliary cause

Amebic Liver Abscess
- Earliest report in Bhrigu-Samhita in 3000 BC—bloody diarrhea
- James Annesley—'hepatic dysentry'
- Ameba discovered by—Friederich Loech—he named ameba after his patient
- E. histolitica—pathogen
- E. dispar and E. moschovskii—not pathogenetic

E. histolytica
- Protozoan
- Cysts—survive gastric acid—travel to terminal ileum and colon—trophozoites emerge
- Cysts—survive under fingernails—for 45 minutes, in soil for 1 month at 10 degree C
- Destroyed by drying, iodine and heat
- Not killed by chlorination
- Similar to E. dispar—need PCR and genetic sequencing to identify

Screening
- Microscopic examination of stool
- Ritchie's fecal concentration
- Staining of alcohol fixed stool
- Robinson's in vitro culture
- Screening stool antigens
- Serology—indirect hemagglutination test (IHAT)
  – ELISA
- Isoenzyme electrophoresis of stool for zymodeme identification
- Gold standards—Robinson's culture and zymodeme identification
- Breast fed neonates—low incidence–due to IgA

Pathogenesis
- Three virulence factors
  – Lectin—surface protein which helps trophozoite adhesion to host cell cause caspase activation and cell necrosis
  – Ameoba phores are inserted into cell causing osmotic lysis of cell
  – Cysteine proteases—degradation of extracellular matrix and cell layer
- Proteophosphoglycans (PPG) in amebic glycocalyx is related to pathogenecity
- In sinusoids—low blood flow, low RBC velocity, lack of tight junctions which allow parasites to breach the sinusoids into parenchyma
- Mucosal IgA against lectin is protective
- E. histolytica cyst enters through fecooral ingestion
- Human are principal host and cyst carrier
- Trophozoite is released and passed to colon, invades mucosa and causes disease
- Reach liver through portal vein, causes abscess formation principally by enzymatic cellular hydrolysis
- Secretory immunoglobulin IgA antibodies have been shown to inhibit adherence to colonic epithelium
- The appearance of fluid is **anchovy sauce** like, the progression of disease is till Glisson capsule
- Most common site of colitis—cecum
- Right lobe of liver is more common because from right side of colon to right branch of portal vein and then to right lobe posterosuperior aspect of right lobe
- Colitis and ALA rarely occur together
- Starts as hepatitis—liver cells undergo liquefactive necrosis—starting in center—spread to periphery—produce cavity full of blood and liquifies liver tissue—anchovy sauce
- No odour and it is sterile
- Fluid contains no ameba—only seen at the periphery of cavity

- Secondary bacterial infection can occur
- Due to lack of fibrotic response—centrifugal extension to Glisson capsule which is resistant to amebae
- Usually solitary, large and in right liver
- Left lobe abscess more prone to rupture—because of lesser volume of left liver
- Vascular and biliary structures cross abscess which are resistant to infection but may be broken while drainage and lead to bile leak/bleeding
- Resolution take 6 months to 2 years—develops fibrous wall
- DD—tumor (PLA—resolve in 2–4 months)

Amoebic vs pyogenic liver abscess		
Clinical features	Amoebic abscess	Pyogenic abscess
Age	25–45	>50
Male:female	>10:1	1.5:1
Solitary lesion	80%	50%
Site	Usually right liver	Usually right liver
Jaundice	Uncommon	Common
Elevated ALP	Common	Common
Positive amebic serology	Yes	No
Positive blood culture	No	Common
Alcohol use	Common	Common
Diabetes	2%	27%

Clinical Features

- More in tropical and developing countries
- Hispanic men, 20–40 years, history of travel, poor socioeconomic status, male:female—10:1
- Heavy alcoholic are more susceptible
- Diarrhoea seen in only 30%
- Concomitant colitis and ALA—in 30%
- Anorexia, fever with chills, pain
- Biliary communication seen in—27%
- Right lobe lesion produce pleural signs
- Left lobe lesion produce pericardial irritation
  - Rupture—peritonitis

Diagnosis

- Mild to moderate leucocytosis, anemia, decreased albumin
- Most common LFT derangement is—**PTINR**
- Antiameobic antibodies seen in 90–95%
- Enzyme immunoassay has reported sensitivity of 99% and specificity 99%
- *E. histolytica* lectin antigen testing
- **Plain chest radiograph**—50% abnormal—elevated right diaphragm, pleural effusion, atelectasis
- **USG**—90% accuracy. Round lesion abutting the liver capsule, without significant rim echoes, interpreted as an abscess wall
  - Hypoechoic with distal enhancement
  - In 80% single, right lobe
  - 10%—left lobe single
  - 6%—caudate lobe—single
  - The rest—multiple
- **CT**—more sensitive than USG, helpful in differentiating from pyogenic abscess with a rim enhancement noted in pyogenic abscess
- **MRI**—not superior to CT
  - Helpful to differentiate from tumor
  - Hypointense in T1 weighted and hyperintense in T2 weighted
- **Nuclear studies**—gallium scanning or technetium Tc 99 liver scan, can be helpful in differentiating pyogenic from amebic, because amebic typically do not contain leucocytes and therefore do not light up on these scans.

Serology

- ELISA and IHAT—most reliable
- Antibodies detectable 7–10 days postsymptoms
- Titers peak by 2–3 months—revert to negative by 12 months
- PCR—detect *E. histolytica* DNA in pus and saliva

Complications

- Rupture
  - Into peritoneum
  - Gastric, colonic fistula
- Sympathetic right-sided pleural effusion:
  - Most common chest complication
  - No treatment needed
- Rupture to bronchus, effusion—thoracocentesis

Treatment

- Oral metronidazole 750 mg three times for ten days curative in 90% patients
- Other—secnidazole, tinidazole

- Emetine hydrochloride is effective against invasive amebiasis, but requires intramuscular injections and is cardiotoxic
- Chloroquine—less effective
- After treatment of liver abscess treat with luminal agents—iodoquinol, paromomycin, diloxanide furoate
  - To eradicate intestinal infection
- Metronidazole
  - Crosses placenta and BBB
  - Contraindicated in first trimester
  - Breast feeding discontinued
- Emetine hydrochloride
  - Effective against trophozoites
  - Ameobicidal action in tissues—not in intestine
  - IM/deep subcutaneous injections
  - In hepatopulmonary disease
- Chloroquine
  - No luminal action
  - In pulmonary ameobiasis
  - Contraindicated in retinopathy
- Diloxanide—in asymptomatic carriers

Aspiration
Indications

- Serology inconclusive and DD is PLA
- Pregnancy—antiamebic inappropriate
- Secondary infection—in 15%
- Fever and pain persisting 5–7 days after treatment
- Rupture imminent if >10 cm especially on left lobe
- Age >55
- Size >5 cm

- Mortality—5%
- If rupture mortality—6–50%
- Factors for poor outcome
  - Elevated serum bilirubin level (>3.5)
  - Encephalopathy
  - Hypoalbuminemia <2
  - Multiple abscess cavity
  - Abscess volume larger than 500 ml
  - Anemia
  - Diabetes

- Average time of radiological resolution is 3 to 9 months

4.8 HYDATID CYST

- Echinococcosis is zoonosis—*E. granulosus*
- Dog is definitive host
- Middle East, South American, Australia, New Zealand, East Africa
- No human to human transmission
- *Echinococcus granulosus* is the most common, *E. multilocularis* and *E. ligartus* account for less number of cases
- Sheep—intermediate host
- Human—accidental intermediate host
- In humans—reach duodenum and embryo releases an oncosphere containing hooklet that penetrates the mucosa, allowing access to bloodstream
- Adult worm—sexual stage
- Cystic or infiltrative larva-metacestode—reproduce asexually

Adult Worm Features

- Head or scolex
- Body or strobilia with 3 or 4 proglottids
- Proglottids bear—mature eggs
- Eggs contain embryo—called oncosphere or hexacanth—has three pairs of lancet-shaped hooklets
- *Humans are dead end hosts*
- Reach liver (most common), lung where parasite develops its larval stage—the hydatid cyst
- Three weeks after infection, a visible cyst develops and slowly grows in a spherical manner
- Pericyst or fibrous capsule develops around it
- Cyst wall has two layers, an outer gelatinous (ectocyst) and inner germinal membrane (endocyst)
- Brood capsules are small, intracystic cellular masses in which future worms heads develop into scoleces
- In definitive host they develop into tapeworms but in intermediate host they do not develop into tapeworm
- Once in liver—cyst development may take months to years
- Cyst contains clear, hydatid fluid with protoscolex

Three Layers
- Germinal layer (germinative membrane) endocyst
- Laminated layer
- Adventitial layer

- Compression of host tissue around endocyst produces pericyst or ectocyst
- Germinal layer is the living component—produces protoscolices—released into fluid cause invaginations and develop daughter cysts
- Daughter cysts—structure similar to mother cysts—but no adventitial layer
- Laminated membrane—can be separated from pericyst—1 to 2 mm
- Daughter cysts formed by
  - Endogenous vesiculation
  - Ectogenic vesiculation—when there is a leak in laminated membrane, germinal layer passes through and develops exogenous cysts called 'satellite hydatid cysts'—in 16–65%
- Ectocyst—present in liver and spleen cysts
  - Absent in lung and brain cysts
  - Vascular structures in ectocyst—remain intact
- Adventitial layer is vascular and cause vascular rim—not separable from normal parenchyma
- Uncomplicated cyst—fluid colorless odorless
  - Concentrations of Na, Cl, HCO_3—same as in plasma, K, Ca lower than plasma
- Secondary hydatidosis—spillage of fluid—development of cysts in surrounding viscera
- More involvement of right lobe—especially segments VII and VIII

Complications

- Compression—compensatory lobe hypertrophy
  - Budd-Chiari
  - Obstructive jaundice
  - PHT
- Rupture into biliary tract
  - Most common complication
  - Cyst >10 cm—high risk
  - Communication >5 mm is called major biliary communication—may find cyst material in bile duct causing obstructive jaundice/cholangitis—seen in 5–10%
  - CT should be followed by ERCP extraction
- Bronchial rupture
- Rupture into peritoneum—allergic reaction, pain
  - Anaphylaxis occurs in 1%

Clinical Features

- Men = female
- 45 years

- 75% right liver
- Abdominal pain, dyspepsia, vomiting
- Most frequent sign—hepatomegaly
- Jaundice and fever in 8% patients
- Free rupture can result in disseminated echinococcosis or potentially fatal anaphylactic reaction

Diagnosis

- LFT—ALP, bilirubin raised
- Leucocytosis

Serology

- Depends on reaction of test antigen to circulating antibodies
- Immunoelectrophoresis
- Used for post-treatment follow-up—not for epidemiology

ELISA

- For epidemiology
- IgG—remains elevated for 4 years—not suitable for post-treatment follow-up
- IgM—disappears in 6 months after treatment

Immunoblotting tests:

- Western blott
- Immunoblotting-sensitivity—95%, specificity—100%
  - Used as first line test and useful to different from other conditions

WHO Classification

- CL type (cystic lesion)—simple cyst—early stage, not fertile
- CE1—concentric hyperechoic halo, contain free floating hyperechoic foci—hydatid sand, fertile
- CE 2—multivesicular with daughter and grand-daughter cysts—rossette, spoked wheel, honeycomb or clustered appearance
- CE 3—detachment of laminar layer—floating—water lily or water snake sign
- CE 4—contains both cystic and solid—without visible daughter cysts
- CE 5—calcified. completely calcified cyst—egg shell calcification—indictive of dead cyst. Some calcification with hypoechoic lacunar structures—not sure of dead cyst

- CL, CE1, CE2—active fertile cysts
- CE3a—transitional active or inactive
- CE3b—transitional. Biologically active cysts
- CE4, CE5—inactive
- CE4—degenerative, CE5—partial or completely calcified

CT
Better delineation

MRI
- More specific than CT
- Choice for cystobiliary communication
- **Diffusion weighted imaging**
- To differentiate from simple cysts and for characterization of cysts
- In suspected biliary involvement—ERCP or percutaneous transhepatic cholangiography may be necessary

		Gharbi's classification
Type 1	Pure cystic fluid collection (spherical oval walled, thick)	
Type 2	Fluid collection with membrane separation	
Type 3	Fluid collection with septa	
Type 4	Heterogeneous pattern	
Type 5	Completely calcified (reflecting) walls	

Treatment
- Radical surgery
- Conservative surgery
- PAIR
- Medical with benzimidazoles

Surgery
Indications
- Removal of large CE2-C3b cysts with daughter vesicles
- single cyst superficial—may rupture
- Infected cysts—when percutaneous treatments not available
- Communicating with bile duct
- Pressure on structures

Contraindications
- Inactive, asymptomatic cysts
- Difficult to access, small cysts

Surgery
- Proctoscolicide packs and soft injection—without pressure
  - 70–95% alcohol
  - 15–20% hypertonic saline
  - 0.5% cetrimide
- Recommended—20% saline—should be in contact with germinal layer for 15 minutes
- Avoided if BD communication is present

Conservative Surgery
- Only cyst removed
- Injection, suction, removal of laminated membrane and germinal epithelium, unroofing of the protruding part of cyst—the adventitia and thinned liver
- Edge of adventitia sutured—may contain bile duct
- If bile duct communication—bile stain—no scolicides used
- If bile duct communication suspected—cholangiogram is done followed by ERCP or suturing of the communication or HJ or resection carried out
- Cavity packed with omentum

Complications
- Biliary fistula
- Biliary stricture—due to scolicidal contact
- Recurrence—local or disseminated
  - Serology—even with complete removal of cysts—blood titers decrease slowly in months to years
- So—positive test is not diagnostic of recurrence—but, rising titer is indicative of recurrence

Radical Surgery
- Pericystectomy (radical cystectomy, capsulectomy, total pericystectomy, cystopericystectomy)
- Surgical plane is created outside pericyst—without opening the cyst—cyst with adventitial layer excised enbloc
- CUSA used to divide parenchyma—like resection—bile duct and vessels sutured
- Avoided if—impinging on IVC, liver hilum

Liver Resection
- Infrequent
- Only surgical therapy for *E. multilocularis*
- Rarely if—atrophic liver
  - Bile fistula—cannot be managed otherwise

Percutaneous Treatments

- Destruction of germinal layer—PAIR
- Evacuation of entire endocyst—percut evacuation of cyst content (PEVAC)
- Transhepatic approach of needle puncture—US/CT guided

  Contraindicated in:
  - Vascular injury
  - Ruptured into bile duct, peritoneum
  - Insufficient liver tissue

PAIR (Puncture Aspiration of Cyst, Injection of Proctoscolicidal and Reaspiration of Fluid)

- Described by Ben Amor in Tunisia, 1986
- Best done in patient with mebendazole or albendazole
- Indications
  - Cyst >5 cm
  - CE 1 and CE 3a cysts
- Puncture–aspirate—inject scolicidal, wait for 15 minutes and reaspirate

PAIR Catheterization

- After PAIR catheter—left *in situ*—after 24 hours if drainage <10 ml or not bile stained—inject 95% alcohol, wait for 20 minutes and remove catheter.
  - If drainage >10 ml—catheter kept until the drainage reduces
- If bile duct communication, no injection is done

PEVAC

- Catheter introduced, aspirated and left in place
- Second session—14–18F sheath introduced—suction and breakdown of the cysts, aspirated and drainage tube kept and if no bile leak they are later removed

APAIR—Albenadazole with PAIR

- Medical management
- In inoperable liver and lung cysts
- Small CE 1 and CE 3a
- Following surgery or PAIR to prevent recurrence
- Albendazole—choice 10 mg/kg twice daily—continuously—optimal duration not sure
- Perioperative treatment—started 1 week prior—post-treatment 3–8 weeks in uncomplicated
- In complicated 3–6 months

Surgery vs PAIR vs medical treatment for hydatid liver cysts

	Surgery	PAIR	Medical (BMZ)
Indications	Large CE2-CE3b cysts with multiple daughter vesicles	CE1 >5 cm CE3a >5 cm Inoperable patients	CE1 <5 cm CE3a <5 cm Inoperable patients
	Single superficial liver cysts	Refuse surgery	Refuse surgery
	Complicated cysts	Relapse after surgery Failure to respond to BMZ alone	Multiple cysts in >2 organs Peritoneal cysts Prevent recurrence following surgery or PAIR
Contrain-dications	General C/I for surgery Uncomplicated CE4 and CE5 Very small cysts	Biliary fistulae CE2 CE3b CE4 CE5	Pregnancy Uncomplicated CE4 and CE5 Alone if cyst >10 cm Cysts at risk of rupture Chronic hepatic disease Bone marrow depression

Wait and Watch

- CE4, CE5
- CL—no treatment until the parasitic nature is proven
- Hepatic hydatid cyst is primary surgical disease
- In preparation for surgery—preoperative steroids can be used
- Anesthesia—adrenaline and steroids should be ready in case of anaphylaxis
- The cyst is usually aspirated through a closed suction system, flushed with scolicidal agents, such as hypertonic saline
- Cyst is then unroofed followed by excision, marsupialization, leaving the cyst open, drainage of cyst, omentoplasty, partial hepatectomy
- If bile duct communication is identified pre-operatively—simple suturing, sometimes major biliary repair, postop ERCP needed
- Laparoscopic techniques for drainage and unroofing of cyst have been reported

Alveolar Echinococcosis

- By *E. multilocularis*
- Definitive and intermediate hosts are wild animals—rodents—foxes

- There is a PNM classification
  - P—primary lesion
  - N—neighbouring organs
  - M—distal metastasis
- Human are accidental hosts
- Mostly in liver
- Grow and metastasis like malignancy
- Antigen test 95–100% accuracy
- CT/MRI—central necrosis with microcalcifications—large mass with relatively less symptoms—vs malignancy

Treatment

- Radical surgery—R0 resection—first choice
- Albendazole—mandatory—temporary after complete resection—lifelong in others
- Palliative surgery—if bilobar, involving IVC or portal vein
- Liver transplantation. can recur after LT—Albendazole added post LT

4.9 HEMOBILIA

- Bleeding into biliary tree from an abnormal communication between blood vessels and bile duct
- Greek haima = blood, latin bilis = bile
- Bilhemia = bile enters blood stream

Etiology

- Iatrogenic trauma (most common 40–60%)
- Following PTBD, liver biopsy, surgery of biliary tree, after cholecystectomy
- Accidental trauma—liver injury—incidence of hemobilia in major trauma—3%
- Gall stones, tumors
- Inflammatory
- Ascariasis
- Vascular disorders
  - Most common—HA aneurism
- Vascular lesions associated with arterial hypertension—can cause hemobilia
  - Most common organ—gall bladder—"apoplexy of the gall bladder"

Clinical Features

- Major hemobilia is rare
- **Triad of Sandblom (Quincke's triad** 1871)(22%)—upper abdominal pain, upper GI bleed, jaundice—seen in only one-fourth
- Melena (90%)

- Hemetemesis (60%)
- Biliary colic in 70%
- Jaundice (60%)
- Major hemobilia—due to hepatic artery bleed
- Blood clot can cause hemetemesis/melena and can act like calculus and cause biliary colic-cholecystitis-pancreatitis

Diagnosis

- Upper GI endoscopy, to rule out other causes and in 10% bleeding from ampulla is seen
- Investigation of choice—hepatic artery angiography
- Cholangiography shows clots in biliary tree seen
- USG/CECT—biliary dilatation, clots, tumors can be seen

Treatment

- Self limiting
- First line for major bleeding—transarterial embolization
  - Selective embolization—preferred—75 to 100% success
  - If embolise main HA—rebleeding is more and future re-embolization is not possible
- Surgery when embolization is failed
- Ligation of bleeding vessel, excision of aneurysm, nonselective ligation of hepatic artery may be needed
- Cholecystectomy in case of hemorrhagic cholecystitis
- Minor cases—endoscopic coagulation, somatostatin, vasopressin

Biliary Tract

After PTC—do cholangiography—if bilio portal vein fistula easily controlled by upsizing the stent size—tamponade

- Arterial fistula—embolize
- If no fistula seen—remove catheter and do arteriography
- Obstructive jaundice—ERCP—clot removal

Bilhemia

- Bile flow into hepatic blood stream via hepatic vein or portal vein branches
- Causes—reversed flow by inversion of pressure gradient—due to increased bile duct pressure from obstruction or low venous pressure
  - Gall stone eroding into portal vein/hepatic vein (necropsy of Ignatius Loyolain in 1559—3 gall stones found in PV)
  - Accidental or iatrogenic trauma

Clinical Features

- Can be fatal if bile embolization in lungs occur
- Rapidly increasing jaundice, marked direct hyperbilirubinemia without elevation of AST/ALT,
- Septicemia in infected bile

Diagnosis

- ERCP—choice
- Angiogram—may not help

Treatment

- ERCP—stenting or sphincterotomy to lower the intrabiliary pressure
- If higher location—PTBD
- Endostenting
- Resection of the liver segment—definitive cure
- Occlusion of fistula by ERCP/angiography

Hemosuccus Pancreaticus

- Bleeding into pancreatic duct producing GI bleed
- Most common cause—rupture of pseudoaneurysm of celiac trunk vasculature into pancreatic duct secondary to acute and chronic pancreatitis
- Rupture of primary celiac aneurysms—rare

Clinical Features

- High degree of suspicion is required
- Abdominal pain, acute GI bleeding, h/o acute or chronic pancreatitis
- Elevated amylase

Diagnosis

- Selective angiography is the choice shows pseudo-aneurysms
- ERCP—shows bleeding and filling defect in pancreatic duct
- CECT

Treatment

- Choice—angiographic embolisation
- If fails, surgery

Principles of Hepatic Resection

- Lortat Jacob (1952) first true anatomic right hepatectomy
- Most blood loss occurs from hepatic veins, hence maintaining a low CVP
- Position—mild Trendelenburg
- CVP lower than 5
- Perioperative mortality—5%
- Accounts to—blood loss, amount of liver resection, condition of liver
- Average blood loss—600 ml
- Up to 80% of liver can be resected in case of non-cirrhotic functional liver

Complications

- Bile leak 10–20%
- Hepatic dysfunction <25%
- Liver failure, extrahepatic organ failure, death

Gall Bladder and Biliary System

5.1 ANATOMY

- Size 7. 5 × 12 cm
- Capacity 25–30 ml, distended GB has a capacity of 50–60 ml
- Distended bile duct can have up to 300 ml of bile
- 4 parts—fundus, body, infundibulum, neck
  - Fundus—junction of 9th costal cartilage and rectus muscle
  - Covered by peritoneum
  - Body in the GB fossa—has intimate relation with D1 and D2
  - Infundibulum—portion of the body between neck and the point of entry of cystic artery. When this portion becomes dilated, it is called Hartmann pouch
  - Neck is S-shaped—becomes cystic duct
- GB contains 5 layers—epithelium, lamina propria, smooth muscle, perimuscular subserosal connective tissue, serosa
  - GB has no muscularis mucosa or submucosa
- Muscle fibres arranged in criss-cross manner and more in neck. Not well-developed layer
- Rokitansky-Aschoff sinuses—invagination of epithelium into lamina propria muscle and subserosal connective tissue. Present in 40% of normal GB and present in all inflammed GB
- Ducts of Luschka—tiny bile ducts found around the muscle layer on the hepatic side of GB. Seen in 10% of normal GB. No relation to RA sinuses or cholecystitis
- "Crypts of Luschka"—mucus membrane indentation
- GB separated from hepatic parenchyma by cystic plate, which is the compressed connective tissue that extends to the left as hilar plate

Cystic Duct

- 3 cm (1–5 cm) long
- 1–3 mm diameter
- Valves of Heister—do not have any valvular function Arrangement of mucosa in spiral fold
- Wall surrounded by "sphincter of Lutkens"
- Prevent gall stones entering CBD
- Joins CHD in supraduodenal portion in 80%—rarely in retroduodenal or retropancreatic portion.

Common Hepatic Duct—2.5 cm Long

Common Bile Duct

- 7.5 cm (8 cm) long
- Diameter—4 to 9 mm

Four parts
- Supraduodenal
  - 2.5 cm
- Retroduodenal
- Infraduodenal (intrapancreatic)
- Intraduodenal (intramural)

- Terminate by opening into the summit of ampulla of Vater.
- Usually pancreatic duct joins CBD before passing through the wall of duodenum or within wall, but anatomical variations are there
- Union with CHD—most common type—angular in 75%. Other types—parallel (20%) and spiral
- **Absence of cystic duct is an acquired anomaly in cholecystocholedochal fistula**
- CBD—has columnar mucosa surrounded by connective tissue layer. Muscle fibers in bile duct are sparse. Distal CBD and sphincter contain more muscle fibers

Sphincter of Oddi

- Contains both circular and longitudinal muscles
- Common channel of <1 cm is seen in 90%
- 4 portions—superior and inferior sphincter choledochus, sphincter pancreaticus and sphincter of ampulla

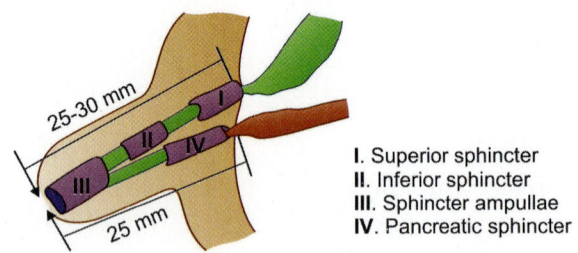

I. Superior sphincter
II. Inferior sphincter
III. Sphincter ampullae
IV. Pancreatic sphincter

- Vascular anatomy
  - Infraduodenal CBD supplied by superior pancreaticoduodenal and gastroduodenal arteries—run in 3 and 9 o'clock positions.
  - Supraduodenal CBD supplied by right hepatic and cystic artery, posterio superior pacreatico duodenal, GDA, retroduodenal artery, they form 3'o clock and 9'o clock arteries provide axial blood supply. 60% blood vessels run upwards, 38% arteries run downwards from RHA and others and 2% provide nonaxial supply from main HA
  - Retropancreatic portion—from retroduodenal artery and pancreaticoduodenal artery—form mural plexus
  - Accessory cystic artery arise from gastroduodenal artery
  - Veins run and for 3 and 9'o clock positions. Veins from GB drain into this venous system, not directly into portal vein. Biliary tree hase its own portal venous pathway to liver
- **Calot's triangle (hepatocystic triangle)**
  - Superiorly—inferior surface of liver
  - Medially—common hepatic duct
  - Laterally—cystic duct and medial part of GB
  - Content—cystic artery, Calot's node
  - Original Calot's triangle described by Calot in 1891 the boundaries are: Cystic artery instead of inferior surface of liver, CHD and cystic duct

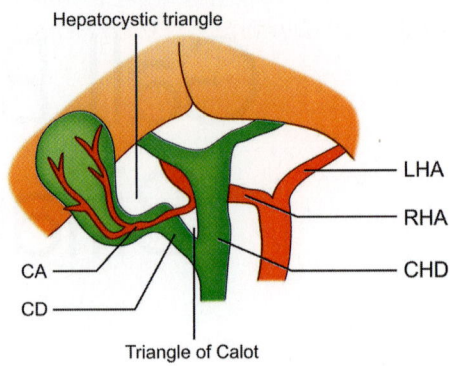

- Moynihan's hump or caterpillar hump
  - Anomaly where the common hepatic artery takes a tortuous course in front of origin of cystic duct or the right hepatic artery is tortuous and cystic artery is short.
  - RHA passes posterior to CHD in 85%.
    - Anterior in 15%
    - Replaced aberrant RHA from SMA in 15%— passes posterior to cystic duct

Physiology

- Bile excretes cholesterol and bilirubin
- Facilitates absorption of lipids and fat soluble vitamins
- Water constitutes 85% of bile volume
- 250–300 mg of bilirubin is excreted in bile daily (75% from red cells and 25% from hepatic heme)
- Normal volume of bile secreted—750–1000 ml/day
- In fasting state pressure in CBD—5–10 cm H_2O
- On feeding GB contract—pressure in GB 25 cm H_2O and CBD pressure 20 cm of H_2O
- Bile gets concentrated in GB 5–10 fold

Enterohepatic Circulation

- Synthesis of bile salts 0.2–0.6 g/day
- Portal venous return—> 95% (reabsorbed)
- Urinary excretion—<0.5 mg/day
- Fecal excretion—0.2–0.6 g/day
- Bile salts are absorbed in terminal ileum
- Excess bile salt causes diarrhoea due to detergent action

- GB wall absorbs water to concentrate bile component
- Concentration leads to cholesterol and calcium concentration
- GB neck and cystic duct produce glycoprotein
- 600 ml bile storage in 24 hours
- Mucus secretion (20 ml/day)
- GB filling is retrograde
- GB contraction is stimulated by CCK (most potent)
- CCK also inhibits tonic sphincter of Oddi pressure
- Vagal action also promotes GB secretion

Cholesterol Saturation

- Cholesterol is highly nonpolar and is insoluble in water and bile
- Made soluble by formation of miccelles, a bile salt—phospholipid—cholesterol complex
- Bile salts have both hydrophilic and hydrophobic portions
- In aqueous solutions, hydrophilic ends are oriented outwards
- Cholesterol is added to the hydrophobic central portion and thus maintained in solution
- Another theory—much of the cholesterol exist in vesicular form—they are bilayers of phospholipid and cholesterol—normally unilamellar.
  - Aggregation leads to multilamellar vesicles. If these exceed the capability to transport cholesterol—crystallisation occurs
- GB secrete mucus and H^+ ions—this reduces hepatic bile in GB pH from 7.5 to 7.8 down to 7.1 to 7.3. This solubilises calcium
- GB mucosa has the greater absorptive capacity per unit of any structure in the body
- Bile is concentrated 5 to 10 fold in GB—water is absorbed—concentrated bile—may promote stone formation
- During fasting, periods—partial emptying of GB may occur (10–15% of its volume), this occurs in MMC phase III
- Sphincter of Oddi relaxation and GB contraction on eating is affected by CCK
- After eating, 60–70% of its contents are emptied in 30–40 minutes—refilling occur over 60–90 minutes

Investigations

- X-ray—10% stones radio-opaque
  - Seagull and Mercedes Benz sign seen in GB stone
  - Calcified GB seen in porcelain GB
  - Emphysematous GB with air in wall and lumen of GB
- USG—investigation of choice
  - Normal GB is anechoic
  - Normal wall thickness <3 mm
- EUS: Accurate in imaging bile duct and detecting choledocholithiasis
- HIDA: Hepatic Immuno Diacetic Acid cholescintigraphy
  - Used to evaluate physiological secretion of bile
  - In 90% patient GB is visualised in 30 minutes and 100% in 1 hour, but nonvisualisation after 2 hours is seen in acute cholecystitis
  - Delayed visualisation is seen in chronic cholecystitis, contracted GB, dyskinesia (confirmed by CCK injection)
  - HIDA scan also detects obstruction of biliary tree and biliary leak
- Tc 99m PIPIDA scan
- MRCP: Uses water in bile to delineate biliary tree
- ERCP: Diagnose stone and stricture, biopsy, stenting and stone removal can be done.
- PTC: Percutaneous Transhepatic Cholangiography
  - Provides anatomic information for biliary reconstruction
  - In malignant stricture at confluence of hepatic duct or high, PTC is preferred over ERCP.
- Cholangiography—for tract anomalies, biliary reconstruction, during cholecystectomy by catheter in cystic duct done at 20 degree angle head down.
- **Choledochoscopy**
  - Flexible fibreoptic endoscope into CBD can aid stone removal intraoperatively.
- Phyrgian cap—seen in 5% (septum of GB)
- Floating GB: GB hanging on mesentry, prone for torsion

5.2 CHOLELITHIASIS

- 80% stones are cholesterol or mixed
- Cholesterol content in stone—50 to 99%
- Pure cholesterol <10%
- Majority—nearly 80%—asymptomatic

- In humans most of the cholesterol found in gall stones are from diet (hepatic synthesis of cholesterol is only 20%)
- **Factors causing stone formation**
  - Supersaturation
  - Concentration of bile in GB
  - Crystal nucleation
  - GB dysmotility
  - Impaired GB function
  - Cholesterol nucleation factor
  - Obesity/high calorie diet
  - Ileal resection
- **Pigment stones**
  - Stones containing <30% cholesterol

Two Types

- Black (large) stones
  - Insoluble bilirubin
  - 20–30% of pigment stones are this type
  - Associated with hemolysis
  - Exclusively seen in GB
- Brown stones
  - Associated with bile stasis and infection
  - Mainly in biliary tree, rare in gall bladder
  - Due to deconjugation of bilirubin glucoronide by enzyme beta gluconoridase
  - Associated with foreign body in biliary tree like stent, parasite

Risk Factors

- Older age
- Females
- Obesity, weight loss—bariatric surgery
- TPN—biliary sludge
- Genetics
- Cirrhosis (black stones)
- Ileal resection
- Ceftriaxone—excreted in bile can cause pseudolithiasis

Complications of Gall Stones

- Biliary colic
- Acute and chronic cholecystitis
- Empyema
- Mucocele
- Perforation
- Biliary obstruction
- Acute cholangitis
- Acute pancreatitis
- Gall stones—ileus

Diagnosis

- Clinical—Murphy's sign
- USG—wall thickness >5 mm (4 mm), pericholecystic fluid
- HIDA scan—demonstrate of absent filling of GB within 60 minutes—indicate CD obstruction—more sensitive and specific than USG in acute cholecystitis

Medical Management

- In unwilling/unable to undergo surgery
- Mild symptoms
- Small stones
- Noncalcified cholesterol stones
- Functioning GB with patent CD
- Hydrophilic ursodeoxy cholic acid is given

Indications of Prophylactic Cholecystetomy

- Haemolytic anemia
- Porcelain GB
- Patient undergoing bariatric surgery
  - Patient with long common channel of bile and pancreatic duct
  - Before organ transplant
  - Diabetes—no increased complications noted—so prophylactic cholecystectomy not recommended (Blumgart)
  - Stones >3 cm high risk of GB cancer

- Cholecystotomy/percutaneous cholecystotomy—in acalculous cholecystitis
  - In patients who are in high risk to undergo surgery
  - Under USG guidance
  - Later cholecystectomy is done in 3–6 months

Tokyo Consensus Grading of Severity of Acute Cholecystitis

- For severity grading
- Grade 1–3
- Grade 1—mild with no organ dysfunction
- Grade 2—moderate leucocytosis with marked inflammation
- Grade 3—severe with systemic complication.

Porcelain GB

- Encountered in 0.8% of specimens
- High risk of cancer

Acute Cholecystitis

- Due to impaction of stone in infundibulum/CD—obstruction—venous congestion—arterial occlusion—gangrene—perforation
- Because fundus is the farthest from artery—most common site of ischemia and necrosis
- Positive bile culture seen in 20%—most common Klebsiella and *E. coli*
- Surgery is considered either within 72 hours or after 6 weeks

Chronic Cholecystitis

- Colic—misnomer—as pain is continuous
- Xanthogranulomatous cholecystitis—mimic cancer—presence of destructive inflammation of GB wall accompanied by proliferative fibrosis—can cause mass formation
- **CA19-9 may be elevated in XGC**

Acalculous Cholecystitis

- In severe trauma, sepsis
- More common in men
- Due to combination of ischemia, biliary stasis, and sepsis
- More common in diabetes and HTN
- More complications like necrosis and perforation—due to disturbance in microcirculation

- **Diagnosis**
  - USG—distended with GB sludge—no stones or thickened wall
  - CT more specific
  - Scintigraphy with morphine—more specific
- **Treatment**
  - Cholecystectomy—definitive
  - Cholecystostomy—in critically ill
  - Percutaneous cholecystostomy—may be definitive as there is no calculous obstruction

Gangrenous Cholecystitis

- More common in diabetes
- More in acalculous type—owing to delay in diagnosis
- Most common site—fundus—may perforate
- Investigation
  CT is the choice:
  - Air in the wall or lumen
  - Intraluminal membranes
  - Irregular wall and collection
  - Lack of contrast enhancement

Emphysematous Cholecystitis

- Due to gas forming bacteria in the bile
- May be seen in association with gangrenous cholecystitis
- More common in men and diabetic
- USG/X-ray can diagnose

Treatment

- Antibiotics with anaerobes cover
- **Emergency cholecystectomy**

5.3 CHOLEDOCHOLITHIASIS

- Gall stones risk factors
  Cholesterol stones
- Demography
  - Northern Europeans
  - North and South Americans
- Increasing age
- Female sex hormones
  - OCP
  - Pregnancy

- Obesity
- Rapid weight reduction
- GB stasis
- Hyperlipidemia
  Pigment stones
- Demography: Asians more common
- Hemolytic syndromes
- Biliary infection
- GIT disorders
  - Ileal disorders
  - Crohn's disease
  - Ileal resection
- Primary CBD stones
  - *De novo* in CBD
  - Usually brown
  - Mixture of bile pigments and cholesterol
  - More common in Asians
  - Associated with bacterial infection and bile stasis

Majority are Secondary

- From GB to CBD
- Seen in 6–12% of patients with GB calculi
- Mainly cholesterol stones
  Primary stones—causes
  - Defective pathophysiology of biliary tree—stasis, dyskinesia
  - Congenital—Caroli's disease, choledochal cyst
  - Infections—clonorchis, ascariasis
  - Others—low protein diet, obesity, females, old age

Risk for CBD Stones

Very strong predictors
- CBD stones seen in US
- Clinical ascending cholangitis
- Bilirubin >4 mg/dl

Strong predictors
- CBD >6 mm
- Bilirubin 1.8 to 4 mg/dl

Moderate factors
- Abnormal LFT
- Age >55
- Clinical gall stone pancreatitis
- High risk—presence of any very strong or both strong predictors
- No predictors—low risk
- All others—intermediate risk

- Retained CBD stones, CBD stones are seen within 2 years after cholecystectomy. Seen in 1 to 2% after cholecystectomy
- Recurrent stones—detected after 2 years of cholecystectomy—20% after second exploration—increases further, after subsequent surgeries
- Retained stones if detected within 4 to 6 weeks, and with no symptoms—observation—10 to 20% pass spontaneously
- After 4–6 weeks—T tube tract extraction
- If no T tube in position—endoscopic sphincterotomy—choice
  - If it fails—reoperation

Clinical Features

- Many are silent
- 1–2% present with retained stones
- Range from biliary colic to obstructive jaundice
- Painful jaundice due to rapid distension of CBD
- Fever, RUQ pain, jaundice—**Charcot's triad**
- Also associated with shock and mental changes—Reynold's pentad

Cholangitis

- Most predictive presentation
- Due to obstruction to bile flow and ascending infection
- Normal bile—sterile

Diagnosis

- LFT
- Conjugated hyperbilirubinemia
- Raised ALP
- Leucocytosis
- USG
  - Stone
  - Biliary dilatation
  - Patients with biliary pain, gallstones, jaundice—dilated duct (>8 mm)—suggestive of choledocholithiasis even without demonstrating stones

ERCP

- Diagnostic and therapeutic
- Sphincterotomy balloon sweep
  Indications
  - Cholangitis,
  - Biliary pancreatitis,
  - Limited surgeon experience with CBD exploration

MRCP

- Preop modality of choice
- >90% sensitive, almost 100% specific
- **Noninvasive**

- Not therapeutic
- A clear MRCP avoids ERCP
- MRCP with lap CBD exploration
- May miss stones <5 mm for this EUS better

PTC
- Invasive
- More effective in dilated biliary tree

EUS
Treatment
- **ERCP**
  - Sphincterotomy, stone extraction
  - If done preoperatively—can avoid open procedure
  - Followed by cholecystectomy
- **Failure of ERCP extraction**
  - Large stones
  - Intrahepatic stones
  - Multiple stones
  - Altered gastric or duodenal anatomy
  - Impacted stones
  - Duodenal diverticula
- Endoscopic balloon dilatation—may result in more pancreatitis
- Indicated in coagulopathy

Lap CBD Exploration
- Intraop cholangiogram to identify stones
- Access using small cholangioscope
- Cystic duct approach using—Segura basket
- Separate CBD incision approach

Contraindications for Trans Cystic Duct Approach
- CHD stones
- Small friable cystic duct
- Multiple (>8) stones
- Large (>1 cm) stone
- Intraop cholangiogram—via cystic duct—water-soluble contrast diluted 1:1 with saline, 5–10 ml with fluoroscopy
- Another method—lap US
- After cystic duct approach of extracting stones, after dilatation. CD is ligated rather than clipping
- Trans cystic balloon dilatation of sphincter of Oddi is avoided in previous pancreatitis, SOD dysfunction
- Trans cystic duct antegrade sphincterotomy
- C tube—cystic duct tube—instead of T tube for drainage postexploration

- In patients with CBD stones after Roux-Y GJ—lap CBD exploration the choice

Sphincterotomy and Sphincteroplasty
- **Choledochotomy**—a catheter or dilator is passed as a guide, generous kocherisation—longitudinal anterior duodenotomy at the level of ampulla—dilator used to guide—ampulla incised antero superiorly—opposite pancreatic duct orifice for 1 cm
- For sphincteroplasty—ampulla and distal CBD divided anteromedially for 1.5 to 2 cm—followed by suture approximation of duodenal and bile duct mucosa
- Sphincteroplasty—in
  - Failed endoscopic sphincterotomy
  - Pancreatitis where drainage of duct of Wirsung is indicated
- **Contraindicated** if
  - CBD >2 cm dilatation and long stricture
  - Duodenal diverticulum
  - Ampullary inflammation
  - Previous Billroth 2 surgery

Subtotal Lower Sphincteroplasty
- Small duodenotomy at D2
- Sphincters of CBD and duct of Wirsung not involved
- Cut is made at 11 o' clock: Can use a Nelaton catheter introduced through cystc duct as a guide. Never use metal instruments—false tracking
- Laterally 10–12 mm long
- Sutures placed between duodenum and CD only laterally—no medial sutures for fear of involving duct of Wirsung
- No need for CBD opening or T tube

Open CBD Exploration
- Indicated when endoscopic or laparoscopic approaches are not feasible or when concomitant drainage procedure is required. Followed by T tube drainage
- Impacted stone in non-dilated biliary tree
  - Transduodenal sphincteroplasty
- **Impacted stone with dilated biliary tree**

Choledochoduodenostomy
- Allows future endoscopic access
- But can cause sump syndrome

Roux-en–Y Choledochojejunostomy
- No risk of sump syndrome
- Does not allow future endoscopic access

- **Intrahepatic stone with/without strictures**
  - Percutaneous drainage
  - Hepaticojejunostomy
- In biliary pancreatitis end to side choledochoduodenostomy is preferred over side to side—prevent stone impaction in future
- Role of T tube is not to prevent leak—but an avenue for removal of retained stones—14 F is the minimum size to use
- **Bilioenteric anastomosis—indications**
  - Stricture distal CBD
  - CBD >2 cm diameter
  - Multiple or primary BD stones
  - Inability to remove all stones
  - Third operation (in second—not mandatory)

- Low risk group—straight away laparoscopic cholecystectomy—with or without IOC (intra operative cholangiogram)—CBD exploration not necessary
- High risk with cholangitis and pancreatitis—preop ERCP
- Intermediate risk—no consensus—first laparoscopic cholecystectomy—IOC OR
- Preop MRCP/EUS

Retained CBD Stone—Management
- May pass spontaneously
- Flush T tube with heparin—saline
- Burhenne technique of nonoperative removal of retained stones
- ERCP after 3 weeks
- Reoperation
- ESWL
- PTC
- Lap choledocholithotomy
- Open choledocholithotomy with or without choledochojejunostomy

5.4 CHOLEDOCHAL CYST
Definition
- Isolated/focal or combined/diffuse congenital dilatation of extra or intrahepatic biliary tree
- Bile duct cyst or biliary cysts more appropriate term—involves whole biliary tree
- Rare
- Occurs in <1/100000 patients
- More in Asians (85%) and women
- Premalignant

- Usually diagnosed in infancy
- Rarely in adults

Pathogenesis
- **Anomalous Pancreatico Biliary Junction (APBJ)—** Babbit
  - PD and BD duct fuse to form a common channel before duodenal wall
  - Pancreatic juice reflux into BD
- PD has higher secretory pressures which can cause inflammation in BD and damage—cystic dilatation
- Anomalous pb junction
  - Associated with type I and IV BD cysts
  - Not with types II and III or isolated intrahepatic Caroli
- Some anomaly—not associated with cysts

Other Pathogenetic Factors
- Family history—hereditary
- Oligoganglionosis—in the distal neck of the cysts
  - Reduction in the ganglion cells in the narrow portion of cyst wall—biliary equivalent of Hirschsprung disease

Choledochal Cyst Classification
- Todani modification of Alonso Lej Classification

Type	Finding	Type	Finding
i	Solitary fusiform extrahepatic cyst	iv a	Fusiform extra and intrahepatic cysts
ii	Extrahepatic supraduodenal diverticulum	iv b	Multiple extra-hepatic cysts
iii	Intraduodenal diverticulum choledochocele	v	Multiple intra-hepatic cysts, Caroli disease

- Type Ia: GB arises from the cyst and extrahepatic biliary tree dilated
- Type Ib: Dilatation of the most distal part of CBD and rest of biliary tree normal
- Type Ic: Smooth fusiform dilatation of CHD and CBD along with pancreatobiliary malunion

- Type Id: Dilatation of cystic duct in addition to dilated CHD and CBD—bicornual configuration of cyst
- Type VI: Isolated dilatation of cystic duct alone without CHD or CBD involvement—very rare only a few cases

Caroli disease with congenital hepatic fibrosis is known as Grumbach disease

- Frequency of bile duct cysts
  - Type I—79%
  - Type IV—13%
  - Type III—4%
  - Type II—2.6%
  - Caroli without extrahepatic component—1%
  - Distribution same in adults and children
  - Except type IV which is more common in adults

Presentation

- Asymptomatic
- Jaundice, RUQ pain, palpable mass, classic—in< 20%
- Most patients have 2 of 3—in 85%
- Jaundice most consistent
- Nausea, pruritus, weight loss
- Long standing—liver injury—cirrhosis (type I and IV—15%)
- Cholangitis, pancreatitis, hepatic fibrosis, malignancy
- Rarely rupture—peritonitis
- Pancreatitis—in 30%
- Cholangitis—the most common initial symptom complex in adults
- Type 3—sometimes incidental on ERCP—also present with pancreatitis
  - Biliary symptoms less common
- Type IV b—'string of beads'
- Matsumoto classification—on configuration of cysts—but management based on location of cysts

Diagnosis

- USG
- CT
- MRCP
- ERCP—for distal BD cysts
- Lab
  - Shows obstructive jaundice
  - Cirrhosis

Criteria for Abnormal PBJ

- PD and CBD connect with long common channel >15 mm
- Ducts unite in anomalous form
- **USG**—absence of septations differentiate from cystic neoplasms—cystadenoma
  - Not useful in choledochocele
- **CT** with IV cholangiography—to demonstrate cyst communication with biliary tract
  - IV cholangiography done 2 hours before
  - CT—can detect accumulation of contrast in cyst.
- **ERCP—procedure of choice in type III—potentially therapeutic**
  - Can assess pb junction
- Scopy—to evaluate inside the cyst
- SpyGlass cholangioscopy—useful adjunct
- PTC—in previous Roux-Y, stricture
  - Cannot visualize pb junction
- **MRCP**
  - Gold standard
  - Initial test of choice
  - Limitation—inability to detect small choledochocele for this ERCP is the choice
  - Also less accurate to detect pb junction

Caroli Disease

- Cholangiography—multiple saccular appearance of IHBR
- CT liver—tiny dots with strong contrast enhancement within dilated IHBR—*Central dot sign*—corresponds to intraluminal portal radicles surrounded by IHBRD

Associated Hepatobiliary Pathology

- Cystolithiasis—most frequent accompanying condition
- Associated with thick bile—form cyst casts
- Soft, earthy, pigmented—bilirubinate
- CBD stone—most common
- Hepatolithiasis—usually in type IV
- GB disease—cholecystitis
- Pancreatitis in 2–70%
- Common channel syndrome or pseudopancreatitis—mimic AP
  - Multifactorial
  - Obstruction of pancreatic duct by stone
  - Bile reflux
- Intrahepatic abscess—result from recurrent cholangitis—more common in left intrahepatic ducts—related to angulation of left main duct

- Portal hypertension—secondary to cirrhosis, PV thrombosis

Bile Duct Cysts and Malignancy

- True incidence not known (10–30%)
- Most common—cholangiocarcinoma—70%
- GB carcinoma—next common
- Others—adenoacanthoma, SCC, anaplastic ca, pancreatic ca
- Age related—increases with age
- Only 57% of tumors are intracystic
- Malignancy may occur after cyst excision
- Greater prevalence in type I (7.6%) and IV (9.2%)
- Type II (4.3%), type III (4%), type V (2.5%)
- **Etiology**
  - K-ras and p53 mutations seen in >60%
  - Bile stagnation—development of intrabiliary carcinogens—epithelial malignant degeneration—most likely mechanism
  - Unconjugated deoxycholate and lithocholate
  - Field defect

Even complete excision of cyst does not eliminate cancer risk

- **Surgical**
  - Resection of entire cyst and reconstruction
  - In asymptomatic children—at age 3–6 months
  - Symptomatic neonates as soon as possible
  - External drainage—no role

Treatment

- **Type 1**
  - Complete excision, cholecystectomy and Roux-en-Y hepaticojejunostomy
  - Excision and hepaticoduodenostomy
  - Roux-Y choledochocystojejunostomy/duodenostomy
  - Proximal extent may be right or left HD
  - If there is substantial dilatation, epithelium is excised leaving outer fibrotic wall: Lilly's operation
  - Hepaticoduodenostomy—associated with increased gastric and biliary cancer—can access biliary tree endoscopically
  - Hepaticojejunostomy—stricture and recurrent cholangitis in 10 to 25%

- Total removal of intracystic epithelium—a must in adults—fear of cancer

- **Type 2**
  - Complete excision
    - If APBJ—hepaticojejunostomy
  - Diverticulum—commonest in upper one-third—58%
  - Similar to cholecystectomy

Neck can be closed primarily

Or via T tube

- **Type 3**
  - Uncommon
  - Approached—transduodenal sphincteroplasty
  - Endoscopic sphincterotomy and drainage is the choice
  - If duodenal/biliary obstruction—transduodenal excision or sphincteroplasty

- **Type 4a**
  - Extrahepatic component
    - Excision, Roux-en-Y hepaticojejunostomy
    - Excision, hepaticoduodenostomy
  - Intrahepatic component
    - Hepatic resection +/– Roux-en-Y hepaticojejunostomy
    - Transhepatic intubation

- **Type 4b**—similar to Type 1: Excision and HJ or hepaticoduodenostomy
  - Transduodenal sphinteroplasty may be done
  - Intrahepatic—one lobe—partial hepatectomy and reconstruction
  - Liver transplantation

- **Type 5—Caroli's**
  - Hepatic resection
  - Roux-Y intrahepatic cholangiojejunostomy
  - Transhepatic intubation
  - Liver transplantation, if diffuse
  - Can develop cirrhosis, PHT, liver failure—liver transplantation best option

- **GB Dyskinesia**
  - Aka—chronic acalculous cholecystitis, functional GB disorder
  - Symptoms of calculus biliary disease with no stone sonologically
  - Associated with IBS, colonic inertia, and gastroparesis
  - Alterations in composition of bile and inflammatory mediators implicated
  - Investigations: CCK stimulated HIDA Scan-ejection fraction less than 1/3rd at 20 mins past CCK administration
  - Treatment-cholecystectomy

Sphincter of Oddi Dysfunction

- Aka—papillary stenosis, ampullary stenosis, post-cholecystectomy syndrome
- A disorder of the contractile function of ampullary sphincter
  - Biliary tract pain with normal LFT and recurrent pancreatitis
  - May be secondarily due to pancreatitis, gall stones, congenital abnormalities
  - Post-cholecystectomy interruption of cholecysto-sphincteric reflex
  - CCK inhibits ampullary sphincter
  - Secretin inhibits pancreatic portion of Sphincter of Oddi
    - **Diagnosis**
- Nardi test—morphine, prostigmine provocation test—evaluation of pain or elevated liver or pancreatic enzymes
- Nuclear medicine biliary transit time studies
- Rome IV diagnostic criteria
- ERCP-based manometry
  - CBD dilated: >12 mm
  - Pancreatic duct dilated
  - CBD diameter increased following CCK administration.
  - Diagnosis: Manometry (if sphincter pressure >40 mm Hg)

Milwaukee classification	
Type	Criteria
I	Pancreaticobiliary pain + Raised liver/pancreatic biochemistries + Dilated bile/pancreatic duct + Delayed contrast drainage (ERCP)
II	Pancreaticobiliary pain + Raised liver/pancreatic biochemistries **or** Dilated bile or pancreatic duct **or** Delayed contrast drainage (ERCP)
III	Pancreaticobiliary pain **only**

Treatment

- **Medical**
  - Smooth muscle relaxants like Nifedipine, phosphodiesterase inhibitors, trimebutine, hyoscine, NO
  - In type I and II—endoscopic sphincterotomy,
  - Type III: ES not useful
  - Surgical transduodenal sphinterotomy/sphincteroplasty—in failed endoscopic treatment and in previous gastrectomy

Cholecytosis

- Chronic inflammatory changes with hyperplasia of all tissue elements
- Cholesterosis
  - Strawberry gall bladder
  - Submucus aggregation of cholesterol crystal and esters
  - Associated with cholesterol stones
- Cholecystitis glandularis proliferans
  - Aka polypadenomyometosis and intramural diverticulosis
    - All layers of GB thickened
    - Incomplete septum
    - Intraparietal mixed calculi may be seen
    - Treatment—cholecystectomy

5.5 BILE DUCT INJURY

- 80% iatrogenic bile duct injury occurs during cholecystectomy
- Factors associated
- Obesity, anatomy, excessive traction of fundus, bleeding
- Intraoperative cholangiogram minimises injury, experience of surgeon
- **Vasculobiliary injury**
  - Most common artery injured—RHA—can result in higher biliary strictures

– Excessive dissection—injury to 3 and 9 o' clock arteries

– Excessive fibrotic reaction

– BD injury—inflammation—fibrosis—stricture

Strasberg Classification

• A: Leak from cystic duct stump or a minor biliary radical in GB fossa

• B: Occluded R posterior sectoral duct

• C: Leak from divided R posterior sectoral duct

• D: Leak from the main bile duct

• E1: Transacted main bile duct with stricture >2 cm

• E2: Transacted main bile duct with stricture <2 cm

• E3: Strictuire of hilus but communication between hilus present

• E4: Stricture of hilus with separation of R&L hepatic duct.

• E5: Stricture of main bile duct and R posterior sectoral branch

• E6: Complete excursion of extrahepatic duct involving the confluence

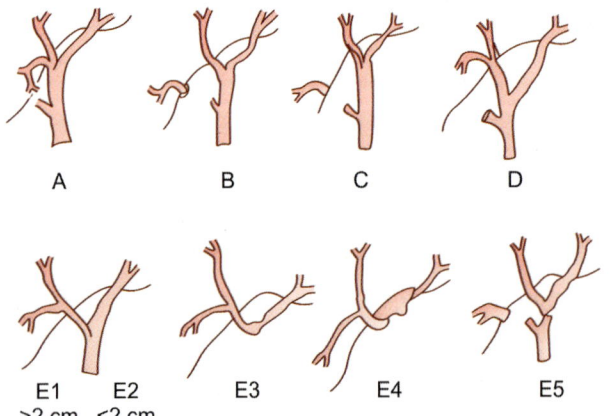

• **Hannover system**

– Another classification system of bile duct injury

– Divided into A, B, C, D, E

Bismuth Classification

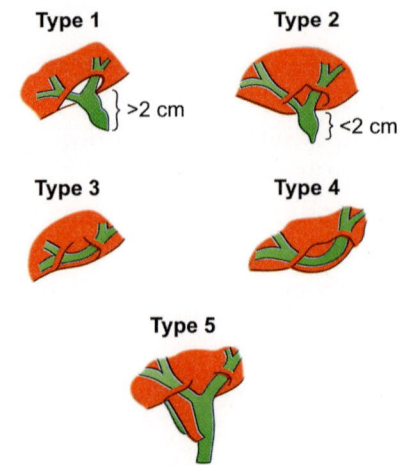

Type 1	Low CHD stricture, stump >2 cm
Type 2	Middle stricture, CHD <2 cm
Type 3	Hilar stricture, no remaining CHD
Type 4	Hilar stricture, confluence involved, loss of communication between RHD and LFD
Type 5	Combined CHD and aberrant RHD injury, separating from distal CBD

• About 15% of bile duct injuries are recognised during surgery

• After open cholecystectomy, the stricture—10% recognised within first week, 70% in 6 months and 80% in 1 year

• Laparoscopic cholecystectomy, 25–30% injury recognised in early post op or during surgery

• Most common bile leak following cholecystectomy is from cystic duct

• **Clinical presentation**

– Early—leak, elevated liver enzymes, bilirubin

– If presents late—most common—cholangitis and then jaundice

Diagnosis

• USG/CT—can detect site of injury, bile duct dilatation and collections

• Gold standard—cholangiography

• PTC is preferred—can assess the proximal ducts, and can drain the bile

- ERCP—less useful in stricture and complete transection. But useful in CD leak and partial injuries

- MRCP—is the Choice as first investigation

- **HIDA scan**

Management

- Recognise at time of surgery

- Convert to open in laparoscopic surgery

- Cholangiography helps in delineating and management

- **Recognised at surgery**—repair or damage control

- **Early postoperative period**—control sepsis and drain the collection—then no hurry to reoperate—proximal biliary decompression and external drainage. The patient can be discharged and allow the inflammation to subside

  - Consider stenting/sphincterotomy

- Early recognition of Strasberg A and D—endoscopic sphincterotomy and stenting

- Presenting late with cholangitis—antibiotics and drainage—PTC better. ERCP also can be done.

- Presenting with jaundice without cholangitis—delineate anatomy with cholangiogram and consider definitive management—early drainage not useful

- In late repair—Left duct can be used for drainage after lowering the hepatic plate—Hepp-Couinaude procedure

- The proximal bile duct is mobilised up to 5 mm—more can produce ischemia

- Goals

  1. <3 mm duct which drains only a single segment or subsegment of liver–simple ligation of duct

  2. Injury to duct >3 mm diameter which drain more than 1 liver segment—reimplant/repair

  3. Injury to larger duct involving less than 50% of wall circumference and not caused by electrocautery—'T' tube is placed

  4. Larger duct >50% circumference or cautery induced injury—resection of injured segment and bilioenteric anastomosis

4a. If defect is <1 cm, not near hepatic duct bifurcation of CBD/CHD—mobilisation and end to end anastamosis with T tube through a separate incision

4b. Injury near bifurcation and >1 cm between ends—Roux-en-Y hepaticojejunostomy reconstruction/choledochoduodenostomy (chance of sump syndrome) with silastic stent

  - If done by an inexperienced surgeon—in complete transection—put a retrograde catheter, abort cholecystectomy and put drain to subhepatic region and refer the case to experts

  - In late repair, HJ is preferred—preop placed PTC catheters can be used as stent

- Goal of treatment of injury recognised after cholecystectomy

  - Control of infection

  - Clear and thorough anastomotic delineation with cholangiography

  - Initial conservative management later to re-establish durable biliary enteric drainage.

- **Interventional radiologic and endoscopic technique**

  - Percutaneous balloon dilation—in a failed bilio-enteric anastomosis

  - Endoscopic dilatation—in primary strictures or with prior repairs or with prior choledocho-duodenal anastomosis

    □ 80% success rate

    □ Done in patient with primary biliary tree stricture and choledochoduodenostomy, not in choledochojejunostomy

- Prevention of bile duct injury can be achieved by adhering to critical view of safety during laparoscopic cholecystectomy

- **Identify structures**

- Lost stones

  - 20–40% cholecystectomies

  - Risk factors

    □ Cholecystitis

    □ Multiple stones (>15)

    □ Inexperienced surgeon

    □ Pigmented stones

– Consequences

  □ Chronic abscess, fistula, wound infection, bowel obstruction

– Management

  □ Conversion to open is not needed.

  □ Extensive irrigation

  □ Documentation of lost stone in surgery notes

• Postcholecystectomy pain due to

– Choledocholithiasis

– Bile leak

– Sphincter of Oddi dysfunction

– Bile duct strictures

– Retained biliary stones

Acute Cholangitis

• **Three factors**—obstruction, colonisation by organisms, elevation of ductal pressure

– Most common pathogens: Klebsiella, *E coli*, enterobacter, pseudomonas, citrobacter

– Clinical feature: Charcots triad: Fever, jaundice, RUQ pain—seen in 50% patients—jaundice is the most common variable

– Raynaud's pentad: Charcots + hypotension and altered sensorium

– **Investigation**s: TC, ALP, OT/PT, bilirubin raised

– USG: Biliary tree dilatation

– CT: Sites of obstruction can be found out

– ERCP/PTC: Not only diagnosis but also biliary drainage and specimen for culture and sensitivity and biopsy.

– Treatment: Medical therapy with antibiotics

  □ Emergency decompression of biliary tree

  □ Percutaneous approach

  □ ERCP

  □ Cholecystectomy done after patient is stabilised

5.6 RECURRENT PYOGENIC CHOLANGITIS

(Oriental cholangiohepatitis, Hong Kong disease, hepatolithiasis, primary cholangitis, oriental infestational cholangitis)

Etiology

• Initiating event—infection by enteric organisms

• Caused by cholangiohepatitis or intrahepatic stones

• Eastern population-low socioeconomic

• Associated with Clonorchis and Ascaris, these parasites form pigment stones (brown)

• Infection—begins in cholangioles—hepatocytes show vacuolisation—necrosis—may spread to larger ducts and CBD—repeated infection—fibrosis—liver abscess

• There may be multiple strictures, dilatations and stones

• Infection in bile duct—changes bile from supersaturated to insoluble precipitate

• Beta glucuronidase from *C. perfringens* and *E. coli*—splits bilirubin diglucuronide—into free bilirubin—bind with ionic calcium—insoluble calcium bilirubinate—stones

• Also increased secretion of mucin

• Small stones may pass

Pathology

• Strictures more common in left hepatic duct branches

• GB affected in 20%

• Stones are calcium bilirubinate—friable-conform to the shape of ducts

• In 10% no stones seen—only debris—biiary mud (composed of mucus, pus, desquamated epithelium, parasites, microcalculi—porridge like)

• Liver surface show atrophy of affected lobe and hypertrophy of other lobe

• Can develop biliary cirrhosis—PHT—liver failure

• CBD stone can cause pancreatitis

• Liver abscess may rupture

• May develop cholangiocarcinoma

Clinical Features

• Charcot's triad

• Liver enlarged in 60%

• Spleen enlarged in 25%

Investigations

- Bloods
- Leucocytosis, obstructive jaundice—mild
- USG: Stones—some stones are isoechoic
  - Pneumobilia—makes it difficult to simulate stones
  - CT
    - Can differentiate stones from pneumobilia
  - Combination of CT/MRCP + ERCP—lobar or segmental atrophy or hypertrophy may be seen
- Contrast from Caroli disease—RPC predominantly affect leftside of liver and has no evidence of ductal plate malformation
  - Bilirubinate stones and chronic proliferative cholangitis—not seen in uncomplicated Caroli disease

Management

- Acute attack
  - Antibiotics, IV fluids

Surgery

- Is indicated in sepsis and failure to improve
- CBD exploration and large T tube drainage
- Stones removed—strictures dilated
- Syringing CBD at high pressure may induce bacteremia and also in choledochoscopy of intrahepatic ducts. So both should not be done. But for lower end of CBD, these procedures can be done
- Cholecystectomy done if patient is stable
- Liver resection of left lateral segment—in multiple liver abscess in a destroyed left lateral segment

Non-surgical Management

- Endoscopic papillotomy and nasobiliary catheter
- Large bore endoprosthesis
- PTC drainage if intrahepatic disease
- If sepsis does not improve, reassess—surgery
- In acute attack—initial intervention of choice—ERCP drainage

Definitive Surgery

- Aim
  - Remove stones
  - Bypass—biliary drainage
  - Enlarge strictures
  - Biliary access
- Simple cases—depending on presence of intrahepatic strictures
- Cholecystectomy
- CBD exploration
- Choledochoscopy/hepaticojejunostomy

Complex Cases

- Hepaticocutaneous jejunostomy
- Stricturoplasty
- Partial hepatectomy

Biliary Tract

- CBD exploration—may have to extend to intrahepatic ducts
- CBD may become posterior to PV, in case of left lobe hypertrophy and right lobe atrophy
- Multiple intrahepatic calculi may be palpated—aproached by hepatotomy and removed
- May use forceps, Fogarty catheter
- Eletrohydrolic lithotriptor/Nd-YAG laser—to break stones
- Cholecystectomy done

Biliary Drainage Procedures

- Transduodenal sphinteroplasty
- CDD
- CDJ
- HJ—in stricture of intrapancreatic portion of CBD or dilated CBD with lost elasticity
- Segment III bypass

Hepaticocutaneous Jejunostomy

- When there are multiple strictures/stones present proximal to HJ—access loop through which choledochoscopic removal of stones achieved

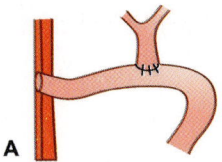 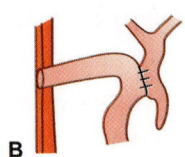

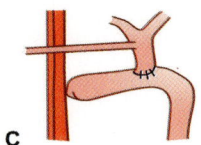 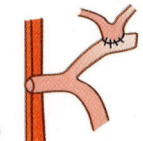

- – **A—standard hepaticojejunostomy**
- – **B—done when separation of CBD from PV is dangerous**
- – **C—when stoma is not required immediately**
- – **D—In previous CDJ**
- Post-op choledochoscopic removal of stones can be achieved by
  - – T tube tract
  - – Stoma
  - – PTBD tract
- Can fragment stones with lithotriptor
- ERCP with Mothe—baby endoscope system—can extract stones

Hepatic Resection
- **In multiple abscesses**
- Destroyed liver segments
- Concomitant cholangio ca
- Mostly left-lateral segmentectomy—sometimes left hepatectomy

Intrahepatic Strictures
- If liver preserved—dilatation—HCJ
- SEMS (self-expanding metallic stent) only when surgery is impossible
- If liver atrophic/multiple abscess—choice—hepatectomy

Liver Transplantation
- In biliary cirrhosis with PHT
- Hepatectomy difficult due to adhesions

- Anterior liver split after vascular control
- Piggy-bag technique

5.7 PRIMARY SCLEROSING CHOLANGITIS
- Idiopathic autoimmune disease affecting both intrahepatic and extrahepatic biliary system
- Associated with ulcerative colitis and Riedel's thyroiditis.
- Antibodies elevated are—pANCA (80%), antinuclear antibodies (53%), anticardiolipin antibodies (66%)
- Antiendothelial cell antibody (35%)
- Most elevated immunoglobulin (IgM) in 45%
  - – Least elevated IgA in 10%
- Anti-smooth muscle antibody and anti-mitochondrial antibodies: Rare
- Causes chronic cholestasis—biliary cirrhosis—liver failure
- 70% cases have associated IBD—less in the East
- Only 3–5% with IBD have associated PSC
- Etiopathogenesis
  - – **Cholangiocytes** upon injury—can release inflammatory mediators
  - – **PSC microbiota hypothesis**

Association with IBD

  - – **Expansion of leaky gut hypothesis**—compromised intestinal barrier—increased enterohepatic circulation of microbial molecules—aberrant response of cholangiocytes—fibrosis

- **Gut lymphocyte homing hypothesis**

  - – Intestinal T lymphocytes—the cell surface receptors alfa-4 beta-7 aberrantly represented in hepatocytes—inflammation—fibrosis

Clinical Features
- Most common symptom—pain abdomen
- May be detected accidentally or with IBD
- Jaundice, hepatomegaly, splenomegaly

Pathology
- Early liver normal later inflammation and cirrhosis
- Liver biopsy—4 stages

LUDWIG STAGING OF PSC

- I: Portal stage—edema, inflammation and ductal proliferation
- II: Periportal stage—periportal fibrosis
- III: Septal stage—septal fibrosis and bridging necrosis
- IV: Cirrhotic stage

- Small duct disease—in 5%—ERCP normal—detected biochemically and by biopsy
- **Diagnosis**
  - Cholestasis—biochemically
  - In some—ALP may be normal
  - **ERCP**—beading or chain of lake appearance due to multifocal diffusely distributed dilatation and stricture of both intrahepatic and extrahepatic biliary tree: Beaded and pruned appearence
- PTC is unsuccessful due to proximal disease
- Four types of PTC
  - Classic—both intrahepatic and extrahepatic strictures
  - Intrahepatic duct only
  - Extrahepatic duct only
  - Small duct
- Cholangiograpy—multiple diverticulum like outpouching of bile duct and multiple short segment stricture
- Mural irregularities
- **MRCP**—diffuse involvement
- **Liver biopsy**—onion skin concentric periductal fibrosis, with progress periportal fibrosis, bridging necrosis and biliary cirrhosis
  - Can differentiate PSC from secondary SC (due to trauma, cancer, IgG4 related)
- **Natural history**
  - Generally progress to end stage liver disease
  - Without LT—medial survival 12–15 years
  - Serum ALP normalisation—good prognostic factor
  - Small duct disease (5%)—better prognosis
- **Associated diseases**

Diseases associated with primary sclerosing cholangitis
Ulcerative colitis
Crohn's disease
Type 1 DM
Autoimmune hepatitis
Hypothyroidism/Riedel's thyroiditis
Sicca syndrome
Sarcoidosis
Celiac disease
Autoimmune hemolytic anemia
Glomerulonephritis

IBD

- Seen in 70% of PSC
- Diagnosis of IBD precedes PSC by 8–10 years—usually
- No direct correlation between the severity of IBD and PSC
- Presence of IBD and intact colon—predictors of post-LT recurrence
- PSC-IBD—more of pancolitis with rectal sparing and backwash ileitis
- PSC—not associated with small bowel only: Crohn's disease
- Colitis is usually milder than usual
- But has a 5 fold increased risk for CRC than IBD alone
- UDCA—has chemopreventive role in CRC
- More chance of pouchitis

Complications
- **Gallbladder**
  - Cholelithiasis—in 30%
  - Choledocholithiasis—in 8%
  - Acalculous cholecystitis
  - Polyps and Ca GB
- **Dominant stricture**
  - Stenosis with diameter <1.5 mm in CBD or <1 mm in hepatic ducts

Malignant Complications
- PSC is premalignant
- Cholangiocarcinoma annual incidence of 1% and lifetime occurrence—15%
- Hilar cholangiocarcinoma
  - In PSC—10–15% chance
  - Detected early due to frequent evaluation
  - Due to multifocality and underlying liver disease
  - No relation to duration of PSC

Resection is not choice, better liver transplant after neo-adjuvant chemo

- CA 19–9 is the primary marker
- Hilar stricture evaluated by brush cytology and FISH
- Percutaneous, EUS guided and trans peritoneal biopsy—not done if transplant is being considered

Other Malignancies

- Intrahepatic cholangiocarcinoma
- HCC
- GB malignancy—due to field defect in 3–14%

Pruritus

- Due to
  - Circulating bile salts
  - Opioidergic neurotransmission
  - Increased activity of autotoxin-serum lysophospholipase and its metabolite-lysophosphatidic acid

Treatment

- Cholesteramine, rifampicin, naltrexone, sertaline
- Antihistamines, gabapentine, ondansetrone
- Extracorporial albumin dialysis, plasmapheresis
- Liver transplant
- Treatment of PSC
  - Pharmacotherapy
- UDCA improves LFT
  - Vit k, cholestyramine, colchicine, immuno-suppressant
  - Tacrolimus, mofetil, vancomycin

Surgical Therapy

- Percut/endoscopic dilatation of strictures
  - Main treatment option is biliary reconstruction and liver transplant
  - PSC with CCA (cholangiocarcinoma)—resection is not an option
    - CCA is multifocal
    - Low hepatic reserve
- Recurrent/concurrent disease results in death in 90%
- Liver transplantation
  - Orthotopic liver transplant 5-year survival (75–85%)—more chance of biliary strictures
    - Due to immunosuppressants and UC—more chance of Colorectal cancers—however, role of prophylactic colectomy is debatable

- Optimal treatment in PSC in endstage disease
- In stage I and II Hilar CCA

In PSC associated ulcerative colitis, proctocolectomy will not affect biliary disease progression.

5.9 MIRIZZI SYNDROME (FUNCTIONAL HEPATIC SYNDROME)

- An inflammatory process involving gall bladder and cystic duct can secondly inflame the CBD causing obstruction.
- Alternatively a large stone in Hartmann pouch can compress adjacent bile duct and cause an apparent stricture
- Prerequisites of Mirizzi
  - A cystic duct runs parallel to CHD
  - An impacted stone in GB neck or cystic duct
  - Obstruction of CHD caused by stones or inflammatory process
- Hallmark of this disease—obstruction of bile duct from an inflammatory process

Types: Csendes classification

- Type I—stone in infundibulum/CD compress CHD
- Type II—stone from GB or CD erode into CHD causing cholecystocholedochal fistula <one-third of circumference
- Type III—involves two-thirds
- Type IV—fistula with complete bile duct destruction
- Type V—cholecystoenteric fistula with or without gallstone ileus, co-existing with any of the other types

Clinical Features

- Like cholecystitis
- Elevated bilirubin and ALP

Diagnosis

- USG
- PTC/ERCP
- MRCP

Treatment

- cholecystectomy—open method gold standard
- Partial cholecystectomy
- Mirizzi I—near total cholecystectomy—leave CBD stent *in situ*
  - Type II—choledochotomy—stone removal—closure of GB or CCD/CCJ
  - In fistula—reconstruction of BD

Cholecystoenteric Fistula

Most common bilioenteric fistula—cholecysto-enteric

- Of these GB to duodenum—55 to 75%

- 15–30%—GB to colon

  – 2–5%—GB to stomach

- Most common cause gall stones. Rarely peptic ulcer

- GB to duodenum or transverse colon fistula formation result in relief of symptoms

- More in women 6–7 decades

- Association with Mirizzi and GB cancer

- Can cause cholangitis and pneumobilia

- 10–15%—Gall stone causes small intestine obstruction—gall stone ileus

In GB: Colon Fistula

- Chronic diarrhea is the most common presentation

  – Cholangitis

  – Cholerectic enteropathy—due to altered enterohepatic circulation—increased bile acids in colon—diarrhea

    □ More fat in colon—fatty diarrhea

    □ **Triad—pneumobilia, chronic diarrhea, vitamin K malabsorption**

    □ **Diagnosis—by barium enema**

    □ **Next—ERCP**

    □ Treatment—surgery—dismantle fistula, cholecystectomy, CBD exploration

- **Proximal choledocho-duodenal fistula—**

  – Most common cause peptic ulcer disease. Then stones, trauma, diverticula, cancers, Crohn's disease

  – Mostly treated conservatively with anti-*H. pylori*

  – If refractory—vagotomy/drainage or duodenal bypass

  – No need to close the fistula

- **Distal choledochoduodenal fistula**

  – Distal 2 cm of CBD

  – Diagnosed by PTC/ERCP

  – Due to stones/operative trauma

Parapapillary Fistulae

- Type I—small opening on the longitudinal fold of duodenum proximal to papilla, due to penetration of small stone through intramural portion of CBD

- Type II—larger opening, large stone eroding extramural portion of CBD

GALL STONE ILEUS

- Most common in terminal ileum—in 70%

- May be in jejunum

- Duodenal obstruction in the bulb—known as *Bouveret syndrome*—in 10%

- Its mechanical block not ileus

- Stone in dependent area of GB fistulised into duodenum passes into ileum and cause obstruction

- 40% may have CBD stones

- Most common in old age

- Features of obstruction

- X-ray: Air fluid level—change in level of obstruction and position of stones called **tumbling obstruction** (only 30% of stones are radio-opaque)

- **Triad-SI obstruction, pneumobilia, ectopic gall stone**

- Barium meal series—seen in 40% in CCD fistula

- ERCP/PTC

- HIDA scan

- USG

- CT/MRI: Pneumobilia—seen in 30–50% only—due to cystic duct obstruction preventing air into CBD

Treatment

- Cholecystectomy is done in young and fit patients in same sitting

- Cholecystectomy, repair fistula, look for Mirizzi

  – Gall stone ileus—enterotomy—stone removal—look for multiple sites for stones—cholecystectomy and fistula repair in the same sitting or later

- Duodenal and high jejunal impaction stone removal can be done by endoscopy and lithotripsy

5.10 BENIGN TUMORS OF BILE DUCT

- Benign bile duct tumors reported in 0.1% of bile duct surgery
- Constitute 6% of all extrahepatic BD neoplasms
- Present with cholecystitis or obstructive jaundice
- Preop biopsy in operable lesions—not indicated

Benign lesions causing bile duct obstruction
Epithelial tumors
Adenoma
Papilloma
Cystadenoma (intrahepatic)
Nonepithelial tumors
Leiomyoma
Lipoma
Hemangioma
Lymphangioma
Granular cell tumor
Osteoma
Neural tumors
Neurofibroma
Schwannoma
Neuroendocrine tumors
Pseudotumors
Idiopathic benign focal stricture
Sclerosing cholangitis
Lymphoplasmacytic sclerosing pancreatitis
Heterotopic tissue

- **Clinical presentation**
  - Jaundice—most common
  - No weight loss
- **Preop diagnosis very difficult**
  - MRCP, ERCP, PTC, EUS, KRAS

Papilloma and Adenoma

- The most common benign tumour—two-thirds of benign
- Most common site–near ampulla or close to vaterian system (47%)
  - Next—CBD—27%
- More in females
- Premalignant

Treatment

- Surgical resection choice—with a portion of duct wall

Multiple Biliary Papillamatosis (Intraductal Papillary Neoplasm of Bile Duct (IPNB))

- **Similar to IPMN**
- Follow multistep pattern and develop cholangio-carcinoma
- Show mucin production and malignant potential
- Jaundice
- ERCP—show open papilla with mucin drainage, filling **defects**
- May be intrahepatic and extrahepatic
- Treatment—during surgery—choledochotomy—scopy—to remove all lesions
  - If confined to one lobe of liver—resection
  - If extensive both lobes involvement—hepatico-jejunostomy with access jejunal loop—multiple scopy—laser ablation
  - Chemotherapy
  - Liver transplant

Granular Cell Tumour (Granular Cell Myoblastoma)

- Most common sites—tongue, breast, subcutaneous
- <1% in bile duct
- In biliary system—most common sites—CBD, CD, GB
  - Ampulla—very rare
- More in females, blacks
- Preop diagnosis—difficult—small lesions may be palpated on surgery
- Arise from Schwann cells—S-100 positive
- Treatment—excision with local BD

NET

- Only endocrine cell in extrahepatic ducts: D cells
- Most common—carcinoid, gastrinoma, somatostatinoma
- **Leiomyoma** of BD—one of the least common
- **Heterotopic tissue** in BD—most common—gastric

5.11 TUMORS OF GB

GB polyps

- Benign masses in gall bladder consist of
- Adenoma—5% of polyps
  - Pseudotumor
    - *Cholesterol polyp—most common—60% of polyps*
    - Adenomyomatosis—25% of polyps
- Cholesterol polyp
  - Appears pedunculated, echogenic lesion <1 cm
  - Usually multiple
- Adenomyomatosis
  - Sessile
  - Usually in fundus, >1 cm

– Characteristic microcysts within the lesion

– In USG: Comet tail artefact seen

• **Adenoma**

– Difficult to differentiate from adenocarcinoma

– Risk factors for malignant disease

  □ Size >1 cm

  □ Age >60 years (50)

  □ Presence of gall stones

  □ Sessile

  □ Single polyp (risk increases with polyp size and reduces with number)

  □ Polyps <1 cm regardless of number—risk of malignancy is very low, except in PSC >0.8 cm resected

Treatment

• <1 cm and asymptomatic—observed—followed up with USG, 6–12 monthly

• >1 cm polyp with no suspicion of malignancy— lap chole—frozen section—low threshold to convert—simple cholecystectomy is curative for T1a lesions

• GB cancer is found in 0.2 to 2% of lap chole

• If found by frozen—liver resection with LN dissection

• For T1a—simple cholecystectomy is enough

• Lesions >T1b—re-resection with liver resection and/or BD resection—if CD stump is involved

  – If risk factors for malignancy present—open cholecystectomy is done to avoid spillage

5.12 CARCINOMA GALL BLADDER

• Ca GB—most common biliary tract malignancy

• Rare and aggressive

• Extremely poor prognosis

• Highest incidence in: Chile, India, Pakistan

• Female > male, 6–7th decade

• Etiology

  – Chronic inflammation and subsequent cellular proliferation

  – GB stone is a primary risk factor (>3 cm)

  – 90% of Ca GB contain stones, incidence of Ca GB in population with calculi—0.3% to 3%—causal

relationship. No malignant risk with pigmented stones

– ABPJ

– Choledochal cyst

– GB polyp (>10 mm)

– Porcelain gall bladder (10% risk)—stippled calcification of mucosa—more risk than diffuse

– Typhoid carrier

– Drugs: Methyldopa, INH, OCP, rubber industry

– PSC

  □ Adenoma—carcinoma sequence

• Pathology

– 90% adenocarcinoma

Others

Squamous carcinoma, melanoma, sarcoma, carcinoid also seen

• Gall bladder cancer usually present late (35%) will already be having liver and lymph node metastasis

• 1% cholecystectomy specimens contain adenomatous polyps

• Risk of Ca GB in cholesterol, hyperplastic and inflammatory polyps—near zero

• Grouped into metaplastic and nonmetaplastic

• Predominant metaplasia—which turn malignant are pseudopyloric and intestinal

Spread

• Invade and metastasise early due to thin wall, narrow lamina propria and single layer muscular layer and no serosa in liver bed

• Lymphatics from GB will not ascend to porta. They follow cystic LN-pericholedochal—retroportal— posterosuperior pancreaticoduodenal—celiac— SMA—interaortocaval. Some directly to interaorto-caval nodes

• The draining nodal basis of gall bladder include hepatoduodenal ligament—paraaortic, pancreati-coduodenal nodes

• Spread directly to segment 4 of liver as gall bladder get direct venous tributaries from liver parenchyma to portal system

• Transperitoneal spread causes carcinomatosis

Gross

- 60% from fundus
- 30% from body
- 10% from neck
- 3 patterns
  - Infiltrative
  - Nodular
  - Papillary—better prognosis—show minimal invasion

Genetics

- Earliest events—mutation of p53 and aberrant gene promoter hypermethylation—ultimately KRAS
- To differentiate cholecystitis from Ca GB—two polymorphisms—CA242 and CA125
- Stage of the disease: Most important prognostic factor (not grade and type)

TNM staging is given in Chapter 15.

Other Staging Systems

- Modified Nevin
- Japanese

Clinical features:

- 90% of the disease start in fundus so symptoms are late
- Most common—pain abdomen
  - Jaundice
  - Weight loss, anaemia
  - Palpable mass

Diagnosis

- USG: Irregular shaped subhepatic lesion, heterogenous mass in GB lumen, asymmetrically thickened GB wall
- CT: For staging and extra gall bladder spread, triphasic CT to diagnose portal, hepatic, arterial involvement.
- Cholangiography: To assess level of obstruction
- Biopsy via percutaneous method, if lesion is operable biopsy not adviced
- CEA— >4 ng/ml

- CA 19-9 elevated in 8%—>20 U/ml
- PET scan

Most are PET Avid

Helpful to detect metastasis than CT

Not helpful to differentiate benign from malignant

- Diagnostic laparoscopy

Treatment

- Operable lesion—not to look for histological diagnosis—for fear of dissemination

Ca GB: Extent of Resection

- T1a—simple cholecystectomy
- T1b—liver resection and LN dissection advised—negative CD margin should be achieved—if not, bile duct resection should be considered
- T2, T3—complete resection of tumour enbloc with segments IVb and V. Bile duct resection if bile duct margin is positive. If involves hepatic vascular structures—extended right hepatectomy—only if no metastasis
- LN dissection of hepatoduodenal ligament also done
- If distal LN (celiac or retropancreatic)—or metastasis found—major resections abandoned

  Liver resection

  - Ideal segment IVb and V resection
  - If intraop, USG is done—can wedge resect liver with 1–2 cm margin
  - Extended right hepatectomy, if margin positive (can consider pre-op chemo)
  - If patient comes back after non-curative chole—segment IV, V resection done
  - Current practice—liver resection done to achieve tumor clearance

LN Dissection

- >T1b lesions: N1 node dissection done (LN on porta hepatitis, gastrohepatic ligament, retroduodenl space). If retropancreatic and aortic nodes positive, N2 resection abandoned
- Adequate LN dissection, if >3 nodes removed
- Bile duct resection only done for negative margin—not for LN dissection
- Extended cholecystectomy—dissection—in T1b lesions, T2
- T1b—extended cholecystectomy

- T2—extended cholecystectomy with liver resection
- T3, T4—vascular resections, extensive LN dissection, extended hepatectomy—poor prognosis

Adjuvant Therapy
- Gemcitabine with platinum agents
- GEMOX (Gemcitabine and Oxaliplatin)
- Ertolimib-EGFRI
- Sorafenib

Palliation
Jaundice
- Segment III bypass—Longmire procedure
- ERCP/PTC—preferred
- Chemo

Treatment is Based on 4 Situations
- Incidental finding of a suspicious polyp

  Polyp >10 mm, open cholecystectomy, as laparoscopy more chance of spread

- GB cancer detected during or after cholecystectomy

  Depends on depth of invasion

  - T1a: Only cholecystectomy
  - T1b: Only muscular invasion without perineural or deep connective tissue involved—cholecystectomy
  - T1b with perineural and vascular invasion—extended cholecystectomy including draining lymph nodes, cystic duct, if CBD Involved—CBD resection with Roux-en-Y reconstruction
    - Liver parenchyma—adjacent 2 cm normal liver also resected
    - Port site excision
  - T2: Extended cholecystectomy
  - Patients suspected of having carcinoma preoperatively
    - Poor prognosis as disease is already advanced
    - In nonmetastatic: Radical resection after preop laparoscopy to look for peritoneal and liver metastasis
- T3 T4 lesions: Radical resection en bloc including at least resection of liver segments 4b and 5. Often central hepatectomy (4, 5, 8) or trisegmentectomy may be required for achieving Ro margins.

- Direct invasion into adjacent structures like hepatic flexure is not a contraindication for surgery, adjacent structure can be resected if a possible negative margin can be obtained
- Advanced disease during presentation
  - For jaundice: Endoscopic biliary stenting, self-expanding biliary metallic provides durable solution
  - Pain: Percutaneous neurolysis of ganglion
  - Intestinal obstruction: Endoscopic duodenal wall stenting or gastrojejunostomy
  - Does not respond to radiochemotherapy

5.13 CHOLANGIOCARCINOMA
- Divided into proximal and distal
- Proximal involving perihilar and intrahepatic regions
- Distal lesion involves periampullary
- >65% involve proximal tree near bifurcation (Klatskin's tumor)
- Distal—20%, 10% intrahepatic, 10% multiple

Risk Factors
- PSC—greatest risk factor

  Others
  - Chronic inflammation
  - Choledochal cyst
  - Caroli's disease
  - Clonorchis, opsithous, liver fluke
  - Recurrent pyogenic cholangitis
  - OCP, diabetes, thoratract
  - Vinyl chloride
  - Cigarette smoking
  - Hepatolithiasis
  - Oriental cholangiohepatitis
  - Hepatitis C
  - Bilioenteric anastamosis
  - Lynch syndrome
- Unilobar—can cause lobar atrophy on affected site, with contralateral hypertrophy

- Cholangiocarcinoma causing obstruction below hepatic bifurcation manifest earlier than intrahepatic cholangiocarcinoma
- Extrahepatic CCA is more common than intrahepatic

Spread

- Characteristically in longitudinal subepithelial manner—along BD—up to 2 cm proximal and 1 cm distal
- Perineural and lymphatic

Pathology

- Majority—adenocarcinoma
- 3 pathological subtypes
- Sclerosing cholangiocarcinoma—most common—70%
  - Occurs in proximal bile duct causing periductal fibrosis in concentric pattern and circumferential duct occlusion
  - Subepithelial causes obstruction—without forming a mass
- Papillary cholangiocarcinoma—5–10%
  - Appears as polypoidal
  - With less periductal fibrosis
  - Good prognosis
  - More common in distal BD
- Nodular cholangiocarcinoma—20%
  - Firm nodular mass based on duct and grows into the lumen
- **Clinical features**
  - Obstructive jaundice in >90%
  - Papillary cause episodic jaundice—tumour may break off—producing distal obstruction due to ball valve mechanism—intermittent obstruction
- **Staging**
- TNM Staging

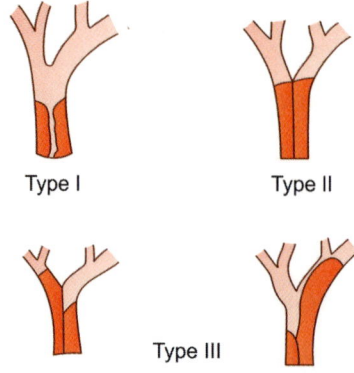

Bismuth-Corlette classification scheme of biliary strictures

Bismuth-Corlette classification	
Type	Definition
I	Limited to CHD, below the level of confluence of right and left HDs
II	Involves the confluence of right and left HDs
IIIa	Type II + extension to right 2nd order ducts
IIIb	Type II + extension to left 2nd order ducts
IV	Extends to both right and left 2nd order ducts

- **Diagnosis**
  - ALP raised, GGT raised
  - CA19 9 and CEA—raised
  - USG: IHBRD, site of obstruction not visualised
  - CT: Triphasic CT—thin 1 to 2 mm cuts
  - Cholangiography: MRCP/ERCP/PTC to determine proximal extend of lesion, but ERCP there is risk of cholangitis
  - MRCP—has more accuracy than ERCP in diagnosis and staging
  - PET CT is indicated to assess metastasis, not for assessment of resectability
- **Preop evaluation—4 factors**
  - Extent inside the ducts
  - Vascular involvement
  - Atrophy of liver
  - Metastasis

Contraindications for Resection

- Bilobar intrahepatic metastasis
- Involvement of secondary biliary radical bilaterally
- Encasement of main pancreatic duct
- Bilateral hepatic lobar artery involved
- Lobar atrophy with involvement of contralateral portal vein or biliary radical
- Encasement of main portal vein
- Metastasis to lymph node outside hepatoduodenal ligament.
- Distant metastasis

- Tissue diagnosis not necessary
- **Preop biliary drainage**—if bilirubin >10—ideally <3 mg/dL
- PTC—preferred in proximal obstruction
- Ipsilateral side of future FLR punctured
- Internal drainage preferred
- Portal vein embolisation—percut transhepatic (previously mini lap and trans ileocolic)
  - If FLR <30%

Treatment

- **40–50% inoperable at operation**
- **Staging laparoscopy**
- For distal/periampullary tumor
  - Whipple procedure
  - 5-year survival (with Ro resection)—50%
- Proximal cholangiocarcinoma
  - Enbloc resection of CBD, with hepatic parenchyma with or without caudate lobectomy with regional lymph nodes based on Bismuth-Corlette/Bismuth-Nekashi classification
  - May be extended right hepatectomy or left hepatectomy, depending on tumor location
  - Resection of caudate lobe advised

Type 1

Common bile duct resection + cholecystectomy + 5–10 mm margin of resection with lymphadenectomy.
  - High recurrence. So liver resection advised—central liver resection/parenchyma preserving liver resection
  - Following this multiple small BD will be open—anastomosis to jejunum—similar to Kasai procedure
- Type 2—may also require partial hepatic resection
- Type 3 and 4—may require complex resection of portal vein, hepatic artery or both with resection of secondary biliary radical, trans anastamosis stenting is done to allow healing and to retain integrity of anastamosis
- Any positive LN found outside hepatoduodenal ligament—metastasis—no resection
- Locally advanced inoperable without LN or distant metastasis—liver transplantation

Associating Liver Partition and Portal Vein Ligation for Staged Hepatectomy (ALPPS)

- To increase FLR
- Typically in right trisectionectomy

Survival

- On negative margins—5-year survival 60% with R0 resection
- Mean survival in unresected patients—5–8 months

Adjuvant Therapy

- After margin negative resection adjuvant therapy—role not clear
- Chemoradiation
- Molecular therapy—cediramib—EGFR
  - GEMOX with cetuximab

Palliation

- In jaundice with cholangitis/pruritus
  - Stenting—SEMS/plastic
  - Segment III bypass
  - Photodynamic therapy
  - Chemo—gemcitabine with cisplatin
  - Intraluminal brachytherapy
- Need >one-third of liver to be decompressed to relieve jaundice
- Decompression of atrophic segment will not relieve jaundice
- Jaundice may be due to—PV obstruction—liver atrophy

Perihilar CCA

- CCA involving perihilar duct, the duct located between right side of the umbilical portion of the portal vein and the left side of the origin of the right posterior PV
- CCA may extend beyond the macroscopic tumor
- Length of microscopic invasive cancer—1 cm in 90%
- Length of noninvasive cancer—2 cm—in 90%
  - So optimal resection line of BD for invasive cancer—1 cm tumor free margin
  - For noninvasive cancer—2 cm
- Residual noninvasive cancer—does not have significant negative impact on survival

- Noninvasive cancer is also called carcinoma *in situ* or high grade biliary intraepithelial neoplasm.

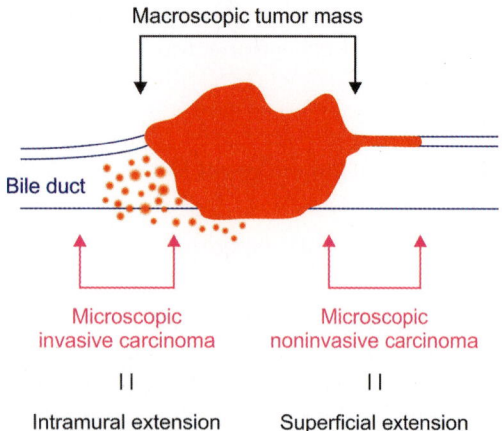

- Superficial spreading CCA—with noninvasive cancer extension >2 cm.

- Less advanced, papillary type
- Complete resection is necessary
- Diffusely infiltrating CCA
  - Extensive infiltration from hilar BD to lower BD
- Entire extrahepatic duct is removed
- Ideal for hepatopancreaticoduodenectomy

Medicines

- Inchikoto: Japanese magic bullet for jaundice
  Cholerectic, induce antioxidants
- **UDCA**
  - On hepatocytes—protection against oxidative stress
  - Inhibition of apoptosis, stimulation of bile flow
- Symbiotics (pro and prebiotics)

Pancreas

6.1 CONGENITAL DISORDERS

Embryology

- Exocrine pancreas begins development—4th week
- Dorsal bud appears first
- During 4–8 weeks—ventral bud rotates posteriorly in clockwise fashion to fuse with dorsal bud
- Pancreas develops from two buds. From endodermal lining of duodenum, forms the dorsal bud, which forms posteriorly within mesentery. Ventral bud is associated with hepaticopancreatic duct.
- There is an avascular plane posterior to pancreas—Todd's fascia
- During second month—stomach rotates, duodenum becomes 'C' shaped
- Ventral pancreas bud migrates dorsally—posteroinferiorly to dorsal bud and forms the inferior part of head and uncinate process
- In majoriity, MPD of Wirsung is formed by entire ventral duct and distal dorsal duct—enters duodenum through major papilla
- Persistence of proximal part of dorsal duct occurs in 25%—accessory duct of Santorini and opens into minor papilla
- Failure of fusion of these two ductal systems is seen in 10%—entire dorsal pancreas (superior head, body and tail)—drain through minor papilla
  - Ventral pancreas which forms inferior part, head and uncinate process and drains through major papilla—**pancreas** divisum

Signalling for Dorsal and Ventral Pancreas

- Dorsal pancreas—signals arise from notochord and dorsal aorta
- Ventral pancreas—the lateral plate mesoderm
- Hedgehog signalling family involved—inhibition leads to endoderm differentiation into pancreatic lineage
- PDX1—pancreatic duodenal homeobox 1, role in exocrine differentiation into pancreatic lineage
- PTF1—pancreatic specific transcription factor 1. Along with PDX1 develops progenital cells to pancreatic tissue

- Notch signalling pathway—suppresses endocrine differentiation and promotes exocrine development
- Wnt signalling—lack of it leads to absence of acinar cells

Pancreas Divisum

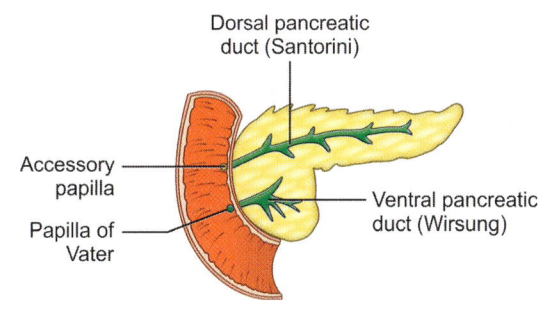

- Incidence 5–10%
- In recurrent acute pancreatitis incidence—25–50%
- There is complete pancreas divisum and incomplete—small branch connect the two ducts
- First description by Josef Hyrtl, 1865
- Small ventral duct can cause obstruction and subsequent symptoms are difficult to differentiate from cancer
- Cannulating major papilla visualize only head—need to cannulate minor papilla to see rest of the pancreas
  - Can cause pancreatitis
- <5% with pancreatic divisum will develop pancreatitis
- Complete variety has no increased chance for pancreatitis compared to incomplete type
- There is cumulative effect of CFTR (cystic fibrosis transmembrane regulator) mutation and pancreas divisum on pancreatitis

Imaging

- EUS sensitivity 87%—superior to MDCT and MRCP
- ERCP shows enlarged/open minor papilla
- MDCT is done in PV phase
- Secretin stimulated MRCP (sMRCP)

Therapy

- Endoscopic procedures on minor papilla
  - Dilatation
  - Papillotomy

Sphincterotomy

- Improvement is seen more in recurrent AP than in CP and chronic pancreatic pain
- Surgical sphincteroplasty of minor papilla
- Frey's procedure
- Lateral pancreaticojejunostomy

Annular Pancreas

- Head of pancreas (ventral bud) completely encircles D2
- Most often seen with congenital duodenal atresia or stenosis
- Data of prevalence
  - ERCP—3 per 1000
  - Autopsy—3 in 20000

Pathogenesis Theories

- Ventral pancreas from two buds—left and right—in mammals left bud regresses
- Lecco—adherence of right ventral pancreatic duct before gut rotation causes a ring of tissue around duodenum
- Baldwin 1910—left ventral bud forms annulus causing obstruction
- Kamisawa 2001—tip of left ventral bud adheres to duodenum and stretches to form a ring. The exact location of this attachment in relation to bile duct determines final arrangement of annular duct

Genetic

- Overexpression of TM4SF3—Transmembrane 4 superfamily member 3—promotes fusion of ventral and dorsal buds
- Hedgehog signalling pathway

Clinical Features

- Seen equally in adults and children
- **Adults**
  - Half to two-thirds are asymptomatic
  - Pain abdomen
  - Pancreatitis
  - Predispose to malignancy
- **Children**
  - Majority present in first few days after birth
  - If complete duodenal obstruction—polyhydramnios seen in mother
  - Primary biliary obstruction and jaundice—not typical
  - Nonbilious vomiting is seen in >90%
  - If obstruction is below ampulla causes bilious vomiting—rare

- Most common associated congenital anomaly—Trisomy 21 (Down's)
  - Others—malrotation, TEF, cardiac

X-ray

- Double bubble sign—air in stomach and D1

Therapy

- No division of annulus—can cause fistula
- In children duodenoduodenostomy—choice—diamond-shaped anastomosis

Cystic Fibrosis

- Autosomal recessive
- In Caucasians—most common inherited disorder
- Mutation of CFTR—chromosome 7—this gene creates a cell membrane protein—control movement of chloride across cell membrane
- Elevated sodium and chloride in sweat—child becomes salty
- Lung—blockage due to thick secretions—COPD
- Meconium ileus
- Pancreatic duct blockage—ectasia—exocrine insufficiency—islets usually normal but later develops diabetes
- Infertility—absence of vas in men—thick mucus in women
- Secondary sexual characteristics—delayed

Diagnosis

- Genetic testing
- Sweat test—sodium and chloride >90 mmol/L

Treatment

- Control consequences
- Pulmonary physiotherapy, antibiotics
- Pancreatic enzyme supplementation
- Low fat diet
- Added salt
- May survive till mid-thirties
- Lung transplantation

6.2 ACUTE PANCREATITIS

Definition

- Defined as acute inflammatory process of the pancreas with variable involvement of other regional tissues or remote organ systems
- Incidence on increasing trend
- Most common GI problem for admission in US

Phases of Pancreatic Secretion

- **Cephalic**
  - Vagal stimulation—acetylcholine mediated
  - Accounts for 20–30% of juice
- **Gastric phase**
  - Triggered by gastric distension
  - Vasovagal reflexes
  - 10% of juice secretion
- **Intestinal**
  - 65–70% of juice secretion
  - Secretin—produced by acidification of duodenum cause—secretion of water, bicarbonate, electrolytes
  - CCK

    Secretion is induced by carbhohydrates, protein, fat in diet-induces secretion of pancreatic enzymes
- Pancreatic enzymes are inactivated at low pH
- Optimum pH for
  - Trypsin 8–9
  - Amylase 7
  - Lipase 7–9

Pathophysiology: Co-localisation

- After 15 minutes of pancreatic injury—lysosomes and zymogens-colocalize
- Lysosomal enzyme Cathepsin B—activates trypsinogen to trypsin
- Activated trypsin causes further release of Cathepsin B—induce apoptosis and necrosis—acinar cell death—induce local and systemic inflammatory cascade

Etiology of Acute Pancreatitis

- Gall stones
  - Most common cause
- Alcohol
- ERCP (overall 5–20%)
- Medications
- Trauma
- Neoplasms 10% of patients
- Anatomic variants—divisum
- Metabolic problems
  - Hypercalcemia
  - Hypertriglyceridemia

- Rare causes of acute pancreatitis
  - Annular pancreas
  - Autoimmune pancreatitis
  - Hereditary pancreatitis
  - Familial adenomatous polyposis
  - Pseudopapillary tumor of the pancreas
- Etiology in children
  - Blunt injury abdomen and systemic diseases— most common

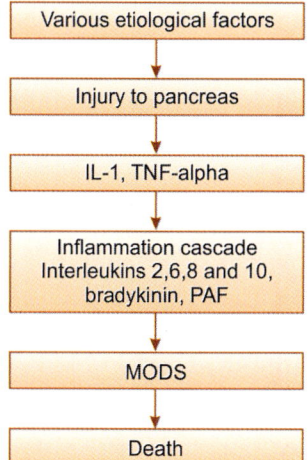

Classification of Acute Pancreatitis

- Revised Atlanta Classification 2013
- Determinant-based classification 2012
- Based on actual factors of severity like
  - Necrosis
  - Organ failure

These factors have a direct causal association with severity

Revised Atlanta classification	
Mild acute pancreatitis	No organ failure
	No local or systemic complications
Moderately severe acute pancreatitis	Organ failure that resolves within 48 hrs Local or systemic complications without persistent organ failure
Severe acute pancreatitis	Persistent organ failure >48 hrs

- **Fluid Collections in AP (Atlanta 2012)**

Collections as defined in the 2012 revised Atlanta classification

Definition	Description
Acute fluid collection (<4 wk after onset and edematous pancreatitis)	• Homogeneous fluid density • Confined by normal peripancreatic fascial planes • No definable wall encapsulating the collection • Adjacent to pancreas (not intrapancreatic)
Pseudocyst (rare, usually >4 wk after onset and necrotising pancreatitis)	• Well circumscribed, usually round/oval • Homogeneous fluid density • Well-defined wall and completely encapsulating the collection • Location: Intrapancreatic and/or extrapancreatic
Acute necrotic collection (usually <4 wk after onset and necrotizing pancreatitis)	• Heterogeneous and nonliquid density • No definable wall encapsulating the collection • Intrapancreatic and/or extrapancreatic
Walled-off necrosis (usually >4 wk after onset and necrotising pancreatitis)	• Heterogeneous and nonliquid density • Well-defined wall and completely encapsulated • Intrapancreatic and/or extrapancreatic

- **Mortality**
  - Mild AP—<1%
  - Severe AP—10–30% (*20–50%—Bailey*)
- Early phase of death—within 2 weeks due to-MODS
- Late period—after 2 weeks due to sepsis
- Most common cause—MODS

Pathophysiology
- SIRS—first 2 weeks
  - Severe inflammation
- CARS (Compensatory Anti-inflammatory Response Syndrome) after 2 weeks
  - Sepsis

Gallstone Acute Pancreatitis
- Most common cause in West (40%)
- Overall incidence of AP in gallstones—3–8%
- More in women—50–70 years
- There are two theories for the pathogenesis—the obstructive theory, which says—due to the obstruction of the pancreatic duct, the pressure increases, thus causing the initiation of the inflammatory process
- The reflux theory—due to the passage of stone and obstruction—reflux of bile can occur into pancreatic duct, thereby initiating the inflammation

Acute Biliary Pancreatitis
- 4–8% of patients with gall stones eventually get AP
- More in women M: F = 3:7
- Recovery may be complete, so there is less endocrine and exocrine deficiency
- Normal pancreatic duct pressure 3 fold higher than CBD. This may be reversed in CBD obstruction—causing reflux of bile into pancreas

High Risk
- Gall stone <5 mm size
- Wide cystic duct >5 mm
- High stone load >20 stones
- Stones—mulberry shape, irregular surfaces
- Excess cholesterol crystals in GB
- Good emptying of GB
- SPINK1 mutation
- ABCB4 gene

Alcohol: Acute Pancreatitis
- Second most common—35%
- More in young men—30–45 years
- 5–10% of patients who drink get AP
- More seen in
  - Heavy abuse (>100 g/day for 5 years)
  - Smoking
    - Genetically susceptible

Pathophysiology-Alcoholic AP
- Triggers inflammatory cascade via NF-κB
- Increase caspases that mediate apoptosis
- Decrease pancreatic perfusion
- Induce sphincter of ODDI spasm
- Precipitation of proteins in the PD
- Fatty acid ethyl esters and reactive oxygen radicles—direct acinar injury
- Alcohol cause increased lithostathine and glycoprotein GP2 result in more stones
- Alcohol increases the trypsinogen, chymotrypsinogen, lipase and Cathepsin B in juice
- Cathepsin B activates trypsinogen and the cascade
- Alcohol metabolism is oxidative and thus releases reactive oxygen species and acetaldehyde
- Nonoxidative metabolism—releases fatty acid ethyl esters
- Both can destabilize zymogen and lysosomes—acinar injury

Rule of 5–10%
- AP in symptomatic gall stone disease—3–8%
- AP in alcoholic—5–10%
- AP in pancreas divisum—5–10%
- AP in ERCP—5%
- Severe disease—5–10%

Metabolic Factors

- **Hypertriglyceridemia**
  - More common in type I, II, V (I, IV, V-Blumgart)
  - Suspect if TG >1000 mg/dL. >2000 mg/dL confirms
  - Hypertriglyceridemia secondary to hypothyroidism, diabetes, and alcohol—do not induce AP
  - Account for 1–10% of AP
  - TG-metabolized by lipase—release FFA—acinar injury—inflammatory cascade
  - Lipoprotein lipase deficiency cause chylomicronemia (autosomal recessive)—high TG levels

Hypercalcemia

- Converts trypsinogen to trypsin
- Precipitates calcium—obstruction
- Increases duct permeability
- PTH—direct toxic effect on pancreas
- Contributes to 1–4% of AP
- Treatment of hypercalcemia—resolves AP

Inborn Errors of Metabolism

- Type 1 glycogen storage disease (von Gierke)
- Maple syrup urine disease
- Cystathione beta synthase deficiency
- 3-hydroxy-3 methylglutaryl co-A lyase deficiency
- Pyruvate kinase deficiency
- Cystinuria

In all these AP is not very common

CRF and Dialysis

- More risk in peritoneal dialysis
- No increased risk in hemodialysis
- Peritoneal dialysis—increase intraabdominal pressure and pancreatic ischemia—AP
- CRF—increase in CCK, GIP, etc. may cause AP

Drug-induced AP

- Incidence 0.1% to 2%
- ACE inhibitors
- Valproic acid, ASA
- Toxins
  - Scorpion Venom
  - Phenol
    - Solvents

Infectious Causes

- Bacteria
  - *Mycoplasma pneumoniae*
  - Leptospira
  - *C. jejuni*
  - Legionella
- Viral
  - Mumps
  - Hep B
  - HIV
  - Cocksackie, CMV
- Fungal/parasitic
  - Aspergillus
  - Ascaris—most common parasitic cause

Increased Risk of Post ERCP Pancreatitis

- 1–3% after diagnostic ERCP
- 2–5% after therapeutic ERCP
- As many as 25% in sphincter of Oddi studies

Patient Factors

- Sphincter of Oddi dysfunction
- Younger age
- Female sex
- History of prior post-ERCP pancreatitis

Procedure Factors

- Low endoscopist's experience
- Small common bile duct diameter
- Pancreatic sphincterotomy
- Difficult biliary cannulation
- Precut sphincterotomy
- Multiple cannulations
- Sphincter of Oddi manometry

Anatomic Obstruction

- Pancreas divisum—most common pancreatic congenital anomaly in 7–12%
  - 5–10% lifetime risk
- Annular pancreas
- Sphincter of Oddi dysfunction
- Anomalus PB junction—reflux
- Choledochal cyst, choledochocele (type 3)
- Duodenal duplication cyst

Tumors

- Acute pancreatitis can be first presentation in periampullary tumors
- Suspected in
  - Older than 40
  - Weight loss
  - Newly onset diabetes
- Most common tumors seen are
  - IPMN, MCN, ampullary tumors, islet cell tumors. PDA, adenoma

Other Causes

- Blunt injury—0.2% (<2%: Blumgart)
- Penetrating injury—1%(12–30%—in gunshot and stab—Blumgart)
- Splenic artery embolization

Assessment of Acute Pancreatitis

- Clinical features
- About 90% of AP patients have nausea and/or vomiting

- Constant pain radiating to back (in 50%)—may last for days
- Grey Turner sign—flank ecchymosis
- Cullen sign—periumblical ecchymosis
  - Due to exudate tracking along falciform ligament and retroperitoneum
- Guarding
- Jaundice

Diagnosis

- Based on 2 or more of the following:
  - Severe abdominal pain and other clinical features
  - Serum amylase or lipase x 3 times the upper limit
  - CECT/MRI/USG s/o acute pancreatitis
  - Lipase is more specific

Amylase

- Elevates within hours and can remain elevated for 4–5 days
- May not be elevated in 15–20% of AP
- High specificity when using levels >3 x normal
- Many false positives
- Most specific is pancreatic isoamylase (fractionated amylase)
- Trypsinogen activation peptide and trypsinogen 2 levels:
  - More specific than amylase and lipase—
  - Not readily available
- Hyperglycemia
- Leukocytosis
- Raised ALT with pancreas enzyme raise—predictive value of 95% in biliary AP

Reasons for Amylase Elevation

- **Pancreatic Source**
  - Biliary obstruction
  - Bowel obstruction
  - Perforated ulcer
  - Appendicitis
  - Mesenteric ischemia
  - Peritonitis
- **Salivary Source**
  - Parotitis
  - DKA
  - Anorexia
  - Malignancies
- **Unknown Source**
  - Renal failure
  - Head trauma
  - Burns
  - Postoperative

Clinical and Radiologic Scoring Systems

- Persistent or deteriorating multi-organ dysfunction in the first 7 days after admission—the most significant predictor of death

Ranson's Criteria

- **Earliest criteria—in 1974**
- 11 parameters
- Mortality rate directly correlates with number of positive parameters
- Severe if >3 parameters positive
- On admission 5 parameters (age, blood glucose, WBC, LDH and AST)
- Main disadvantage—does not severity at the time of admission—as 6 (hematocrit, calcium, base deficit, BUN, fluid requirement and PaO$_2$) parameters are assessed only after 48 hours
- Has low positive predictive value (50%), high negative predictive value (90%)
- Mainly used to—rule out severe pancreatitis
- Predict risk of mortality

Glasgow-Imrie Score

- 9 parameters
- 5 on admission, 4 within 48 hours

APACHE II

- Based on
  - Patient's age,
  - Previous health status
  - 12 routine physiologic measurements
- Predicts general measure of severity
- Score >8 indicates severe AP
- Advantage—can be used on admission and can be repeated at any time
- Complex
- Positive predictive value—43%, negative predictive value 89%

APACHE O—Obesity as a Variable

Bedside index of severity in acute pancreatitis (BISAP) score:

BUN >25 mg/dL (8.9 mmol/L)—1 point
Abnormal mental status with a GCS < 15–1 point
Evidence of SIRS—1 point
Patient age >60 yrs old—1 point
Imaging study reveals pleural effusion—1 point

Assessment of Severity of AP

- Ranson's score 3 or more and APACHE 8 or more—severe disease
- Any organ failure or local pancreatic complication indicates severe disease
- Other markers for severity—procalcitonin, IL-1, IL-6, elastase trypsinogen activation peptide

Harmless Acute Pancreatitis Score (HAPS)

- Abdomen—no guarding/rebound tenderness
- Normal hematocrit
- Normal creatinine

Marshall Scoring System: Parameters

- Respiratory—(PO_2/FiO_2)
- Renal—creatinine
- CVS—systolic BP

Scoring systems in acute pancreatitis	
	Cutoff for predicted severe acute pancreatitis
APACHE II	≥8 in first 24 hrs
BISAP	≥3 in first 24 hrs
Modified Glasgow (or Imrie)	≥3 in first 48 hrs
Ranson	≥3 in first 48 hrs
Urea at admission	>60 mmol/L
CRP	> 150 U/L in first 72 hrs

Laboratory Assessment

C-reactive Protein (CRP)

- Peaks 48–72 hours after onset of pancreatitis
- Correlates with severity
- CRP >150 mg/ml—severe AP—accuracy 70–80%
- Cannot be used on admission
- Sensitivity less if done within 48 hours
- Accuracy of 86%
- Readily available
- Gold standard single marker

Hematocrit

- >44% on admission or absence of fall in first 24 hours
  - Risk predictor for pancreas necrosis, pancreatic infection and organ failure
- Hematocrit >50%—predict severe pancreatitis
- <40% to 44–90% exclude severe AP
- Role—due to fluid loss

Procalcitonin

- A marker of bacterial infection or sepsis
- >1.8 ng/ml—predict severity

Imaging

The role of imaging in acute pancreatitis
- Confirm the diagnosis
- Identify necrosis

- Determine the presence of complications
  - Fluid collections
  - Vascular abnormalities
- X-ray
- USG
- CECT
- MRI/MRCP
- Secretin MRCP
- EUS
- ERCP

X-ray

- To rule out other conditions—DU perforation
- Ileus
- Colon cut-off sign—due to colonic spasm at splenic flexure
- Widening of C loop of duodenum—due to head of pancreas edema
- Sentinel loop (local ileus)
- Renal halo sign—enhancement of perirenal fat due to retroperitoneal exudate collection—may be bilateral suggestive of AP
- Pancreatic, biliary calculi
- Pleural effusion

USG

- Limited use—abdominal gas and fat
- High sensitivity to diagnose gall stones: 95%

Multidetector Computed Tomography (MDCT)

- The imaging study of choice for acute pancreatitis
- Faster image acquisition
- Improved resolution
- Can be converted into three-dimensional reconstructions
- Most valuable is contrast phase to evaluate parenchyma—portal venous phase (60 to 70 seconds after contrast injection)
- Can assess viability, peripancreatic inflammation/fluid

Plain CT—can assess fluid collection or extraluminal air

CT severity index, by Balthazar in 1994

- Focuses on the presence and degree of:
  - Pancreatic inflammation (fluid collections)
  - Necrosis.
- Successfully used to predict overall morbidity and mortality
- **Limitations**

Does not correlate significantly with

- Development of organ failure extrapancreatic parenchymal complications
- Peripancreatic vascular complications

Modified CT Index: Considers

- Pancreatic morphology
- Pancreatic necrosis
- Additional 2 points for extra pancreatic complications

Extra Pancreatic Inflammation on CT (EPIC) Score

Factors

- Ascites
- Pleural effusion
- Retroperitoneal inflammation
- Mesenteric inflammation
- Do not need CECT
- **CT scan should not be routinely performed on admission for assessing severity**
- As clinical scoring systems have equal accuracy

Current Recommendation for CT

- Persistent organ failure
  - SIRS or sepsis
- For those who do not improve in 6–10 days
- Probable infected necrosis
- Diagnostic dilemma

MRCP—severity index

- **Based on the existing Balthazar CTSI**
- **Advantage:**
  - Ability to generate cholangiopancreatography image
  - Detection of pancreatic duct disruption with the use of secretin

---

Imaging in acute pancreatitis

- CECT is the best modality
- Portal venous phase 65–70 seconds after contrast injection is the best phase
- MRI can assess extent of necrosis, inflammation and free fluid
- MRCP—not indicated in acute setting AP
- MRCP useful in idiopathic or recurrent pancreatitis
- Secretin MRCP is useful in pancreatic divisum
- EUS is very sensitive in diagnosing choledocholithiasis
- EUS
  - In gall stone AP

Treatment

- Aggressive fluid resuscitation
- Ringer lactate is preferred initially—reduced SIRS vs NS
- Invasive monitoring
  - CVP
  - Arterial line
  - Foley's catheter
- Pulse oximetry—oxygen—to maintain saturation above 95%
- Analgesia—narcotics preferred
- Thoracic epidural may be tried
- Morphine not ideal but can still be used—it can theoretically worsen symptoms by increasing spasm of the sphincter of Oddi. Other opioids are
  - Demerol
  - Hydromorphone

Monitor Markers

- Urine output
- Serum lactate
- Mixed venous oxygen saturation
- Base deficit

Management

No Proven Benefit

- Antiproteases
  - Gabexate mesilate
  - Aprotinin
- PAF inhibitors
  - Lexipafant
- Octreotide
- Glucagon
- Polypeptide YY
- CCK receptor antagonists

Intraabdominal Hypertension

- IAP >20 mmHg with or without abdominal arterial perfusion pressure <60 mmHg that is associated with new onset organ failure
- Associated with severity and mortality
- Measure the IAP in ventilated patients

Nutrition in Acute Pancreatitis

- Enteral nutrition
  - Less infectious complications
  - Less need for pancreatic surgery
  - Reduced mortality in recent meta-analysis
  - Mild AP: Same day or the next day start oral feeding
  - Severe: Within 3 days oral or nasojejunal feeds
- TPN can cause
  - Mucosal atrophy
  - Decreased intestinal blood flow
  - Increased bacterial overgrowth and translocation
- When tolerated—oral nutrition
- When orally not tolerated—try enteral tube feeding
- Oral/enteral preferred over PN even in severe AP
- Nasogastric drainage only in severe cases initially, when tolerating oral feeds, remove tube

PYTHON Trial

- NG route is tolerated and feasible in 80%
- Majority of the remainder—nasojejunal
- TPN only if enteral nutrition is not feasible or tolerated

Antibiotics

- Sepsis
  - Accounts for >80% of deaths
- Intestinal flora
  - Gram-negative bacteria
- Mechanism—translocation of the bacteria across the gut wall

No proven benefit for prophylactic antibiotics even in necrosis mainly advised only as treatment

- Antibiotics indicated in cholangitis
- No role for probiotics
- Selective gut decontamination—uncertain

Early ERCP

- Nontherapeutic ERCP—avoided—more complications

ERCP Indicated in

Severe Acute Biliary Pancreatitis

- Cholangitis
- Persistent bile duct obstruction
- If contraindication for surgery—ERCP—sphincterotomy
- Jaundice with SIRS—cholangitis
- Not indicated in mild AP—where bile duct obstruction may be transient

Role of Urgent CT

- In diagnostic uncertainty only
- Thereafter only in assessment and follow-up of local complications
- USG is enough—to see gall stones
- MRCP/EUS–in cholestasis in the absence of cholangitis
- In AP—no gall stones found and alcohol is not apparent—EUS should be done—to exclude microlithiasis/neoplasm

Diagnostic Criteria in Biliary Pancreatitis

- Abnormal LFT—raised ALT
- USG—gall stones or dilated CBD >8 mm in young or >10 mm in old patients

Cholecystectomy in Biliary Pancreatitis

Mild Disease

- Early cholecystectomy (once symptoms subsides and cholestatic enzymes normalize)

Severe Disease

- Delayed cholecystectomy—after 6 weeks

Complications

Acute Fluid Collection

- Acute fluid collection—seen in 30–57%
- Fluid collections are not surrounded by epithelium or fibrotic capsule unlike cystic neoplasms/pseudocysts
- Most fluid will be absorbed
- If infected—percutaneous aspiration

Pancreatic Necrosis and Infected Necrosis

- Necrosis—presence of nonviable pancreatic parenchyma or peripancreatic fat
- CECT—choice
- Low attenuation (<40–50 HU)—(normal pancreas 100–150 HU)
- Up to 20% of AP—develops pancreatic necrosis
- Pancreas necrosis seen in 80% of autopsies after death due to AP
- Inflammation—48–72 hours—bowel mucosal ischemia and reperfusion injury—increased permeability initiated in 72 hours, peaks in 1 week cause bacteremia—pancreatic necrosis infection
- Infections from other sources and interventions can also cause pancreatic infection

Pancreatic Necrosis

- **Sterile necrosis**—Systemic Inflammatory Response Syndrome (SIRS) (first 2 weeks)
  - Mortality rate of 10–20%
- **Infected necrosis (CARS)**—Sepsis (after 2 weeks)
  - Mortality—20–30%

Infected Necrosis

- Risk directly related to amount of necrosis—45–50% if >70% gland involved
- Mainly *E. coli*, klebsiella, pseudomonas
- Role of CT guided FNA with gram stain and culture as a confirmatory test is debatable
- Even if aspiration culture negative—40% have infected necrosis
- Evidence of air within pancreatic necrosis is suggestive of possible infection
- Air by itself not an indication for intervention. Spontaneous enteric discharge may cause air inside necrosis—may improve clinically
- Once infection demonstrated—antibiotics given
- Carbapenems—choice
- Overall mortality—25–30%

Indications for Necrosectomy

- Failure of non-operative management (at least 48 hours of maximal ICU support)
- Infected necrosis
- Extra visceral air
- Uncontrolled hemorrhage (failed endovascular)
- Colonic complications
- Intervention by endoscopic or operative methods is better delineated and tolerated after optimizing the patient with antibiotics and nutrition—preferably after 2 weeks
  - Fluid collection becomes more mature

Minimally Invasive Approaches

- Percutaneous Minimally Invasive Retroperitoneal Necrosectomy (MIRP)
- Video Assisted Retroperitoneal Debridement (VARD)
- Endoscopic cystogastrostomy
- Laparoscopic cystogastrostomy
- Laparoscopic debridement
- MIS—less SIRS and less ICU care

PANTER (Pancreatitis, Necrosectomy Versus step-up Approach) Trial: Dutch van Santvoort: 2010

- Open necrosectomy vs step-up based on endoscopic/ percutaneous as initial with progression to RP debridement if no improvement

- Significant benefit with step-up approach
- Consensus—early optimization—followed by delayed minimally invasive approach
- Solid, infected—MIRP or VARD
- Later when well-organized predominantly fluid collections develop—endoscopic or lap transgastric drainage.

Intervention for Pancreatic Necrosis Step-up Approach: VARD

- Catheter drainage.
- 5 cm incision at the site of catheter at mid-axillary line on left side and necrosectomy by suction and 0 degree laparoscope assisted drainage is done
- Drains placed—lavage

Step-up—MIRP

Percutaneous drain placed—drain tract dilated with balloon—operating nephroscope is used for percutaneous necrosectomy

Transmural Drainage

- **NOTES**—Natural Orifice Transluminal Endoscopic Surgery—even for solid necrosis
- **PENGUIN** (Pancreatitis Endoscopic Transgastric vs Primary Necrosectomy in Patients with Infected Pancreatic Necrosis) trial—Bakker (2012)
  - Equal benefit
- **TENSION** (Transluminal ENdoscopic vs SurgIcal necrOsectomy in patients with infected pancreatic Necrosis) trial van Brunschot (2013)—awaited

Transmural Drainage

- First drainage
- If no improvement—tract dilated to 15–18 mm via endoscope
  - Necrosectomy done using snares
- Debris left in stomach
- Similar to step up
- Necrosectomy achieved in 91%

Management of Late WOPN (Pseudocysts)

- Indications for intervention
  - Infection
  - Nutrition failure
  - Persistent abdominal pain

EUS Guided Cystogastrostomy/Necrosectomy

- True pseudocysts are rare—collections requiring intervention are considered—WOPN

- EUS guided puncture with cystotome—guidewire-tract dilated to 12 mm—two pigtail cathters 7 FR—nasocystic catheter introduced for irrigation

Multiple Gateway technique (Varadarajulu)

- Two or three transmural stents (SEMS) placed—one for nasocystic irrigation—others for drainage

Endoscopic Necrosectomy (Seifert)—difficult

Intracavitary Hydrogen Peroxide Irrigation

- May need multiple sittings
- Fully covered SEMS with flanges are used
- Lumen apposing metal stent (LAMS)—lumen apposed to cyst wall, hence causes less migration

Laparoscopy

- Necrosectomy with cystogastrostomy
- In biliary pancreatitis—cholecystectomy is also done

Open Surgical

- Midline/BL subcoastal incision
- Transgastric approach—to reduce contamination

Procedures

- **Open necrosectomy with open packing**—abdomen left open
- **Open necrosectomy with closed packing**
- **Open necrosectomy with continuous postop lavage—Beger**
  - Peripancreatic compartment reconstituted by suturing gastrocolic and duodenocolic ligaments—drain placed inside—irrigated 1 to 10 liters per day
- **Programmed open necrosectomy—Bradley**
  - Repeated planned laparotomies—debridement

Necrosectomy technique	Anatomy	Advantages	Limitations
Open	Pancreatic head, disrupted duct, mesentery, collections	Direct access, more complete, concurrent procedure	Higher morbidity, fistulas
PCD	Anterior pararenal, retroperitoneal	Less invasive	Limited utility, long drains
Endoscopic	Central retrogastric, duodenal	Less invasive	Limited necrosectomy
Laparoscopic	Anterior, paracolic, lesser sac	Multiple areas, GB	Difficult in bleeding
Lap transgastric	Retrogastric	Direct debridement	Only retro gastric
MIRP	Posterior, lateral, pelvis	Continued lavage	Repeated procedures

Pancreatic Pseudocysts

- Occur in 5–15% of patients who have peripancreatic collections after AP
- Capsule lined by collagen and granulation tissue
- Fibrotic reaction—requires 4–8 weeks to develop
- 50%—develop symptoms
- Pain, early satiety, weight loss, elevated pancreas enzymes
- Most common location—lesser sac
- Chronic pancreatitis form pseudocysts in 40%

CT/MRI

- Cannot reliably exclude neoplasm
- Neoplasm—may be macrocystic

EUS FNA

- If diagnosis is in doubt and pseudocyst shows
  - High amylase
  - Absence of mucin
  - Low CEA

Pseudocyst Classification D' Egidio and Schein Classification

Type 1—Postnecrotic pseudocyst after AP, rarely involving ductal disruption

Type 2—Postnecrotic pseudocyst after exacerbation of CP, sometimes showing ductal disruption

Type 3—Retention pseudocyst always related to obstruction and dilatation of PD

Nealon Classification

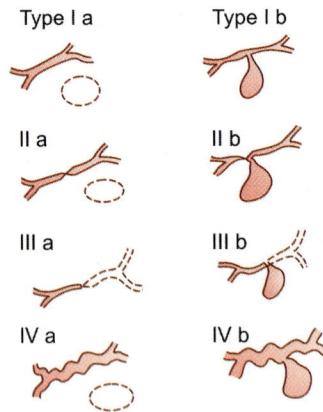

Type I a Type I b

II a II b

III a III b

IV a IV b

- **Type I**—normal main pancreatic duct
- **Type II**—PD stricture
- **Type III**—PD occlusion (disconnected pancreatic duct syndrome)
- **Type IV**—chronic pancreatitis
- **Subtype a**—no radiological communication of cyst with pd
- **Subtype b**—radiological communication present

Treatment

- Observation as below:
  Asymptomatic—70% spontaneous regression occur in
  - <4 cm size
  - Located in tail
  - No evidence of duct obstruction or communication with MPD—Nealon I

Endoscopic

- **Transduodenal/trans gastric drainage**
  - If in close contact (<1 cm)
- Large vessel or varices—contraindication
- Trans papillary if cyst is communicating to MPD
- In stricture—endoscopic dilatation and stenting

Endoscopic

- LAMS
- Stents can be removed after 4–6 weeks, if there is no pseudocyst to main pancreatic duct communication—after pseudocyst has been completely drained

Surgical

- Cystogastrostomy
- Cystoduodenostomy—rarely done—high complications
- Cystojejunostomy
- Successful immediate cyst drainage in 90%
- After initial resolution—12% chance of recurrence
- Percutaneous drainage—in infection

Resection Indicated

- Disconnected pancreatic duct syndrome with narrow duct
- Splenic parenchymal involvement by pseudocyst
- Cannot rule out PCN

External Drainage

- In hemorrhage/peritonitis—as a temporary procedure
- Too thin wall
- Infected cyst

Pancreatic Ascites

- Complete disruption of pancreatic duct
- Abdomen distention
- Paracentesis—raised amylase and lipase
  - SAAG >1.1

Treatment

- Abdominal drainage
- Pancreatic stenting
- Failure—surgery—distal resection

External Fistula

- Drain tract fistula
- Fistula tract jejunostomy may be attempted after 6–12 weeks (ideal 6 months)
- Distal pancreatectomy

Internal Fistula

- Due to
  - Localized peripancreatic necrosis
  - Microvascular compromise
- Most common—pancreaticocolonic fistula
  - High bacterial load—sepsis
  - Early colostomy/resection has to be done to control fistula and sepsis.
- In other fistulas a longer period of nonoperative management

Pancreato-pleural Fistula

- Posterior disruption of PD—into pleural space
- Negative IT pressure—draw retroperitoneal fluid into mediastinum
  or
  - A reactive pleural effusion
- Causes cough, chest pain
- More common in alcoholic AP
- 70% associated with pseudocyst
- Large left-sided effusion—amylase >50000 IU—confirm
- **CT, CXR—diagnostic**

Treatment

- Intercostal drainage, parenteral nutrition, octreotide
- 60% respond
- Endoscopic stenting or surgery may be indicated
- MRCP if shows
  - Duct is normal or dilated—transpapillary stenting may be done
  - If complete blockage/disruption of duct—ductal drainage/resection is indicated

Vascular Complications

- Most commonly involved—splenic artery
- Elastase—damages vessels—pseudoaneurysm—spontaneous rupture—massive bleeding
- Most common symptom—abdominal pain

Treatment

- Arterial embolization
- Refractory—ligation of vessels
- Mortality—28–56%
- If bleeding is from CHA—stent
- Pancreatic inflammation—vascular

Thrombosis of Splenic Vein

- May extend into PV

Imaging Shows

Splenomegaly, gastric varices, splenic vein occlusion

Treatment

- Early acute phase—thrombolytics
- Conservative
- Recurrent UGI bleeding caused by venous hypertension—splenectomy
- Less consequential than in cirrhosis and cancer
- Not recommended are
  - Routine anticoagulation
  - Splenectomy
- If bleeding from varices—left-sided PHT—splenectomy—splenic artery embolization

Bleeding

- Primary bleeding—venous in origin
- Delayed—arterial—due to sepsis

6.3 CHRONIC PANCREATITIS

- A continuing inflammatory disease of the pancreas characterized by irreversible morphologic changes that typically cause abdominal pain and/or permanent impairment of pancreatic function

CHRONIC PANCREATITIS IS CHARACTERIZED BY

- Persistent inflammation
- Irreversible fibrosis
- Atrophy of parenchyma

TIGAR-O classification for chronic pancreatitis					
Toxic-metabolic	Idiopathic	Genetic	Auto-immune	Recurrent and severe acute	Obstructive
Alcoholic Tobacco smoking Hyper-calcemia Hyper-lipidemia Chronic renal failure Medi-cations (phenacetin abuse) Toxins (organotin com-pounds)	Early onset Late onset Tropical (tropical calcific and fibro-calculus pancreatic diabetes) Other	Auto-somal dominant. Cationic tryp-sinogen gene Auto-somal recessive/modifier genes CFTR SPINK 1 Alpha 1 anti-trypsin deficiency	Isolated auto-immune chronic pan-creatitis Syn-dromic auto-immune chronic pan-creatitis (Sjögren/IBD/primary biliary cirrhosis)	Post-necrotic (severe acute pan-creatitis) Recurrent acute pan-creatitis Vascular disease/ischemic Radiation injury	Pancreas divisum Sphincter of Oddi disorders Duct obstruction per-iampullary duodenal wall cysts Post-traumatic pancreatic duct scars

- **M-ANNHEIM—another classification of risk factors**
- **Manchester classification system**
  - Mild pain abdomen, no functional deficit, ERCP evidence
  - Moderate pain, needs analgesics, impaired function, no peripancreatic complications
  - End stage—extra pancreatic features, functional deficit, pain may or may not be present (**burn out**)

Risk Factors

- Heavy alcohol consumption—most common—70–80% cases
- Smoking

Two Hit Hypothesis

- Susceptible patient—hit by acute pancreatitis by alcohol, gall stones, etc.—either the pancreas recover—or hit by another insult—fibrosis, irreversible damage—loss of exocrine and endocrine functions
- Pancreatic stellate cells are major mediators for dense fibrotic extracellular matrix around acini and ducts.

Alcohol

- CP develops in 3–7% heavy drinkers (5–10 Blumgart)
- 70% CP—associated with alcohol
- Usually after 10–15 years of heavy drinking
- Rarely in short course drinking—in puberty
- Critical threshold of alcohol intake daily—40 g for women
  - 80 g for men
  - Regardless of quality or type of beverage
- May be only a cofactor along with smoking
- Cause—fibrosis, atrophy, calcifications
- Alcohol induced—necrosis and pseudocyst more common

Pancreatic Stellate Cells (PSCs)

- Specialized quiescent fibroblasts found at the base of acinar cells
- Once stimulated, PSCs differentiate into activated myofibroblasts
- Which synthesize proteins that form the extracellular matrix (collagen I and III, fibronectin, laminin, and matrix metalloproteinases)
- Inflammatory mediators, such as PDGF, TGF-β, TNF-α, IL-1, and IL-6 activate PSCs
- Ethanol and some of its metabolites (e.g. acetaldehyde) activate PSCs and induce pancreatic fibrosis

Smoking

- Independent risk
- Dose related
- Tobacco—oxidative stress—alters secretion and composition of juice—decreased juice and bicarbonate secretion and inflammation

Calcium

- Central role in trypsinogen secretion and trypsin stabilization
- Hypercalcemia (PTH)—reccurent AP—progress to CP
- Calcium—intraductal stone and protein plugs

Idiopathic

- 30% CP—no known risk factors—idiopathic
- Early idiopathic—in first 2 decades of life
  - Pain predominant
  - Calcifications, endocrine and exocrine deficiency—rare
- Late idiopathic—5th decade
  - Relatively painless
  - With calcifications, endocrine and exocrine deficiency

Tropical Pancreatitis/Nutritional

- Genetic type
- Mutations—SPINK1, cathepsin chymotrypsin C, carboxypepsidase A1

- 45–50%—have SPINK1 mutation
- Severe fibro calculous pancreatic diabetes
- Calcifications
- Pain abdomen
- Pancreatic endocrine deficiency
- Earlier in young—now seen in older also

Causes

- Malnutrition, ingestion of cyanogenic glycosides in cassava
- Exposure to hydrocarbons released by kerosene, paraffine lamps
- Role of malnutrition/cassava toxicity—debatable

Genetic

SPINK1 Pancreatic Secretory Trypsin Inhibitory (PSTI)—responsible for encoding for SPINK1

- PSTI inhibits activated trypsin
- SPINK1—deactivator of activated trypsinogen and malfunction of this induce prolonged action of trypsin.
- Mutation of cationic trypsinogen gene—protein serine 1 (PRSS1) leads to pancreatic enzyme activation—in hereditary CP
- CFTR gene regulate bicarbonate, chloride and pancreatic secretions—mutation decrease juice volume, augment enzyme concentration inside duct

Tropical Pancreatitis Clinical Features

- More in males, 2, 3 decades
- Diabetes seen in >90%
- Calculi in >90%—in large ducts
- Very high association with cancer
- No association with alcohol

Autoimmune Pancreatitis

- Present with obstructive jaundice with or without pancreas mass
- Lymphoplasmocytic infiltration and fibrosis
- Seen in 2–3% of pancreatic resections for pancreas cancer
- Causes painless obstructive jaundice—stricture
- Diabetes in 60%

Two Types

Type 1: Lymphoplasmocytic sclerosing pancreatitis
- In older men
- Elevated IgG4
- Extra pancreatic involvement—Sjögren's syndrome, RA, PSC, orbital pseudotumor, IBD
- Swelling of salivary and lacrimal glands precede pancreatic involvement

Type 2
- In younger, both sexes
- Often absent elevation of IgG4
- Other involvement—only IBD
- Idiopathic duct—centric CP

Imaging
- Diffusely enlarged
- Sausage-shaped pancreas
- Absent ductal dilatation, calculi, pseudocysts
- Most common site—head, distal bile duct
- Inflammatory myofibroblastic tumors

Diagnosis—Type 1
- Lymphoplasmacytic infiltration
- Fibrosis of peripancreatic adipose tissue around ducts
- Obliterative phlebitis
- IgG4 positive

Diagnosis—Type 2
- More challenging
- Duct lumen obliteration seen
- Lack IgG4 positivity

Clinical features	Type 1 AIP	Type 2 AIP
Synonyms	Lymphoplasmacytic sclerosing pancreatitis, AIP without GEL	Idiopathic duct centric chronic pancreatitis, AIP with GEL
Age at diagnosis	Old age, 7th decade	Young age, 5th decade
Gender	3/4th males	½ are males
Presentation	Painless obstructive jaundice	Painless obstructive Jaundice, abdominal pain, pancreatitis
Serum IgG4 level	Often elevated 68%	Normal, occasionally elevated 26%
Extrapancreatic involvement	Proximal bile duct, salivary gland, retroperitoneum—50%	No
IBD, association with UC	Rare	More common
Response to steroids	Good	Good
Recurrence	High (around 50%)	Low
a/w IgG4 related disease	Yes	No
Histology		
IgG4	Abundant (>10 cells/HPF)	Scant (<10/HPF)
GEL	Absent	Present
Lypmhoplasmacytic infiltration	Present	Present
Storiform fibrosis	+++	+

GEL: Granulocytic epithelial lesion

Treatment
- Corticosteroids .6 mg/kg: 2 weeks
- Maintenance dose: Prednisolone 2.5–5 mg/day
- Falling IgG4—good response
- Rituximab—in relapse on steroids

Pathogenesis of Chronic Pancreatitis
Necrosis-Fibrosis hypothesis Comfort etal
- Several attacks of AP—inflammation—fibrosis, duct obstruction—stone formation—further obstruction—fibrosis—CP
- Origin in acini

Protein Plug (Stone/Ductal Obstruction Hypothesis—Sarles)
- Origin of CP in duct lumen
- Eosinophilic proteinaceous plug obstruct ductules—become rich in calcium—due to deficiency of Lithostatin or pancreatic stone protein which are important in avoiding calcification in ductules—form stones and later ulcerations of ductules produce inflammation—fibrosis—obstruction—further calcification—CP

Oxidative Stress Theory Braganza 1983
- Hepatic mixed function oxidases—detoxify and produce waste products like epoxides, free radicals get released into systemic circulation or bile—reach pancreatic parenchyma—inflammation of acini and ductules—fibrosis, calcification also reduction in lithostatin—CP

Toxic Metabolic Theory
- Toxic metabolites of alcohol—accumulation of intracellular lipids and fatty acid ethyl esters—damage acinar cells—inflammation—fibrosis
- Activated Kupffer cells induce fibrosis—similar to cirrhosis

Primary Duct Hypothesis Cavallini—1993
- Immunologic attack to a specific genetic, structural or acquired antigen of periductular epithelium—inflammation—fibrosis—outflow obstruction
- Similar to PSC

Sentinel Acute Pancreatitis Event Hypothesis SAPE—Whitcomb—1999

- Final common pathway of all theories
- Various factors cause membrane and mitochondrial injury and release of cytokines and cause AP and CP and activation of stellate cells—fibrosis—calcification

Sustained Intraacinar Nuclear Factor-κB Activation

- NF-κB activation occurs early in CP independent of trypsinogen activation causing inflammation and fibrosis

Diagnosis

- M:F = 4:1, mean age 40
- Abdomen pain—most common
  - Absent in 15% alcoholic CP
- For steatorrhea—90% exocrine function must be lost
  - Change in bowel habits, bloating if 60–90% function lost
- Fat soluble vitamin deficiency—osteopenia
- Diabetes in 40–80%—develops many years after exocrine deficiency and pain
- Weight loss
  - Initial due to fear of eating due to pain
  - Later—malabsorption
- Exocrine deficiency seen in—80–90% long standing CP

Mechanism of Pain

- Ductal obstruction—pressure
- Periductal fibrosis—ischemia
- Fibrosis—parenchymal compartment syndrome
- Neural factors

Chronic Pancreatitis and Pancreatic Cancer

- 4 fold increase in pancreatic cancer
- Late presentation
- Cumulative risk—nonhereditary CP—2% per decade
- Hereditary—40% by age 70 starting at 35
- More in alcohol CP

4 Scoring Systems

- Luneburg—more complete—US, EUS, CT, PFT
- Mayo clinic
- Milwaukee
- Rosemond—EUS based

Pathology

- Lesions affect lobules produce ductular metaplasia
- Atrophy of acini
- Hyperplasia of duct epithelium
- Interlobular fibrosis

Imaging

- ERCP—still gold standard
- But being replaced by EUS/MRI as the choice

Plain X-ray

- Calcifications seen in 30–40%—in late disease

USG

- In late disease—limitations
- Useful as an early investigation
- Irregular contour
- Duct dilatation
- Echo rich and echo poor areas
- Cysts or cavities
- Calcification

CT

- Dilatated pancreatic duct—most common finding—70%
- Stones—50%
- Atrophy—54%
- Cystic lesions, peripancreatic lesions
- Cannot detect
  - Early parenchymal changes
  - Changes in small ducts
- Optimum slice thickness 5 mm
- Most sensitive to detect calculi in noncontrast phase

Features of Chronic Pancreatitis

- Intraductal or parenchymal calcification
- Lack of obstructing mass
- Irregular dilatation of duct
- Limited atrophy of gland

Neoplasia Features

- Appearance dilatation with obstructing mass
- With associated atrophy
- Vascular invasion, metastasis

ERCP

- Gold standard for diagnosis and staging
- Currently low—used as therapeutic
- Chain of lakes—in late disease
- Dominant stricture—suggestive of cancer
- Multiple stenosis, irregular side branches, calculi are suggestive of CP

EUS

- Can visualize subtle changes before other investigations
- Can detect early changes and late
- More accurate than ERP
- Can't diagnose solely on EUS
- Most accurate in minimal change disease and early disease

Cambridge—ERCP classification of chronic pancreatitis

	Main duct	Side duct abnormality (number)	Other features
Equivocal	Normal	<3	
Mild	Normal	>3	
Moderate	Abnormal	>3	
Severe	Abnormal	>3	Presence of cavity, severe dilatation

MRCP/sMRCP

- Secretin MRCP—can assess duct and exocrine function
- MRI: More sensitive than CT/US—in early disease
- Can detect main duct, stenosis, calculi
- Not so good in visualizing side branches
- Calcifications not well visualized
- Histologic evidence—gold standard in CP
- EUS guided FNAC/Tru-cut—not supported

Tests for Exocrine Function

Invasive—Secretin stimulation test

Duodenal intubation/scopy—inj secretin—measure volume and concentration of bicarbonate and enzymes by 60 minutes continuous aspiration—bicarbonate <50 mEq/L consistent with CP

- Gold standard

Noninvasive

- Stool estimation of fat, chymotrypsin and fecal elastase
- Fecal elastase 1 >200 micr gm/g feces—normal
  - 100–200 mild to moderate insufficiency
  - <100 severe exocrine deficiency
- Fecal fat estimation—100 g of fat per day is given for 3 days—stool content of fat >7 g/day indicative of steatorrhea

Management

Conservative

- To avoid fat maldigestion

Fat digestion affected more due to

- Impairment of lipase synthesis occurs early
- Impaired bicarbonate—acidic duodenum—destruction of lipase
- Proteolytic degradation of lipase
- Extra pancreatic sources of lipase are inadequate
  - Acidic duodenum—precipitation of glycine conjugated bile acids—deterioration of fat metabolism
- So steatorrhea is a major symptom

Pancreatic Exocrine Enzyme Supplementation

- For
  - Weight loss and steatorrhea
  - Dyspepsia, diarrhea, meteorism
  - Pain
- Aim is to deliver adequate lipase to duodenum
- But steatorrhea cannot be totally corrected
- Azotorrhea (protein malabsorption)—can be corrected

Substitution Therapy in CP

- 80% managed by diet and enzyme supplements
- 10–15% need oral supplements (polymeric or semi-elemental diet)
- 5% require enteral tube feeding
- 1%—TPN
- Total abstinence from alcohol
- Rich in carbohydrates, can aggravate diabetes
- 30–40% calories should be from fat
- Medium chain FA used—directly absorbed even in absence of lipase and bile salts
- Enteral nutrition in
  - Unable to eat
  - Weight loss
- TPN—in fistula, GOO

End Points

- Weight control
- Relief of diarrhea
- Decrease in 72 hours fecal fat excretion

Pain-treatment

- Abstinence from alcohol—reduces pain in 50%
- Alcohol—worsens results after surgery
- Enzyme therapy
  - Uncertain
  - Somatostatin
- Antioxidant
  - Anticipate study
- Analgesics
- Paracetamol—NSAID—narcotics—antidepressants

Interventional

- Celiac plexus neurolysis—EUS guided better
- Lithotripsy

Endoscopic

- Stone extraction, dilatations, stenting—have to be repeated
  - Surgery—superior

Recommendations

- Proximal ductal stenosis with no calcifications—two attempts of endoscopic therapy followed by surgery
- Distal duct obstruction, stone—surgery better
- Pancreatic pseudocysts—endoscopic—fails—surgery
- Biliary obstruction in CP—occurs in 10%—surgical bypass choice
- Temporary bypass with stent in cholangitis/malnourished

CBD Stenting

- High rate of obstruction, migration
- So in young with CP—surgery is preferred
- Nonsurgical candidates—can be stented

PD Stones—Endoscopic

- Pancreatic stones are harder—calcium carbonate
- May be upstream to stricture
- "Pseudodivisum"—Ventral PD is obstructed by a large stone or stricture. Access and drainage are achieved through minor papilla
- ESWL to fragment stone or LASER probe
- "Pseudotumor"—small stones in pancreatic head

ESWL: Contraindications

- Extensive stones in MPD
- Multiple strictures in MPD
- Isolated stones
- Ascites
- Pseudocysts
- Pancreatic mass

Surgery: Indications

- Intractable pain
- Symptomatic local complications

- Failed endoscopy
- Fear of malignancy

Drainage Procedures

- **Roux-Y-cystojejunostomy**
- **Lateral pancreaticojejunostomy (Partington-Rochelle)**

Roux-Y-Cystojejunostomy

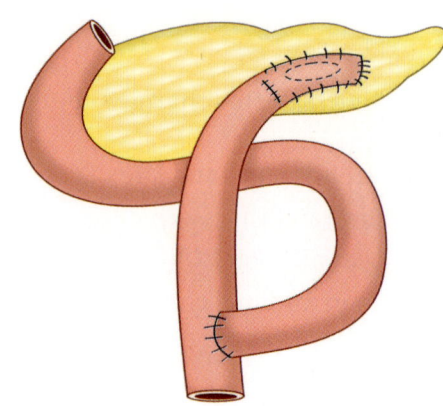

In isolated pseudocyst and following severe AP—procedure of choice

Duval Procedure

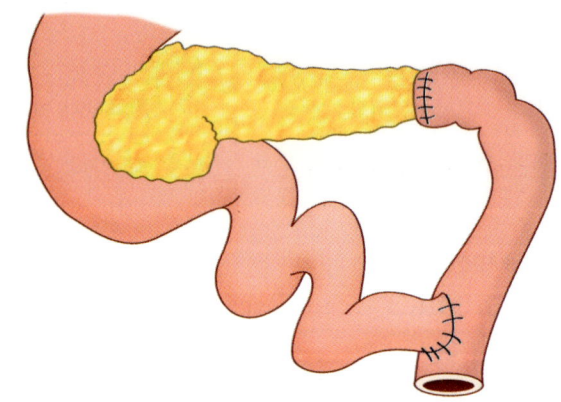

- Resection of tail—PJ at the tail
- Effective only if a single stricture
- Proximal stricture—would not be drained

Puestow-Gillesby Procedure

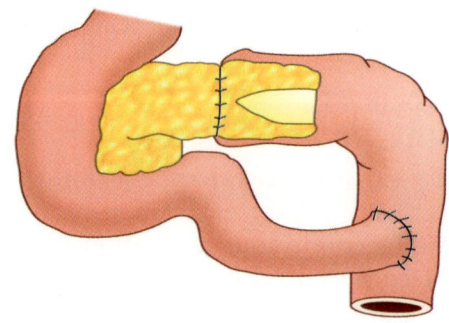

- Resection of tail and spleen
- Longitudinal opening of PD to the right of mesenteric vessels
- Invaginate pancreas in to Roux-en-Y jejunum
- Take care of multiple strictures

Partington-Rochelle

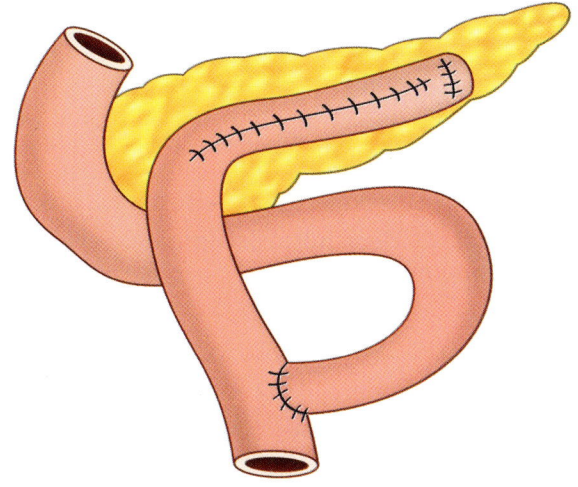

- In dilatation of duct
- No inflammatory mass
- No tail resection
- Lateral—lateral PJ
- Duct unroofed—resected sent for HPR
- Proximally 1 cm from duodenum—distal 2 cm of the end of pancreas
- Conserve parenchyma
  - Conserve endocrine function and exocrine function
- Pain relief—in 80%
- Recurrence 30% in 3–5 years
- Do not alter natural history of disease, it can progress

Resection Procedures

- Head mass—pancreaticoduodenectomy (Kausch-Whipple) or PPPD (Traverso-Longmire)
- **Duodenum preserving**—organ preserving, good long-term results
  - **Frey**
  - **Beger**
  - **Bern**

PD/PPPD

- In head mass
- PPPD—delayed gastric emptying in 30%
- Less reflux, dumping

Duodenum Preserving Pancreatic Head Resection
Beger, 1989

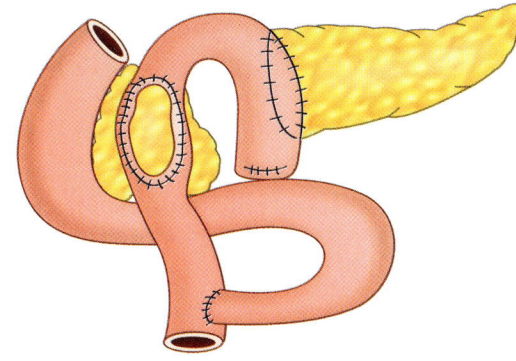

- CP with head mass
- Pancreas divided at the level of PV
- Pancreas head excavated
- BD exposed—in case of biliary obstruction—CBD opened—bile drained into head cavity
- Uncinate process removed
- PJ and pancreaticoduodenostomy to the cored head
- Mortality <1%, morbidity 15%
- Better weight gain
- Better glucose tolerance
- Higher insulin secretion capacity
- Better pain control

Imaizumi Procedure

- Removal of more pancreatic head than Beger including intrapancreatic bile duct—in CP with BD stenosis in pancreatic head

Frey Procedure, 1994

- Hybrid between Beger and Partington-Rochelle
- Head resection smaller than Beger
- Head coring
- PJ—extended up to tail
- Single anastomosis
- Done in less inflammation in head with obstruction to the left side of pancreatic duct

Bern procedure 2001

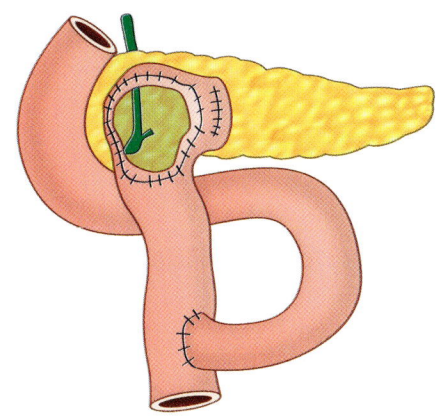

- Head excavation same as in Beger
- Pancreas is not divided—bleeding reduced
- Single anastomosis
- BD—if obstructed—internally anastomosed to jejunum
- Done in inflammatory mass in head—with no stenosis in left-sided duct
- Duct should be probed—if found obstructed may need to converted to Frey or Partington-Rochelle procedure—2–3%

Izbicki-Hamburg Modification of Frey

- V-shaped excision of anterior aspect of pancreas
- In small duct disease
- PD <3 mm
- **No** pancreatic head mass

Segmental Involvement—Segmental Resection/Tail

Left-sided Resection

- In pseudocyst, fistula, isolated left-sided disease
- Spleen preserving
- Stump stappled or sutured
  - Roux-en-Y—PJ if dilated duct, or stenosis in head
- Distal resection—40–60% of gland

Surgical treatments for chronic pancreatitis
Resection procedures
- Pancreaticoduodenectomy
- PPPD
- Beger procedure
- Near total or total pancreatectomy

Decompression procedures
- Duval
- Puestow-Gillesby
- Partington-Rochelle
- Izbicki

Hybrid
- Frey
- Hamburg modification
- Berne modification

Total Pancreatectomy with Islet Cell Transplantation

- CP in the absence of main duct pathology
- Pain relief
- Use their own islet cells—to prevent diabetes

Biliary stricture significant in 6%, more in intrapancreatic portion

Child's Resection

- Spleen, tail, body and uncinate process resected—cuff of head preserved—protects vascularity and bile duct. Done when other procedures fail
- **Duodenal stenosis**
  - In 1.2% of CP
- **Pseudocyst**
  - In 30–40% of CP
- Only 10% regress spontaneously—due to stricture
  - Endoscopic/surgical

Complete pancreatic denervation—**Hirokawa procedure**

Transthoracic/video thoracoscopic denervation for **greater splanchnic nerves**

6.4 NEUROENDOCRINE TUMORS OF PANCREAS

- Pancreas = Sweet bread (Greek) = All flesh
- Endocrine cells—first described by medical student Paul Langerhans in 1869—islets of Langerhans
- Frederick Banting and Charles: Best discovered insulin in 1922—Nobel Prize
- PNET originate from dedifferentiation of an immature pancreatic stem cell
- May secrete more than one hormones

Aggressive Tumors are

Glucoganoma, somatostatinoma, VIPoma, non-functioning
- Features
  - Liver metastasis
  - LN metastasis
  - Local invasion
  - Size >2 cm
  - Nonfunctioning
  - Incomplete excision
  - c-MET expression—malignant
- PNET are vascular tumors
- Appear bright in arterial phase of CECT
- Majority sporadic

Histomorphology

- Adult pancreas contains 10^6 islet cells (1 million)
- Each containing 3000 cells of size 40–900 µm
- Endocrine cells comprise <2% pancreas mass
- Combined weight 1 to 1.5 gm
- In fetus islets comprise one-third of pancreas mass

A, B, D, F cells

- B cells secrete insulin comprise 70% of islet mass
  - Located centrally in islets
- A cells secrete glucagon, located in the periphery—10–15% of islets
- F cells—periphery secrete PP—1%
- D cells—evenly distributed in islets
- D2 cells—secrete VIP
- B and D cells—in body and tail
- F cells mainly—uncinate process
- A cells—evenly distributed

- Arterioles enter periphery of islets—nonbeta—mantle of cells
- Order of perfusion is B cells to A cells and then D cells
- B cells inhibit A cells which stimulate D cells

Islet—acinar axis

- Insulin stimulates exocrine secretion, amino acid transport, synthesis of protein and enzymes
- Glucagon counter regulatory

Embryology

- A cells appear at 3-week embryo
- Organized islets appear by 10 weeks
- B cell formation occurs before birth—proliferate up to first 2 years only
- A and D cells—no postnatal proliferation
- B–A ratio doubles neonatally
- Seven fold increase in B–D ratio in childhood—due to loss of D cells

ACTIONS

Insulin

- Glucose transport into cells
- Inhibition of glycogenolysis and FA breakdown
- Stimulates protein synthesis

Glucagon

- Increase blood glucose glycogenolysis, lipolysis, gluconeogenesis

Insulin

- Anabolic hormone—56 aa…6kDa
- Promotes glucose transport into all cells except
  - **B cells**
  - **Hepatocytes**

- CNS cells
- RBC
- Glucose induce B cells stimulation and proinsulin is synthesized in ER which is transported to Golgi complex and cleaved into insulin and residual C peptide
- Insulin has two polypeptide chains (A and B) bound by disulfide bridges
- Insulin released into blood stream by exostosis
- C peptide and insulin are secreted in equimolar amounts
- B cells are maximally stimulated at glucose 400–500 mg%
- Insulin has 7 to 10 minutes half life
- Primarily metabolized in liver
- Brain cells and RBCs do not take up insulin
- Insulin receptor is a 300 kDa glycoprotein. On stimulation by insulin facilitates entry of glucose into cells
- *Orally administered glucose has a greater effect on insulin secretion than IV*
- Insulinotropic factors called **Incretins**—directly act on B cells
  - Gastric inhibitory polypeptide
  - Glucagon
  - Glucagon like peptide-1
  - CCK
  - Amino acids (arginine, lysine, leucine)
  - FFA
- Humoral inhibitors of insulin secretion—somatostatin, amyline, leptin, pancreostatin

Ghrelin

- Inhibits insulin release
- Prevents glucose disposal in muscle
- Produce hyperglycemia and impaired glucose tolerance
- Inorectic hormone

Leptin

- Inhibits food intake—satiety hormone
- Inhibits insulin secretion
- In obese, leptin resistance occurs but leptin levels may be elevated lead to hyperglycemia

Somatostatin

- Actual function—not known
- Endogenous somatostatin does not inhibit other hormones
- Exogenous—inhibit glucagon, insulin, GH

PNET

- Functional—with symptoms
- Insulinoma 10% malignant
- Glucagonoma, somatostatinoma—nearly 80% malignant
- Malignancy is determined by metastasis
- Poorly differentiated = Neuroendocrine carcinoma (G3)
  - Account for <3%
- Most are well-differentiated (G1 and G2)

Molecular Genetics

- Most are sporadic
- Most common genetic syndrome with PNET is MEN 1

  Due to allelic deletion of TSG menin on chromosome 11q13
- von Hippel-Lindau
  - RCC, pheochromocytoma, inner ear tumors, NET, pancreas cysts
- PNET usually indolent can be observed—until 2–3 cm in size
- In well differentiated—G1 and G2—chromogranin A and synaptophysin—strong positive
  - In poorly differentiated and G3—weak positive

Tumor and pancreatic ductal adenocarcinoma		
Genes	PNET%	PDAC%
MEN1	44	0
KRAS	0	100
CDKN2A	0	25
TP53	3	85
TGFBR1, SMAD3, SMAD 4	0	38
DAXX,ATRX	43	0
Genes in mTOR pathway	15	0.8

- Functional tumors are about 20% of PNET
- >50% of functional tumors located in tail—except gastrinoma

Diagnosis and Management

- History for functional tumors
- Cross sectional imaging to localize
- Evaluation of metastasis

- Nonfunctioning PNET have elevated
  - Chromogranin A
  - Neurotensin
  - PP

Localization
CECT

- Hyperattenuating
- Most PNET can be detected except insulinoma, gastrinoma due to small size
- For them
  - Thinner 1.25 mm cuts, multiphase imaging
  - Vascular blush in arterial phase
  - Less pronounced in venous phase
- Water is used as contrast in duodenal gastrinoma
- Sensitivity—70 to 95% related to size and location

MRI

- CEMRI sensitivity 80–90%
- If cannot be seen with CT/MRI do EUS

EUS

- Sensitivity 90% for all tumor size and location
- Better sensitivity in <3 cm lesions than CT/MRI
- Best in insulinoma
- Small duodenal tumors—sensitivity 50%

Somatostatin Receptor Scintigraphy (SRS)

- Useful adjunct if not seen with CT/MRI
- Sensitivity >80% in PNET, except insulinoma
- Gastrinoma—abundant somatostatin receptors
  - Sensitivity 80–100%
  - Specificity 90%
- Useful in glucagonoma and nonfunctioning
- Useful in liver metastasis except from insulinoma
- Insulinoma and PDAC—do not possess somatostatin receptors
- Cannot show exact location of tumor—only show vicinity
- Gallium 68 labelled somatostatin—combined with PET CT
- Ga DOTA-Tyr3—Octreotide—DOTATOC
- Ga-DOTA Na3—Octreotide—DOTANOC
- Ga-DOTA-Tyr3—Octreotide—DOTATATE

SPECT/CT

- Better sensitivity in localization
- 88% sensitive, 95% specific
- SPECT and SRS—potentially can replace biopsy in recurrence and response to therapy

Angiography

- **In insulinoma** >5 mm
  - Vascular blush
  - Calcium stimulated portal venous sampling
- Secretin test—in gastrinoma
  - Localizes the region
  - Sensitivity >90%
- Very rarely done

Treatment
Nonmetastatic—Localized Preop

- Surgical excision with regional LN
- Head resection, distal pancreatectomy, enucleation
- Most common complication due to soft gland
- Doubtful value of lymphadenectomy

Nonmetastastic—Not Localized Preop

- IOUS—choice
- High resolution—7.5 to 10 MHz—greater depth of penetration
- Islet tumors are seen as sonolucent masses, uniform consistency
- Color Doppler addition—detect vasculature and duct
- If still cannot localize—fully mobilize pancreas—palpate, visualise and utilise USG

Metastatic

- In metastasis—after resection can expect good prognosis
- Low grade tumor 5-year survival >50%
- High grade about 10%
- Liver resection can be done if all the disease can be removed
- If not amenable for resection and symptomatic disease
  - RFA
  - TAC, TACE
  - TARE-yitrium
- Resection has improved survival
- No survival benefit in cytoreduction in non resectable liver disease
- **Chemotherapy**
  - In poorly differentiated tumors respond better

- PROMID study—somatostatin analogue
  - Prolonged survival
- RADIANT-3 trial
  - Everolimus—mTOR inhibitor
  - Sunitinib—tyrosine kinase inhibitor

Liver resection is the choice
- Synchronous resection vs later—depend on complexity
- Metastatic tumor not resectable—still resection of primary indicated
  - Respond better to somatostatin therapy
- Metastasis often does not spread beyond liver
- Recurrence in liver common
- Liver transplant—only metastatic indication

Metastatic Disease, Criteria for Liver Transplant
Milan Criteria

- Age <55
- WD tumor
- Ki proliferative index <5%
- Completely resected primary with portal drainage
- <50% liver involvement
- No extra hepatic disease

Incidental Small Tumors

- Controversial
- If observed—no clear guidelines about surveillance
- Strongest predictors of survival after resection
  - Tumor grade
  - Metastasis

Familial Syndromes

- Four familial diseases
  1. MEN1
  2. VHL
     - Autosomal dominant
     - RCC, pheochromocytoma, hemangioblastoma cerebrum, retinal angioma
     - Cystic and solid tumors of pancreas
  3. Tuberous sclerosis 1/2-mTOR—defects in TSC gene:
     - Hamartoma brain, eyes, lung, skin, kidneys, pancreas
  4. Neurofibroma 1
     - Multiple neurofibromas, pheochromocytoma, sarcomas, PNET pancreas, duodenum

Insulinoma

- Most common functioning PNET
- First reported by Whipple and Frantz—1935

- Whipple's triad
  - Neuroglycopenic symptoms consistent with hypoglycemia
  - Low plasma glucose when symptomatic
  - Relieved by administration of glucose
- Average age—45
- Distributed equally throughout pancreas
- Small—average size 1 to 1.5 cm
- Most are benign—85 to 95% and solitary—curative surgically
- Approximately—10% malignant
- 5% associated with MEN1, they are multiple and more chance of to be malignant, and >3 cm (5–10% shack)
- Most (>80%) are sporadic and <2 cm, solitary

Symptoms

- *Sympathetic overactivity due to hypoglycemia*
  - fatigue, tremor, hunger, tachycardia, diaphoresis
- *CNS symptoms*
  - Apathy, anxiety, confusion, blurred vision, stupor, coma, seizures
- Symptoms worse during exercise and fasting
- Weight gain
- Episodic hypoglycemia—due to intermittent nature of insulin secretion

DD for Symptomatic Hypoglycemia

- Insulinoma
- Noninsulinoma pancreaticogenous hypoglycemia syndrome
- Exogenous insulin/OHA
- Insulin autoimmune hypoglycemia
- IGF mediated hypoglycemia

Diagnosis

- During hypoglycemia—insulin level high
- Measure
  - Plasma glucose
  - Insulin
  - C-peptide
  - Pro-insulin
  - Beta-hydroxy butyrate
- 72-hour fasting
  - Can drink non-caloric caffein-free drinks
  - Glucose, insulin, C-peptide, butyrate estimated every 6 hours till blood glucose reaches 60 mg%—then 1–2 hours
  - Fast stopped when glucose <55 mg% or symptomatic

- 60–75% become symptomatic in 24 hours
  - 95% in 72 hours

INSULINOMA

- Insulin/glucose ratio—0.3 suggestive of—insulinoma
- In obese with insulin resistance—can get 0.3—but not hypoglycemia
- C-peptide >1.2 microgm/mL with glucose <40 mg/dL—highly suggestive of insulinoma
- Blood sugar <45 and insulin >5 microgm /L

Localisation

- US—sonolucent
- EUS—most sensitive 65% cases detected
- CECT thin cut—the choice—hypervascular
  - Can pick up 80% lesions
- MR—sensitivity similar to CT
  - Bright on T2 weighted images
- SRS scan (*only 30% possess somatostatin type II receptors*)
  - DOTA scan—a type of SRS scan—better
- IOUS—can detect 2 to 3 mm tumor
  - Sensitivity 70–90%, specificity 100%
  - More in head lesions
  FNAC can be done
- GLP-1 radioligands (glucagon like peptide) Scintigraphy—better than somatostatin scintigraphy

Localisation and Treatment

- Surgery—mainstay
- Somatostatin—not indicated—no receptors
- Preop glucose, diazoxide (prevents insulin release)
- Enucleation is preferred as 90% are benign
- When tumor is within 2 mm of MPD, and in deep tumors—no enucleation—resection is done
- Distal pancreatectomy, central pancreatectomy or Panreaticoduodenectomy—for larger and abutting pancreatic duct
- If could not localize preop
  - IOUS
  - Mobilize pancreas—palpate, US

Can localize most tumors

- If still could not localize
  - Biopsy from tail—to evaluate nesidioblastosis—if found proceed with distal pancreatectomy

- If could not localize—no blind resection—risk of iatrogenic diabetes
- *Most common complication after insulinoma excision—pancreatic leak*

More after enucleation

- Life expectancy good after benign resection
- Complete excision in malignant
- Debulking in metastasis—may get biochemical cure
- Persistent hyperinsulinism in metastasis after surgery:
  - Somatostatin analogues, though not very beneficial
  - Hepatic artery embolisation, diazoxide
    - Streptozotocin + 5FU
- Long-term medical therapy is indicated in <5% in
  - Unlocalized tumors
  - Unresected
  - Metastatic, unresectable tumors

VIP SECRETING PNET

- Also known by various names like VIPoma,
  - Verner-Morrison syndrome 1958,
  - WDHA (watery diarrhoea, hypokalemia, achlorhydria) syndrome
- Arise from pancreatic D2 cells
- >Two-thirds—malignant
- >70 % have metastasis at presentation
- Lesions—90% in pancreas
- 10% in colon, bronchus, liver, adrenal, sympathetic ganglia
- Most seen in middle aged
- Elevated VIP in young—most commonly due to—ganglioneuroma, neuroblastoma, or ganglioblastoma—not VIPoma
- Usually solitary
- >3 cm
- Located in pancreatic body and tail in 75%
- Easily seen in imaging
- Sporadic in 95%
- MEN1—5%

Diagnosis and Treatment

- Normal VIP—<200 pg/ml
- In VIPoma 225–2000—measured after overnight fasting
- VIP—acts on intestinal epithelial cells—increase cAMP in colonocytes—hypersecretion of fluid—watery diarrhoea

- Profuse, watery, iso-osmotic, secretory diarrhea—most common feature
  - 3–5 litres/day
- Diarrhea persists—despite fasting shows its secretory nature
  - Persists despite NGT aspiration—contrast from gastrinoma
- Hypochlorhydria—due to inhibition of gastric acid secretion by VIP
- In some show hyperglycemia—(25–50%)—due to glycogenolytic action of VIP
- Diarrhea—in 70%
- Hypochlorhydria—in 75 %

Treatment

- Fluid and electrolyte balance
- Somatostatin to control diarrhoea—if not controlled, add steroids
- Formal resection—not enucleation—with LN dissection—the choice
- After resection 5-year survival—68%
- Debulking—no evidence

Glucagonoma

- Rare
- More common in females
- Larger tumors—average size 5–10 cm
- Almost always arise in pancreas
  - Body and tail—65–75%—alfa cells
- Malignant in 50–80%
- Of the malignant—80% have liver metastasis at diagnosis
- Most are sporadic—5–17% associated with MEN1

Clinical Features

- 4Ds—**Diabetes, Dermatitis, DVT, Depression**
- Catabolic, weight loss
- Necrolytic migrating erythema—seen in two-thirds—often appear first
  Intertrigus areas—groin

Due to amino acid deficiency and trace elements
Parenteral amino acids—relieve

- Diabetes—in 75–90%—usually mild

Diagnosis

- Fasting glucagon >1000 pg/ml—diagnostic (normal <100)
- Easily localized with—CT

Treatment

- Improve nutrition
- Amino acid infusion, to reverse dermatitis

- IV octreotide—for catabolism
- DVT—prophylaxis—pulmonary embolism—major cause of morbidity and mortality
- Resection—the choice
- Chemotherapy with—5 FU, Oxaliplatin, Bevacizumab
- Liver, pancreas transplantation—reported
- If no metastasis—5-year survival—85%
- If metastasis—60%

Somatostatinoma

- Very rare
- Full syndrome described in 1977
- Diabetes, gall stones, steatorrhea, hypochrohydria
  - Nonspecific symptoms—rarely diagnosed preop
  - Fasting somatostatin >160 pg/ml—diagnostic
- Diabetes: 60%, Gall stones: 70%, diarrhea, steatorrhea—30–68%, hypochrolhydria 80–90%
- Solitary from duodenum and pancreas
- 85% >2 cm, 75% >5 cm
- >60% seen in pancreas—usually head
  - Remainder—duodenum and SI
- 90% malignant with metastasis to liver and LN at diagnosis
- Rarely seen in MEN1
- But associated with von Recklinghausen disease (duodenal disease) and pheochromocytoma
- 5-year survival with metastasis—30–60%

Treatment

- Surgical resection
- In metastasis—debulking

GH Releasing Factor Producing Tumor

- GRF secreting
- Most common site—bronchus—then pancreas, jejunum, adrenals
- 50% have gastrinoma
- 33% in—MEN1
- Acromegaly and pancreatic mass—the feature
- One-third has metastasis at diagnosis
- Large >6 cm
- CT diagnostic
- Surgical resection—the choice
- Debulking—if not resectable advised
- Octreotide

Other Tumors

- **ACTH secreting**
  - Not resectable
  - Elevated cortisol
  - Debulking/BL adrenelectomy
- **Neurotensinoma**
- **PTH related protein**—most malignant
- **Ghrelinoma**

Non-functional PNET

- 10–25% of all PNET (75% Blumgart)—30–50%—Bailey
- Calcitonin—secreting
- Neurotensin secreting
  - they have little biologic consequence
  - rarely symptomatic
- All PNET secrete neurotensin—tumor marker
- Chromogranin A—correlate with tumor burden—posttreatment decrease—favorable outcome
  - Prognostic significance
- Pancreastatin (PST)—post-translational product of CgA—more powerful marker in surgically managed PNET
- Neurokinin A—less accurate
- Serotonin—elevated in foregut NET 43%
- IHC cannot differentiate them from functional tumors—as they also express gastrin, insulin, etc

Clinical Features

- >5 cm, solitary except in MEN1
- More common in head

Pancreatic Polypeptide Tumors (PPomas)

- Large >5 cm
- >80% malignant with metastasis
- Malignancy more than functioning PNET
- Present with pain, cachexia, pancreatitis
- Sometimes incidental finding

Diagnosis

- CT/MRI
- PP assay
- To differentiate from PDAC—chromogranin A and DOTA scan

Nonfunctioning

- >2 cm resected
- <1 cm with no signs of invasion—observed
- Worse prognosis than functioning

Treatment

- Most in the head—Whipple
- Debulking—if not resectable
- Hepatic embolization, dopamine agonists—reduce PP and chromogranin A
- Everolimus—m-TOR inhibitor

- SRS tagged RT—peptide related RT(PRRT)
- Liver transplantation—reported
- Survival less than functioning tumors
- Ki67 index—most important predictor

	Pancreatic cancer	Non-functioning pancreatic endocrine tumors
Tumor size	<5 cm	>5 cm
CT scan	Hypodensity	Hyperdensity
	No calcifications	Calcifications possible
Chromogranin A in blood	Negative	Positive
Somatostatin receptor scintigraphy	Negative	positive

MEN 1 and PNET

MEN1

- Four gland clonal parathyroid adenoma—94%
- Pituitary adenoma 35%—most common prolactinoma
- PNET—malignant—75%
  - Knudson two hit model
  - Inherited mutation in one chromosome—unmasked by mutation of another chromosome
- Long arm chromosome 11
- PNET seen in 30–80% in MEN1
  - Most common cause of tumor related death
- Seen in younger patients
- More likely to be malignant
- Multicentric
- 50% present with metastasis
- Most common pancreatic endocrine syndrome—gastrinoma—54%
- Insulinoma—**21%**
- Glucagonoma—3%
- VIPoma—1%, GR fomas—33%, somatostatinoma—5%
- PP secreting and nonfunctioning seen in—80%—most common tumor (100%—Blumgart)

Screen for

- Gastrin, insulin, proinsulin, chromogranin, PP, glucagon, serum calcium, sestamibi scan
- Hyperparathyroidism if present—treated first
  - Correction of hypercalcemia—improves outcome of PNET and ZES

- Family history
- May have lipomas

Gastrinoma in MEN1

- 20% ZES have MEN1
- Develop 5–10 years younger
- More in duodenum, multiple
- Metastatic to LN in 85 at presentation
- Tend not to metastasize to liver vs sporadic
- PPI therapy
- Surgery—if appear malignant—rapid growth or new appearance, >2 cm—Whipple or distal pancreatectomy

Noninsulinoma Pancreatogenous Hypoglycemia Syndrome (Nesidioblastosis)

- Excessive pancreas B cell function
- Islet hyperplasia and dysplasia
- B cell budding from and in apposition to ductal structures
- Usually in infants
- Rarely in adults—difficult to differentiate from insulinoma
- Postprandial hypoglycemia—within 4 hours—hallmark vs insulinoma
- 72-hour fasting test positive
- Hypoglycemia with elevated insulin, C peptide and proinsulin
- Diagnosis of exclusion
- Final diagnosis on HPR and clinical response to treatment
- **Treatment**
  - 95% distal pancreatectomy
  - Dietary control
  - Diazoxide
  - Somatostatin
- Seen after RYGB for morbid obesity
- Postulations
  - Obesity induced B cell hypertrophy not reversed after RYGB
  - Inappropriate GF release
  - Persistent altered gut hormonal signalling

Nesidioblastosis in RYGB

- Treatment
  - Continuous glucose monitoring
  - Acarbose
  - Ca channel blockers
  - Diazoxide
  - Somatostatin
- Surgery—pancreatic resection

PNET

- Benign or uncertain behavior
  - Size <2 cm
  - Mitotic rate <2/10 hpf

– Ki67<2%

– Absence of vascular or perineural invasion

WHO grading mitotic index and Ki67
- **Low grade—mitotic index**
  - **<2/10 hpf**
  - **Ki67<3%**
- **Intermediate**
  - **MI 2–20/10 hpf**
  - **Ki67—3–20%**
- **High grade**
  - **MI and Ki67>20**

Postop Surveillance
- Regardless of tumor type—all express—chromogranin A
- In addition to the hormones

Metastatic PNET
- Liver metastasis resection indicated—it can reduce tumor burden by 80–90%
- 20% have LN metastasis at diagnosis
- >10 LN needed for formal lymphadenectomy—improve biologic cure
- Radiotherapy
- Somatostatin
- Transplant
- In metastasis—most amenable for treatment with Octreotide are gluagonoma, VIPoma
- Lesser extent—gastrinoma, insulinoma

Biologic Therapies
- M-TOR inhibitor—everolimus (RADIANT-3 trial)
- Sunitinib—inhibit c-KIT, VEGF

Systemic
- CAPTEM—capecitabine +temozolamide
- Poorly differentiated—etopuside + cisplatin
- Not very effective

NET of Stomach
- Comprise 5% of all NET of GIT
- **4 types**
- **Type 1**
  - Most frequent—80%
  - Mostly in elderly women
  - Chronic hypergastrinemia—due to atrophic gastritis and achlorhydria which induce alkaline pH which is a stimulus for secretion of gastrin
  - <1 cm, involving mucosa and submucosa
  - Benign, nonfunctional and well-differentiated tumors
  - Normal pancreostatin
  - Asymptomatic—detected accidentally on OGD
  - Treatment—endoscopic resection
  - Surgical resection—in recurrent, multiple (>6) with at least one >1 cm and extending into submucosa

Type 2
- Similar to type 1
- Cause of hypergastrinemia is MEN1 and multiple gastrinomas in duodenum and rarely in pancreas
- 1–2 cm, with angioinvasion and involvement of mucosa/submucosa
- Benign or low grade malignant and differentiated
- Pancreaostatin is elevated

Type 3
- Rare, solitary
- Serum gastrin—normal
- Most common symptom—UG bleeding
- Size larger >2 cm and invasion beyond submucosa
- Caused by sporadic ECLomas, not related to hypergastrinemia
- Often with LN and liver metastasis at diagnosis
- Low grade malignant, differentiated tumor
- Gastrectomy + LN dissection and resection of liver metastasis—choice

Type 4
- Large ulcerating malignancy like adeno ca, high grade malignant.
- Size varies and poor prognosis
- Treated accordingly
- Types 3 and 4—poor prognosis
- Types 1 and 2—benign, small arise from ECL cells in the gastric mucosa
  - Grow nodular or linear fashion
  - Endoscopic resection
- Types 3 and 4
  - Are malignant and resection is indicated

Investigations
- Type1 <2 cm—OGDscopy and EUS
- Type 1>2 cm, type 2 and type 3—MRI and CECT for liver metastasis and extrahepatic metastasis respectively
- Somatostatin scan

6.5 ZOLLINGER-ELLISON SYNDROME (GASTRINOMA)

- In 1955 Zollinger and Ellison at Ohio state described
- Gregory and Tracy in 1960—identified gastrin as the hormone responsible
- Second most common functional PNET—most common insulinoma
- More common in men, mean age 38 years
- Sporadic—75%
- MEN1 association—25%
- Approximately 50% of pancreatic endocrine tumors are functional
  - Of these, 50% are gastrinomas
- Gastrinomas—60–90% are malignant with high risk for metastasis potential
- All gastrinomas have malignant potential
- Gastrinoma—20% of all PNET
- 0.1% of duodenal ulcer—have ZES
- Gastrinomas: Most are sporadic
  - Most in head
- >70% of gastrinomas in MEN1 and most sporadic cases are located in D1 and D2
- All gastrinoma should be tested for MEN1
- Gastrin produced by islet cell tumors—not subject to normal stimulation by amino acids and peptides in stomach or gastric distention
  - And not suppressed by high intraluminal pH
  - And stimulated by secretin (instead of getting inhibited)

Clinical Features

Triad

- Acid hypersecretion
- Severe PUD
- Non-beta cell pancreatic tumor
- Tumor produces gastrin—hyperacidity and other symptoms
- Abdomen pain and PUD—in >80%—most common symptom
- Diarrhea—in 65%—in 10–20% only symptom
- Steatorrhoea, esophagitis,
- Weight loss

Suspect ZES

- Recalcitrant PUD
  - DU—most common
  - Jejunal ulcers—suspect ZES
- Diarrhoea—relieved by NG aspiration
- *H. pylori* negative
- Failure to improve after eradication and PPI
- They have very high BAO
- No marked response to pentagastrin—as parietal cells are already maximally stimulated by gastrin

Endoscopy

- Prominent gastric rugal folds due to trophic effect of gastrin
- PUD
  - **Fasting gastrin** level >200 pg/ml
    - >1000 pg/ml—diagnostic
- For evaluation of fasting gastrin—to stop PPI 72 hours (ideal 7 days)
- Two-thirds have value 150–1000 range—equivocal
  - Seen in, chronic PPI use, renal failure, *H. pylori*, short bowel syndrome

Secretin Test

- In equivocal values do **secretin test**
- Gastrin level assessed before and after injection of secretin 2 U/kg (0.4 µg/kg)
- No need to stop PPI or H2B
  - Assessed at 5 minutes intervals for 30 minutes
- Elevation >200 pg/ml above basal value diagnostic of gastrinoma

Calcium Provocative Test

Calcium given 5 mg/kg/hr—rise in gastrin level >395 pg/ml

- **Elevated gastrin + pH <2 in gastric aspirate—diagnostic of ZES**

Excluded Antrum Syndrome

In distal gastrectomy + Billroth II—part of antrum left attached to duodenum is not exposed to gastric acid and thus uninhibited and produce hyper-gastrinemia and shows negative secretin pro-vocative test

Causes of hypergastrinemia	
High gastric aid output	*Normal or low gastric acid output*
ZES	H2 receptor antagonist therapy
GOO	PPI therapy
G cell hyperplasia	Prior acid reducing procedure
Retained gastric antrum	Atrophic gastritis, pernicious anemia, gastric cancer, vitiligo, achlorhydria, vagotomy, renal failure

MEN and ZES

25% of ZES are part of MEN1 syndrome (Wermer)– autosomal dominant

- 10–15% with von Hippel-Lindau—autosomal dominant

Gastrin

- From G cells of antrum and duodenum
- Release stimulated by gastric protein, distension, calcium, achlorhydria, epinephrine
- G cells are not normally present in pancreas
- Pancreatic gastrinoma—from multipotent stem cells

Gastrinoma

- Slow growing
- Malignancy determined by histology and invasion and metastasis
- Metastasis to LN and liver
- Liver metastasis—most important predictor of long-term survival

Biologic Markers Predicting Aggressive Behavior and Metastatic Disease

- HER2/neu expression
- Size> 2 cm
- p16/MTS1 tumor suppressor gene inactivation
- Ki67 proliferative index
- Cytokeratine (CK) 19 expression

Preop Localization

- Pancreas gastrinomas are usually >1 cm
- Duodenal lesions are smaller—nearly impossible to localize preoperatively
- Pancreas gastrinoma localized by
  - EUS 80–90%
- EUS/CT + SRS-better results

Management

- High dose PPI in
  - Preoperative
  - Also in unresectable/metastatic lesions
  - Keep basal acid output <10 mEq/hr in men and <5 in women
  - Somatostatin analogues
- Localisation
  - Gastrinoma triangle—most are localized here
  - CECT/MRI done with—water as contrast
  - EUS
  - Not good if <1 cm and small liver metastasis

Gastrinoma Triangle: Passaro

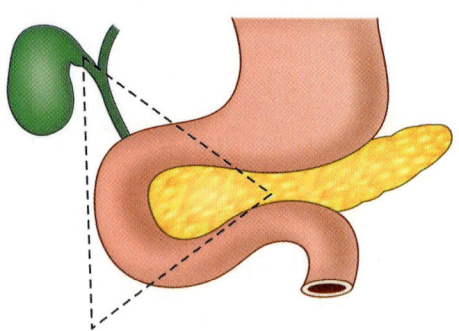

- Superiorly junction of cystic duct and CBD
- Inferiorly junction of D2 and D3
- Medially junction of neck and body of pancreas (SMA)
- 90% located in this triangle
- >60% located in duodenum—most in D1
- Many are found in the duodenal loop—from G cells found in Brenner glands
- Tumors found outside this triangle—worse prognosis
- Somatostatin scintigraphy is done in small tumors which are not detected by CT/MRI
- Radionucleotide labelled Octreotide
  - Detects liver metastasis 85–90%
- CT/MRI detects liver metastasis only—70–80%
- EUS—useful in previous pancreatectomy

Selective Secretin Arteriography

- Cath in RHV
- Inject secretin into GDA, splenic artery, SMA, proper HA

- Can localize depending on gastrin level in RHV
- PET—no localizing role
- PET DOTATOC scan—better than CT and SRS scan

Treatment
- Resection—only 40% cure
- Preop localization not necessary
- If Gastrin level suggestive—surgery—on table localization possible in 98%
- Oncologic resection is done and not enucleation
- LN metastasis in 43–82%
- In MEN 1 after resection gets more recurrence
- Recurrence/metastasis are treated with chemotherapy with Streptozotocin with or without 5FU and Doxorubicin

Pancreas Gastrinoma
- Most in head and uncinate
- In tail—distal pancreatectomy
- Even if tumor is seen in pancreas—duodenotomy is done to look for additional tumors, in MEN1

Surgery
- Kocherisation
- Duodenotomy is a must to inspect duodenum
- Frozen section is done
- Intraop localization—not possible in 5–8%
- Search for entire abdomen, LNs, transilluminate duodenum, palpate. Do duodenotomy
- Duodenotomy detects 25–30% tumors not detected preop
- In MEN1—Whipple—improve survival—prevents local recurrence
- LN dissection improves survival
- 50% show recurrence by 5 years

Unresectable, Symptomatic Metastatic Disease
- PPI 60–80 mg pantoprazole/day—symptom control in 90%
- To keep BAO <10 mEq/hr or <5 mEq/hr, if prior acid reducing surgery done
- Total gastrectomy—in gastric carcinoid
  - Or those who cannot tolerate PPI
  - But has no effect on disease progression

Unresectable, symptomatic metastatic disease: Aggressive form—25%

- Present with larger pancreas tumors and liver metastasis

- 90% seen in pancreas
- 10-year survival—30% (nonaggressive form—90%)
- Best predictor of survival—liver metastasis
- LN metastasis—not predictive

Prognosis
- 5-year survival 65%
- 10-year 51%
- Pancreas gastrinoma worse prognosis than duodenal
- No marker to predict biological behavior

6.6 PANCREATIC CYSTIC NEOPLASMS
- Not very uncommon
- Increasingly recognized these days
- 1978 Compagno and Oertel—distinction between serous and mucinous lesions
- 1982 Ohashi et al described IPMN

Incidence
- Identified in 1% of CT abdomen
- Comprise 15% of pancreatic neoplasms
- SCN, MCN, IPMN comprise 90%
- Mostly in women

Serous Cystic Neoplasms
- Represent 1% of nonendocrine pancreatic neoplasm
- >30% of all cystic neoplasms of pancreas
- Most common in female
- 50%—in head and uncinate
- 5–10 cm in size

4 Types
- Serous microcystic adenoma
- Macrocystic (oligocystic) adenoma
- von Hippel-Lindau associated
- Serous cystadenocarcinoma

Microcystic (Honeycomb)
- Cysts <2 cm, no atypia, mitotic figures
- Clear, watery fluid
- Thin translucent wall
- Lined by glycogen rich cells
- No mucus
- Central stellate/starburst calcification
- Not communicating to duct
  - Oligocystic (macrocystic)
- Cyst spaces >2 cm
- Fewer number of cysts

- More in head and can cause biliary obstruction
- Microscopically similar to microcystic
  - von Hippel-Lindau associated
- Autosomal dominant
- Chromosome mutation 3p25.3
- Multiple
- Similar in nature

Serous Cystadenocarcinoma

- **Very rare**

Malignant SCN

- Extremely rare
  - SCN—are practically benign
  - >4 cm have some malignant potential

Mucinous Cystic Neoplasms

- 40–50% of PCN—*most common PCN*
- 90% seen in female
- Mean age 50 years
- 95% near body and tail
- In perimenopausal women
- Macrocystic
- Cyst spaces >2 cm
- Spherical
- <6 cysts in number
- Do not communicate with duct
- No pericystic inflammation/reaction
- Peripheral egg shell calcification
- Mucinous columnar epithelium
- Ovarian stroma and epithelium—differentiation (*ovarian corpora albicantia*)
- Can have atypia, dysplasia, *in situ* or invasive cancer
- Contain mucin
- Size 6–10 cm
- Epithelium shows immunoreactivity to
  - Cytokeratin 7, 8, 18, 19
  - CEA,
  - MUC5AC
  - CA 19–9
- Stroma cells stain for
  - Estrogen 50%
  - Progesterone—60%
  - Alfa-inhibin—60%

Risk of Malignancy in

- Large tumor size >4 cm
- Associated mass, mural thickening

- Asymmetrically thickened cyst wall
- Eggshell calcification
- Older age
- Symptomatic
- Splenic vein thrombosis

Intraductal Papillary Mucinous Neoplasm (IPMN)

- Intraductal proliferation of mucinous cells
- Form papillae and cystic dilatation of ducts
- Contain mucus—exudes from ampulla
- Comprise 25% of PCN
- More common in males, 6–7 decades
- Devoid of ovarian stroma

Main Duct IPMN (25% of IPMN)

- Dilatation of main duct >5 mm
- Diffuse or segmental
- Usually body and tail
- Adjacent pancreas fibrotic due to c/c pancreatitis

Branch Duct IPMN (50–60% of IPMN)

- From side branches. Cysts >5 mm, grape-like
- Communicate with main duct but do not involve them
- Usually from head and uncinate
  - Adjacent pancreas normal
- Branch duct—larger lesions
- Wide spectrum of changes like—normal, metaplasia, atypia, dysplasia, *in situ* and invasive carcinoma seen in same lesion
- Similar to adenoma—carcinoma in Ca colon

Mixed Type (18%)

In IPMN—papillary changes—5 types
- Gastric type—majority of branched type
- Intestinal type—may develop into colloid carcinoma better prognosis—mainly in main duct type
  - Pancreatobiliary—worst prognosis
  - Oncocytic
  - Null cell

Genetics

- K-Ras point mutations
- Loss of heterozygosity of 9p21 and 17p13
- Overexpression of cyclo-oxygenase 2
- Increased expression of
  - Metalloproteinase-7
  - VEGF
- Increased telomerase activity
- KRAS, p16, TP53 mutations seen in IPMN and PDAC
- SMAD4/DPC4—inactivated in PDAC—preserved in noninvasive IPMN—lost in 10% colloid type carcinoma

- GNAS mutations—prominent in colloid ca
- KRAS more common in tubular ca
- IPMN is a field defect—can develop recurrence or cancer—at remote areas

Risk Factors for Malignancy

- Main duct disease—risk 40–50%
- Main duct dilatation >1 cm
- Branched duct cyst >3 cm
- Mural nodules
- Advanced age >70
- Presence of symptoms—pain, weight loss, jaundice
- Increased telomerase activity in pancreatic juice

Worrisome and high risk features of IPMN	
Worrisome	High-risk
Main duct 5–9 mm	Main duct >1 cm
Nonenhancing mural nodule	Enhancing solid component
Thickened, enhancing cyst wall	Jaundice
BD-IPMN size >3 cm	
Abrupt caliber change in main duct with upstream atrophy	
Lymphadenopathy	
Pancreatitis	

- All IPMN with worrisome features on CT/MRI should consider EUS
- With high risk features—resected

Diagnosis

- Confirm pancreatic origin
- Exclude pseudocyst
- Decision on resection of potentially malignant tumors

PCN: Clinical Presentation

- Incidental
- MCN, IPMN—75% symptomatic
- SCN—50% asymptomatic
- Pain abdomen
- Fullness, mass
- Jaundice
- Symptoms more with MCN

IPMN

- Recurrent pancreatitis
- Idiopathic chronic pancreatitis
- Malignant—painless jaundice, weight loss
- Amylase, lipase—usually normal
- CA19-9, CEA, CA125—limited diagnostic value

MD-IPMN

- Most common—pain abdomen—50%

Mixed Duct-IPMN

- Side branch IPMN—which involves MD which cause dilatation of MD
- Behaves like MD-IPMN

Cancer risk 30–50%—so resected.

Cross Sectional Imaging: CECT, MRI in SCN

- Polycystic—70%
  - Multiple cysts, <2 cm
  - Central 'stellate'/'starburst' scar—in 30%
- Honeycomb—20%
  - Subcentimeter cysts
  - May appear solid
- Macrocystic—2%
- Small cysts
- Stromal hypervascularity
- Lack of metastasis/invasion
- SCN—diagnostic if 3 out of 4 features are present
  - Location head
  - Lobulated
  - Lack of wall enhancement
  - Wall thickness equal to or <2 mm

CECT, MRI-MCN

- Macrocystic and unilocular—80%
- Multilocular—20%
- Spherical
- Do not communicate with duct
- Extrinsic pressure on duct
- Cysts—thick, irregular walls with papillary excrescences unlike SCN
- Lack of perilesional inflammation
- Peripheral eggshell calcification: 20%
- Malignancy suspected when:
  Calcification
  - Multiple papillary structures
  - Wall enhancement
  - Mass/nodules
  - Invasion/metastasis
    - Biliary obstruction, ascites

CECT, MRI-IPMN

- Dilatation of main duct
- Side branch dilatation in head
- Mucinous globules cause—filling defects
- MRI—better to see side ducts
- Malignancy suspicion
  - Main duct involvement
  - Mural nodules
  - Dilated bile duct

ERCP Shows

- Communication with duct
- Little role in SCN, MCN
- IPMN
  - Communication with duct

- Dilated duct with nodules, papillomas
- Invasion
- Copious egress of mucin
- Differentiate MCN from Branch duct IPMN
- Fish mouth deformity of ampulla

Triad of Ohashi in IPMN

- Bulging of ampulla of Vater
- Mucin secretion
- Dilated pancreatic duct

MRCP

- Better to determine duct connection with a cyst
- Side branch lesions—'bunch of grapes'
- Better in cysts not communicating
- Suggestive of malignancy
  - Mural nodules
  - Main duct >1 cm
  - CBD dilatation

MRI

- Better to assess cysts
- To assess relation with duct and to differentiate MCN from pseudocysts and IPMN

EUS

- Through stomach or duodenum
- Can do FNAC
- Determine cyst—duct communication
- Can differentiate between SCN, MCN, IPMN
- Can determine malignancy

PET

- Role in evaluating pancreatic cystic lesions has not been established precisely

Intraductal Pancreatoscopy

- IPMN: 'Fish egg' like appearance

Virtual Pancreatoscopy

- Shows the cyst and ducts

Intraductal US

- IPMN: Branched duct with mural nodules

FNAC

- Under image guidance: CT/EUS
- EUS guided FNAC is preferred
- Aspirate as much fluid as possible
- Viscous fluid—less aspirate
- Less cellular
- Contamination with GIT epithelium
- **CEA in MCN and IPMN → >192 ng/ml**
- SCN:
  - Cuboidal epithelium with glycogen

- MCN
  - Columnar cell sheets
  - With mucin
- IPMN
  - Papillary clusters lined by columnar cells with atypia
- Pseudocyst
  - Cellular debris with macrophages
- FNAC fluid—telomerase activity to determine malignancy

Characteristics	Pseudocyst	SCN	MCN	IPMN
Epidemiology	F = M	F:M (4.5:1)	F:M (10:1)	F = M
Age	50–60	60–75	55–60	65–70
Imaging				
Site	Equally distributed	More in head and uncinate	Head<< body/tail	Head > diffuse >body/ tail
Description	Round, thick walled large cyst; calcification	Multiple small cysts separated by septations with central starburst calcification	Thick walled with septations, microcyst with smooth surface having solid component and eggshell calcifications	Poorly delineated, lobulated polycystic mass with dilation of the mass or branch ducts
Communication with ducts	Yes	No	Rare	Yes
Cyst fluid study				
Cytology	Inflammatory cells	Scant (PAS +, glycogen rich)	Sheets/ clusters of columnar, mucin containing cells	Tall, columnar mucin containing cells
Mucin staining	–	–	+	+
Amylase level	Very high	Low	Low	High
CEA value	Low	Low	High	High

Treatment

SCN

- Conservative
  - Asymptomatic
  - Head lesion
  - <4 cm
  - Unfit patient
- Follow-up by serial imaging 1 or 2 yearly
- Indications for surgery
  - Symptoms
  - Size >4 cm, rapid growth
  - Not sure SCN or MCN

Procedures

- Whipple
- PPPD
- Distal pancreatectomy
- Segmental pancreatectomy
- Enucleation
- No role for lymphadenectomy

MCN

- Potentially can turn malignant
- All MCN better removed
- Regardless of size and location
- Pancreatoduodenectomy
- PPPD
- Distal pancreatectomy with spleen
- If not suggestive of malignancy, spleen preserving
- If frozen section shows malignant lesion, spleen removed with LN

Spleen Preserving Distal Pancreatectomy

Kimura—splenic artery and vein not divided
Warshaw—splenic artery and vein divided, vascularity depends on short gastric vessels.
- Segmental pancreatectomy—if no invasion
- Suboptimal procedures
  - Enucleation
  - Duodenum preserving resections
- Only peripancreatic LN removed
- Malignant MCNs are 'pushers' not 'invaders'
- Frozen section—not accurate
- Cysts may lack epithelium

MCN-Watchful Waiting in

- Small, benign, <3 cm
  - No mural nodules, no BD, PD dilatation
  - Regular follow-up
    - Accepting risk of future malignancy
- Early surgery is preferred
- MCN—malignancy
  - Slower growth than PDA
  - Less LN involvement than PDA
  - Less aggressive than PDA

IPMN: Treatment

- Surgery—choice
- Main duct disease should be resected
- Aim—to remove all adenomatous/malignant epithelium to reduce recurrence
- It is a field defect
- Total pancreatectomy—may be required
- Determined by—main duct or mixed or branch duct
- Branch duct
  - Pancreatoduodenectomy
  - PPPD
  - Conservative if <3 cm

- Multifocal disease (20–30% of BDIPMN): Total pancreatectomy or resection of most significant lesion and follow-up and later surgery—if indicated

Main Duct IPMN

Less controversial
Surgery
- Body and tail (approx. 33%)—DP with splenectomy
  - Frozen section—if positive—'creeping' resection
  - If tumor positive after two resection—total pancreatectomy
- Main duct IPMN
  - Head lesion: Whipple or PPPD
  - Creeping resections with frozen section and total pancreatectomy (5%)
  - Prophylactic total pancreatectomy—unacceptable
- **Risk of malignancy in**
  - **BD-IPMN: 10 to 15%**
  - **MD-IPMN: 30–50%**

Adjuvant Therapy

- In LN and margin positive malignancy
- Postop chemoradiation and RT
- Gemcitabine the drug
- Neoadjuvant therapy—role not clear

IPMN

- Inj. Alcohol, Paclitaxel in unfit patients and in small cysts
- Contraindicated in MDIPMN alcohol—zymogen activation—pancreatitis

Prognosis and Follow-up

- **SCN and MCN** benign and noninvasive lesions
  - Cured after resection
  - Regular CT not necessary
- **MCN invasive lesions**
  - 5-year—15–35% survival
  - CT/MRI 6 monthly for 2 years
- **Nonresectable MCN**—very poor prognosis

IPMN

- Branched duct localized—resection curative
- Main duct may be multifocal
  - Noninvasive—5-year survival 70%
  - Invasive—5-year 30–50%
  - Recurrence very common in pancreas or distant 50–90%
- Can have other malignancies and
- Adeno Ca pancreas

IPMN

- Tubular type aggressive

Poor prognosis seen in

- Tubular, LN metastasis, vascular invasion, positive margins
- **Better prognosis** in colloid type

Solid Pseudopapillary Neoplasms

Other names
- Solid pseudopapillary tumor of pancreas (SPT)
- Solid pseudopapillary neoplasm (SPN)
- Solid pseudopapillary epithelial neoplasm (SPEN)
- Papillary cystic neoplasm
- Hamoudi tumor
- Gruber-Frantz tumor

- Accounts for 5–12% of PCN, 3% of all pancreatic tumors
- Young females—third decade—mean age 22 years.
- Encapsulated, large >10 cm
- Anywhere in pancreas
- Start as solid later cystic degeneration
- Present as large fleshy tumor with cystic areas
- Has a fibrous capsule
- Most common presentation—pain abdomen 45%
- Incidental
- Abdominal mass
- No ductal dilatation

Imaging
CECT
- Large heterogenous
- Peripheral enhancement with central calcification
- Solid and cystic areas

MRI
- Low signal intensity on T1, and high on T2
- Cystic areas—not truly cystic—necrotic areas
- Differential diagnosis—MCN, SCN, PNET
- Under age 30—PNET and SPT likely
- Under age 20—SPT more likely
- FNAC—inconclusive
- FNAC—myxoid stroma, branching papillae
- Cells similar to neuroendocrine tumor
- **IHC**—positive for vimentin, CD10, beta-catenin, neuron-specific enolase

- Positive for progesterone receptors, estrogen receptors—variable
- Positive for—alfa-methylacyl-CoA (AMACR)
- Surgery—curative
- Role of adjuvant therapy—not used routinely
- Most common sites of recurrence—liver, mesentery, peritoneum
- In unresectable and with metastasis—gemcitabine

6.7 PANCREATIC ADENOCARCINOMA
History
- Halsted did the first successful resection of pancreatic tumor in 1898
- Codivilla did the first enbloc resection
- Kaush reported the first successful two-stage pancreaticoduodenectomy in 1909
- Hirshel reported the first single stage surgery in 1914
- Whipple and colleagues reported 3 cases in 1935

Overview
- Fourth and fifth most common cause of cancer deaths in men and women in the West respectively.
- Men are affected slightly more
- Peak incidence in age 60–80, mean age 72 years
- African Americans with slightly higher incidence compared with caucasians

Pancreas Lymph Nodes
- **Regional LN—head neck**—Along CBD, CHA, PV, pyloric, posterior and anterior pancreatoduodenal, SMV and along right lateral wall of SMA
- **Body and tail**—along CHA, CA, splenic A, splenic hilum
- Other LNs—metastatic

Ampulla
- Epithelia lining pancreas duct, bile duct and common channel are pancreaticobiliary type
- Papilla is intestinal type

Adenomas
Adenoma of Ampulla
- Two types
  1. From duodenal surface—similar to colonic polyps, may occur in FAP
  2. Arise within ampulla—intestinal type, similar to colonic

Duodenal Surface Adenomas
- Carcinomas outnumber adenomas
- Adeno ca arise from adenomas
- Many adenoma contain ca
- In FAP multiple—mean age 41
- Sporadic—solitary mean age 62

- Initial symptom—biliary obstruction
- Similar to large bowel polyps—tubular, villous, mixed
- Treated by endoscopic resection and frozen section is done to confirm malignancy

IAPN: Intra Ampullary Papillary Tubular Neoplasm

- More in men in 60s
- Exophytic masses ampulla—protuberant ampulla with widened orifice
- 75% intestinal type
  - Rest have gastro pancreatobiliary features
- In >75% invasive carcinoma seen

Flat Intraepithelial Neoplasia—Flat Dysplasia

- Does not form ampulla mass
- Carcinoma *in situ*

Pancreatic Carcinoma (Pancreatic Ductal Adeno-carcinoma, PDAC)

- >85% Ductal adeno ca (tubular)
- PDAC—most common site—head
- Solid, scirrous, desmoplastic
- Infiltrate locally, nerve sheath, lymphatics and blood vessels
- Undifferentiated carcinoma
  - Anaplastic giant cell
  - Sarcomatoid spindle cell
  - Carcinosarcoma
- Sarcomatoid
  - Osteoclastic giant cell with osteoclast like giant cells
  - Large tumors

Risk Factors

- Obesity (up to 3 fold)
- No clear dietary factors—high fat, processed food
- Increased BMI associated with increased risk
- Occupational exposures, chronic pancreatitis, alcohol, cholelithiasis, postcholecystectomy.

Cigarette smoking (1–3 fold)

- Linear association with pack years
- Risk persists after cessation of smoking
- Most consistent risk factor
- Nitrosamines in smoke—DNA damage

Diabetes

- New onset diabetes—more risk
  - In elderly
  - Having low BMI
  - Having weight loss
  - Not having a family h/o diabetes
- May be caused by cancer
- Long duration of diabetes
- 80% PDAC—have diabetes

Familial Pancreatitis

- Peutz-Jeghers syndrome, familial atypical mole and multiple myeloma syndrome, cystic fibrosis, Lynch syndrome, FAP, BRCA2 mutation
- Most cases are sporadic

Hereditary Risk Factors

- Hereditary pancreatitis
- PJS
- Familial atypical mole and multiple myeloma syndrome
- Hereditary breast and ovarian cancer syndrome
- Cystic fibrosis
- Ataxia—telangiectasia
- These genetic syndromes responsible for 20% of hereditary cancers
- Remaining 80%—called familial pancreatic cancer—with an inherited predisposition—but no genetic syndromes

Hereditary Pancreatitis

- PRSS1 and SPINK1 gene mutation
- Mutation of cationic trypsinogen gene PRSS1—responsible for 80% of hereditary pancreatitis—elevated trypsin activity—c/c inflammation
- SPINK1 gene—codes for serine protease inhibitor—mutation cause hereditary pancreatitis
- HP—50 fold increase—pancreatic cancer

PJS

- STK 11 gene mutation (TSG)
- Higher risk for lung, ovary, breast, uterus, testes cancers
- Pancreatic cancer risk >100 times than unaffected
- More IPMNs

Cystic Fibrosis

- CFTR gene mutation
- >30 times more risk
- Thickened secretions—partial ductal obstruction—c/c inflammation—risk

Familial Atypical Mole and Multiple Myeloma Syndrome

- CDKN2A mutation
- CDKN2A—encodes for p16—mutation causes uninhibited cell proliferation
- 20 fold more risk of PDAC

BRCA2 Mutation

- 10 times more risk
- 10% of high risk pancreatic cancer family (at least two first degree relatives with PC) has BRCA2 mutation

Lynch Syndrome

- MMR gene MLH1, MSH2, MSH6
- MSI also seen on pancreas
- 8 fold increase in PC

FAP

- APC gene
- 4 fold increase in PC

Familial Pancreatic Cancer

- Unknown gene
- 2 or more first degree relatives with pancreatic adenocarcinoma, who do not fulfil any other criteria
- 18 fold increase in PC
- More first degree relatives affected, before age 50—more risk
- Autosomal dominant

IPMN (Pancreatico Biliary, Gastric, Intestinal, Oncocytic)—More Risk for PDAC

IPNB—intraductal papillary neoplasm of biliary tract—equivalent to IPMN-(Pancreaticobiliary, gastric, intestinal, oncocytic)-more risk of cholangiocarcinoma

- **Ampullary ca** more risk in
  - HNPCC, FAP, PJS
- Screening test of choice for familial/hereditary **PDAC-EUS**

Pathogenesis of Sporadic PC

- Mostly sporadic
- A sequential pathway has been observed in development of PDAC
- Pancreatic intraepithelial neoplasia to invasive cancer
- Tumor suppressor and oncogenes involved are PDX1, KRAS2, CDKN2A/P16, P53, DPC4 (SMAD4)

Pancreatic Intraepithelial Neoplasia (Pan IN)

- Pan IN 1A—columnar metaplasia without atypia
- Pan IN 1B—papillary architecture, no atypia
- Pan IN 2—papillary growth to nuclear atypia
- Pan IN 3—complete atypia carcinoma *in situ*
- KRAS 2 oncogene mutation is seen in 95% of pancreatic cancers—initiating event

- KRAS 2 mutation seen in, 87% of Pan IN 3
- *CDKN2A/P16, DPC4—tumor suppressor genes*
- CDKN2A/p16 Mutation in 90% of PDAC
- *P53* mutation rare in Pan IN,
  - But in 79% of PDAC
- DPC4—related to TGF-beta
- Loss of DPC 4
  - 20–30% Pan IN—3
  - 78% in metastatic

Periampullary Neoplasms

- They are group of neoplasms arising in the region of ampulla of Vater
- Rarely cystic neoplasms, endocrine tumours, GIST, sarcomas, lymphomas,
  - Metastases from breast, lung, colon, stomach, melanomas.

Ampullary Cancer

- 20% of carcinomas after Whipple are ampullary
- Intestinal, pancreaticobiliary type or mixed
- Infiltrative clusters at advancing edge of tumor called tumor budding
- Perineural invasion less common than PDAC
- LN also less common

Clinical Features

- Jaundice (75%)
- Weight loss 50–55%
- Abdominal pain > pain can suggest neural plexus, tail lesion, unresectability, poor prognosis (39%)
- Nausea, vomiting (11%)
- Pruritis (11%)
- Fever (3%)
- Gastrointestinal bleeding (1%)
- Courvoisier's sign, Virchow's node, sister Mary Joseph's nodes, Blummer shelf
- Palpable GB seen in one-third of patients with periampullary cancer

Atypical Presentations Like

- GOO
- A/C pancreatitis
- New onset DM
- Anemia

Pathology after surgery
- PDAC—(40–60%),
- Ampulla of Vater—(10–20%),
- Distal bile duct (cholangiocarcinoma)10%,
- Duodenum—(5–10%),
- Benign—10–20%

Diagnosis
- Hemogram,
- Tests for hepatic function including coagulation profile
- Nutritional assessment
- CEA, CA 19.9, AFP may be done as initial evaluation
- Of these, CA 19.9 most sensitive 79%, specificity 82%.
- 10–15% do not develop elevated CA 19.9 in Lewis antigen –ve blood

CA 19-9
- Is a sialylated Lewis A blood group antigen
- Commonly expressed and shed in pancreatic and hepatobiliary disease,
- Not tumor specific
- Elevated in benign conditions of pancreas, liver and bile ducts
- When significantly increased, can assist in differentiating between PDAC and inflammatory pancreatic disease
- Decrease in serial CA 19–9 correlates with survival of pancreatic patients after surgery or chemotherapy
- Debatable as to whether this is useful as early treatment of recurrences have not been shown to improve outcomes
- 5–10% cannot express CA19–9 due to Lewis antigen variability (presence or absence of a fucosyltransferase)

Screening is Indicated in
- First degree relatives relatives
- PJS
- BRCA2
- HNPCC
- EUS and MRI preferred
- Starts at age 50
- In hereditary—before 50

Imaging Investigations
- **Ultrasound abdomen** to identify pancreatic mass, liver metastasis, peripancreatic nodes, etc. but sensitivity less

- **MRI with or without MRCP**—more useful in imaging hepatobilliary tree, MRA in assessing vasculature
- **MDCT**—the choice
  - 3 phase—noncontrast, arterial, portal venous phase
- Oral water, IV contrast
- 3 mm slices
- PC—hypoattenuating lesion in portal venuos phase
- 85% sensitivity
- Pancreatic phase ~45 sec
- Portal venous phase ~70 sec
- Adeno Ca—typically hypodense/intense
- Double duct sign—upstream pancreatic and biliary ductal dilatation
- Periampullary
  - 3 phase
  - 3 mm
    - Coronal 3D reconstruction
- MD CT has 90% sensitivity,
- Accuracy of 93% in involvement of peripancreatic tissues,
- 95% in vascular involvement,

ERCP
- Can do biopsy, palliation
- Doubtful utility in operable cases
- Preop decompression—increase wound infection caused by bacteribilia
- Overall mortality and morbidity unchanged

EUS
- EUS FNAC—accuracy 92–95%
- Better than CT in <2 cm lesions
- Peritumoral vasculature and LN—no advantage over CT
- Better to see venous invasion than CT
- Less useful in arterial invasion

PTC
- More chance of hemobilia than ERCP and EUS
- Same accuracy for HPR as ERCP

MRCP
- For luminal pancreatic anatomy
- Cystic lesions
- MDCT with 3D reconstruction is preferred

PET
- FDG-PET to differentiate between autoimmune pancreatitis and other benign conditions from adenocarcinoma

- Routine use—not recommended
- Useful in liver mass evaluation

Staging Laparoscopy

Periampullary Carcinoma

Adverse Factors

- Size
- Perineural invasion
- Lymphovascular invasion

Resectable Lesion: Head and Uncinate

- Localized to pancreas
- No SMV/PV involvement—no abutment, distortion, thrombus or encasement, or <180 degree contact without vein contour irregularity
- Preserved fat plane surrounding SMA and CA branches, hepatic artery—no contact
- Stage IA to IIB

Borderline Resectable Head and Uncinate

- *One of the following*
  - Severe UL/BL—SMV/PV impingement—<180
  - <180 degree tumor abutment (contact) of SMA
  - Abutment/encasement of HA—if reconstructible
  - SMV occlusion, thrombus >180—short segment and reconstructible
  - Contact with IVC
  - T4 lesions
  - Contact with variant arterial anatomy—accessory RHA, etc

Unresectable: Head and Uncinate

- Metastatic
- LNs outside field of resection
- Ascites
- Vascular involvement beyond described earlier
- SMA >180 degree
- CA >180 degree
- Unreconstructible SMA/PV involvement
- Contact with most proximal jejunal branch to SMV

Borderline Operable: Body and Tail

- Tumor contact with celiac axis <180
- Contact with celiac axis >180 without involvement of aorta and uninvolved GDA

Unresectable: Body and Tail

- Tumor contact >180 with SMA or CA
- Contact with CA with aorta involvement
- Unreconstructible SMV/PV

Laparoscopy

- Detects 30% additional unresectable disease
- Indicated in high risk cases to detect occult metastasis
  - >3 cm tumors (4 cm: Blumgart)
  - Significant high CA19–9 >1000 u/ml
  - Uncertain findings on CT
  - Body, tail lesions
- Clinical indicators of widespread disease—weight loss, pain, malnutrition
- Peritoneal cytology—role unclear
- If positive, behave like metastasis
- Mainly to detect occult metastasis
- For tumor vascular relationship—imaging better
- More advised in distal pancreatic tumor where carcinomatosis is more common

Treatment

- Pancreaticoduodenectomy—the choice
- First described by Kaush in 1909
- First successful resection—Whipple and Parsons—1935—two stage—biliary decompression followed by pancreaticoduodenectomy
- First one stage Whipple-Trimble, et al—1941 John Hopkins
- First step—evaluation of peritoneal surface
- Cattel-Brach—mobilization of right colon exposing infrapancreatic SMV
- Kocherisation—up to lateral border of aorta with clearance of lymphatics on vessels
- RGEV divided, middle colic vein—may be divided

Lymphadenectomy

- Minimum of 12 LN should be studied
- Standard lymphadenectomy in Whipple includes—lymph node stations—8a/p, 12a/b, 12c (gb), 12p, 13a/b, 14a/b, 17a/b
- In distal pancreatectomy—lymph node stations—10, 11p/d, 18
- Standard lymphadenectomy—peripancreatic, portal, pyloric LN
- Extended lymphadenectomy—also hilar, retroperitoneal LN from celiac origin to level of IMA, laterally between two renal hilum
  - But currently not favoured
- Antecolic DJ—may improve gastric emptying

Not Contraindication for Resection

- Tumor size
- Continuous involvement of duodenum, stomach, colon
- LN involvement in the operative field

Preop Stenting in

- Cholangitis
- Level of bilirubin—no clear value
- Long wait for surgery
- Use plastic or covered metal stent preferred
- If naked metal stent used—use short one which does not extent to confluence
- >85% tumors unresectable at presentation
- Biological rather than chronological age should be considered
- Cystic lesions no matter how big—should be resected because there is more chance of cure

Whipple Resection

- GDA—before division—occluded to see hepatic artery flow—in CA atherosclerosis—retrograde flow through GDA from SMA sustains hepatic artery flow
- If so GDA spared or aortohepatic conduit done
- Classic PD—30–40% stomach removed
- PPPD—duodenum divided 2–3 cm distal to pylorus
- Jejunum divided 10–20 cm distal to Treitz
- PV/SMV involvement <50%—resected and closed primarily—>50% grafted using IJV/left renal vein

Standard Whipple Preferred in

- Tumor encroaches D1 or distal stomach and in FAP

Specimen Marked for HPR

- Pancreatic neck margin
- Uncinate margin
- CHD margin

Anastomosis

- PJ duct to mucosa—if duct <5 mm stent placed
  - 6 cm stent is used—infant feeding tube
  - 3 cm inside PD, 3 cm inside jejunum
- HJ—If <5 mm—spatulated
  - 5–10 cm distal to PJ
- DJ/GJ—10–15 cm distal to HJ
  - Retro/antecolic
- FJ—if malnutrition (albumin <3.5 g/dl)

PDAC of Body and Tail

- Worse prognosis than head—late presentation
- Distal pancreatectomy with splenectomy is the choice
- Involvement of splenic artery or vein—not contraindication
- Involvement of celiac artery—contraindication for resection

Appleby Procedure

- Distal pancreatectomy + resection of celiac artery with reconstruction
- Hepatic arterial supply will be through GDA retrograde

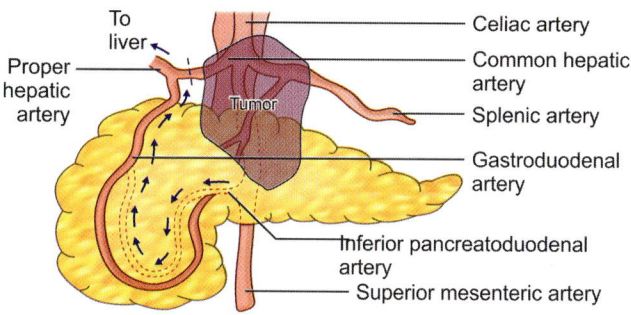

- Retrograde approach—first spleen and pancreas mobilized lateral to medial
- Radical antegrade modular pancreatico-splenectomy (RAMPS)—pancreatic neck divided—medial to lateral approach with lymphadenectomy—LN dissection is reported to be more complete

PDAC: Prognosis

- Perioperative mortality—2% (3–5%)
- Morbidity—30–50%
- After sugery and adjuvant therapy—mean survival 22 months
- 5-year survival 15–20%
- In most patients relapse as metastasis (85%)
  - Local recurrence—40%

In the Absence of Surgery

- Locally advanced with chemo—survive 10–12 months
- With metastasis—6 months

5-year Survival After Resection

- Pancreatic adeno ca—15%
- Distal BD ca—25–30%
- Ampullary adeno ca—35–40% (small lesions)
- Duodenal adeno ca—55–60%

Pathological Bad Prognostics

- LN metastasis
- Poor differentiation

- Size >3 cm
- Positive resection margins

Morbidity

- Most common complication—delayed gastric emptying—5–15%
- Pancreatic fistula—output via drain of any measurable volume after postop day 3, with amylase >3 times
  - Occur in 5–22%
  - Most predictive factor is texture of gland—soft, fatty—more chance

International Study Group of Pancreatic Surgery (ISGPS)

- Delayed gastric emptying—inability to return to standard diet by end of first week postoperative, necessitating NGA
- Grade A—unable to tolerate oral on day 7, requiring NGA on day 4–7—vomiting not seen
- Grade B—cannot tolerate oral by POD14, NGT required on days 8 to 14. Vomiting seen
- Grade C—cannot tolerate oral by POD 21, NGT beyond day 14. Vomiting

Delayed Gastric Emptying: Treatment

- Prokinetics
- Dietary changes
- TPN
- Majority settle

Postop Hemorrhage—ISGPS

- Mild—<3 g/dl Hb drop
- Severe—>3 g/dl drop
- Early—within 24 hours
- Late on or beyond day 5—caused by pseudo-aneurism—formed by pancreas fistula or infection
- Interventional radiology treatment of choice
- **PPPD—mainly to reduce dumping and bile reflux**
- **Non-PPPD preferred**
- Duodenal involvement
  - Duodenal vascular compromise
  - Pasireotide—11 hours half life
  - Role of somatostatin analogues
  - Blocks somatostatin receptors subtypes 1, 2, 3 and 5
  - Lowers fistula occurrence
- Octreotide
  - Blocks receptors 2 and 5
  - Half life 2 hours

Adjuvant Therapy

GISTG-GI Tumor Study Group

- Adjuvant 5FU with 40 Gy RT
- Showed survival advantage

ESPAC-1—European Study Group for Pancreatic Cancer

- Adjuvant CRT (5FU, 20 Gy RT) vs Chemo vs observation
- Chemo was better

Charite Onkologie (CONKO-001)

- Used Gemcitabine—improved survival

RTOG 97-04 RT Oncology Group

- Compared 5FU and Gemcitabine before and after 5 FU based CRT
- Gemcitabine found to be better

ESPAC-3

- 5 FU vs Gemcitabine after curative surgery
- Gemcitabine found to have less toxicity, better compliance

ESPAC-4

- Gemcitabine + capecitabine—better survival

Others

- Folfirnox-5FU, irinitecan, leucovrin, oxaliplatin
- Nab-paclitaxel-Gemcitabine + albumin bound paclitaxel
- No long-term results

Current Recommendation

- Gemcitabine or 5 FU alone or in combination with 5 FU based CRT after surgery

Neoadjuvant

- In borderline resectable
- SMV/PV—>180 degree
- Short segment encasement
- HA, SMA abuttment <180 degree
- In others neoadjuvant indication—unsettled

In metastasis

- >80% present with metastasis
- Gemcitabine Vs Folfirinox (folinic acid, 5FU, Irinotecan, Oxaliplatin)
- Folfirinox has better and progression free survival
- Erlotinib—EGFR antibody + gemcitabine
- VEGFR—bevacizumab
- EGFR—cetuximab

Palliation

Jaundice

- ERCP stenting
- Percutaneous stenting
- Surgical HJ, CCJ
- No clear difference in superiority between operative and endoscopic palliation

GOO

- 20 % develop (15%—bailey)
- Stenting/GJ
- Pain—opioids, celiac ganglion block
- 3 ml .25 bupivacaine + 10 ml absolute alcohol
- Most patients for HJ may undergo GJ also—without added morbidity
- If stent placed for GOO and jaundice—biliary one is placed first

Recurrence

- Typically within 1 year
- Most common sites
  - Retroperitoneum (57%)
  - Liver 51%
  - Peritoneum 35%
  - Lung 15%

Pancreatoblastoma

- Most common malignant pancreatic tumor in children
- <8 years of age
- Associated with Beckwith-Wieldmann syndrome and AFP
- SMAD4 and CTNNB1 mutations seen
- No KRAS mutation
- Predominantly acinar tumors
- Squamoid nest (morules)—typical pathology
- Can have acinar, ductal, NEC differentiation—acinar most common
- Malignant 5-year survival: 25%

Pancreatic Cancer—Duodenal Adenocarcinoma

- Represent 0.3% of GI malignancies
- Represent 25–45% of SI tumors (length represents 10% of total length of SI)
- 50% occur near ampulla
- 50% present with pain abdomen, GOO
- Present as circumferential—napkin ring type lesions

Risk Factors

- FAP
- Gardner's syndrome
- PJS

Treatment

- Endoscopic in superficial lesions
- Invasive ca—Whipple
  - Segmental resection-depend on proximity to ampulla
- Minimum 15 LN removed

- Most powerful independent predictor—perineural invasion
- Recurrence—locoregional—20–40%

6.8 UNUSUAL PANCREATIC TUMORS

Acinar Cell Carcinoma

- Account <1% of pancreatic cancers
- Arise from acinar elements—not duct
- So retain exocrine properties—secrete enzymes—trypsin, chymotrypsin, lipase
- M:F = 2:1
- 6–7 decades
- 50%—asymptomatic
- 10% have paraneoplastic syndrome—due to enzymes (lipase hypersecreting syndromes)
  - Subcutaneous fat necrosis
  - Bony infarcts
  - Arthritis
  - Eosinophilia
- No specific serum markers
- S. lipase elevated in 25%
- CA 19–9. CEA, AFP—variable
- S lipase and AFP are equally helpful

Imaging—CECT

- Large solitary—7–10 cm
- Head 47%, tail 47%, neck 3%, uncinate 3%
- Exophytic circumscribed mass, capsular enhancement
- No PD and BD dilatation
- FNAC can distinguish from PDAC
- Difficult to differentiate from PNET and pancreatoblastoma
  - Need IHC-synaptophysin and chromogranin A to differentiate
- Acinar cell carcinoma—stain negative for CEA and mucicarmine

Acinar Cell Adenoma

- Always cystic
- Solid—more carcinomas
- Better prognosis than PDAC—5-year 40%
- Can have NEC cells
- If NEC cells >25 % of tumor—called mixed acinar-neuroendocrine carcinoma
- If >25% ductal elements—mixed ductal acinar carcinoma

Treatment

- Well circumscribed—amenable to resection
- Distant recurrence more common—liver and lung

- Adjuvant gemcitabine
  - Less responsive than PDAC
  - Combination with oxaliplatin, irinotecan—better response

Primary Pancreatic Lymphoma

- NHL—most common DLBCL
- Represent <0.5% of pancreatic tumors
- And <2% of extranodal lymphomas
- No specific biochemical markers
- Elevated LDH and beta 2 macroglobulin with normal CA 19–9

Imaging

- Large mass head of pancreas
- No ductal dilatation
- Extensive LN involvement
- Vascular involvement—very rare
- CT—low attenuation, minimal enhancement
- PET avid—uptake—focal, nodular or segmental

Diagnosis

- On core biopsy
- CD20, leucocyte core antigen positive
- Flow cytometry

Treatment

- Chemo—CHOP, RCHOP, CVP, MACOP-B

Metastatic Tumors

- Represent <2% of malignant lesions
- RCC—most common tumor—40% and most amenable for resection
- Synchronous in 20–30%
- Metachronous in 40%
- Can happen many years later
- No relation with site of primary and location of metastasis in pancreas
- 34% have extra pancreatic metastasis
- Some form metastasis in pancreas in the absence of other metastasis—RCC—most common
  - Lymphoma
- RCC—polypoid ampullary lesion—may even grow inside ducts
- Most commonly resected metastasis—RCC
- Symptomatic—worse prognosis
- CECT—enhancing (RCC)—lesions
- Multifocal

In Metastasis from RCC

- LN metastasis 10–30%
- Multifocality 60–70%
- Synchronous have worse prognosis
- Resection preferred over enucleation

Imaging

- CT—hypervascular with central low attenuation in arterial phase—similar to PNET
- Biopsy usually not needed—but if want exclude PNET

Treatment—isolated—surgery—RT

Pearls

- Acini constitute most of the organ
- Ducts—most of the neoplasm
- At least 12 LN should be identified in Whipple specimen—most on pancreas and p-d grove
- In pancreaticoduodenectomy, most important margin retroperitoneal margin also termed uncinate, SMV, or vascular margin
- Low grade Pan IN—common in normal population—presence does not need any further evaluation
- Pan IN 3—associated with PDAC—should be evaluated

Paraduodenal pancreatitis, groove pancreatitis, cystic dystrophy of heterotopic pancreas

- Men 50s
- Mucosal irregularity proximal to ampulla—inflamed mucosa—pseudotumors—centered around minor papilla—between CBD, duodenum and pancreas—groove region
- Some may form duodenal cysts—paraduodenal cyst—mimic pseudocyst

6.9 PANCREATIC TRANSPLANTATION

- First transplantaion—William Kelly and Richard Lillehei—1966

Patient Selection

- Type 1 diabetics with C peptide deficiency
- SPK: Simultaneous pancreas and kidney—80% done this way
- PTA—pancreas transplant alone—in non-uremic with brittle diabetes—in 5%
- PAK—pancreas after kidney—15%
- Patients with minimal secondary complications are the candidates for PT

- PTA—need good renal function
  - PTA is an independent risk factor for renal failure
- PAK—may be from different donors
- SPK—done in type 2 diabetes also
  - Criteria for SPK in T2DM
    - Insulin therapy and C peptide <2 ng/ml or
    - Insulin therapy with C-peptide >2 ng/ml and BMI <28

Donor

Contraindications

- Type 1 DM
- Relative—contraindication
  - Previous disorder/procedure on pancreas
  - Chronic pancreatitis
  - IPMN
- Hyperglycemia—not a contraindication

Donor should be

- Neither fatty nor edematous
- Donation after cardiac death—DCD—warm ischemia time 45 minutes
- Younger, leaner hemodynamically stable deceased
- Liver and pancreas dissected together
- Spleen is retained—to act as a handle to minimize manipulation of gland
- Duodenum is flushed with povidone iodine solution
- Heparinize: Abdominal aorta ligated at bifurcation
- Liver is perfused via IMV—perfused with UWS at 4 degree
- Liver is dissected first
- Pancreas—duodenum divided—to avoid any gastric tissue
- Done in ice cold saline
- Spleen removed
- Has two arterial source—body and tail via splenic artery, head from branches of SMA
- SMA is divided close to origin from aorta
- Splenic artery divided at origin—rest of the celiac axis retained with liver
- Arterial reconstruction using donor iliac artery—bifurcated Y graft—IIA joined to splenic artery, EIA to SMA
- CIA of donor—to recipient iliac artery
- PV is divided 1 cm cephalad to pancreas

- In replaced RHA from SMA—SMA with carrels patch of aorta remains with liver—distal SMA for pancreas

Recipient

- Exocrine drainage—duodenum to bladder or intestine
- Bladder—easy to monitor amylase—but can cause cystitis, hematuria
- Preferred enteric drainage—to jejunum directly side to side or into a jejunun Roux-Y
- Venous drainage—into PV or systemic circulation—into iliac vein or IVC
  - Systemic—preferred

Locations

- Based on type of venous drainage
- Pelvis on right side for systemic drainage—donor PV anastomosed to EIV, IIV or IVC
- Pelvis—duodenum oriented in inferior position for bladder drainage—superior for enteric drainage
- Mid-abdomen for PV drainage—PV of donor to major branch of SMV found in small bowel mesentery—end to side manner
- Venous drainage may be to PV or systemic vein but arterial anastomosis always to CIA or EIA end to side
- Most common enteric drainage—in 80%
  - Most common systemic venous drainage—in 90%

Complications

- Major—technical
- Thrombosis—5–10%
- Pancreatitis in 10–20%—reperfusion injury. Managed non surgically with octreotide
- Anastomotic leak in bladder anastomosis may be managed with Foley's
- Enteric anastomosis leak may need surgery

Rejection—Indicators

- Elevated serum amylase, lipase, low urine amylase in bladder drainage, tenderness over allograft, biopsy
  - Hyperglycemia—a late feature—once develop—pancreas unsalvageable
- Total amount of immunosuppression in pancreas transplant—highest of any solid organ transplant
- SPK has highest graft survival
- Euglycemia develops
- Retinopathy, neuropathy and nephropathy—slows down/improves

Living Donor

- Ideal with identical twins
- Splenic artery and vein—to EIA and EIV
- Duct to bladder/bowel

Pancreatic Islet Transplantation

- Islet auto transplantation
  Total pancreatectomy in chronic pancreatitis—infusing the pancreatic digest/islet into PV
- Need islets from multiple donors for a single recipient
- Loss of islet cell mass after engraftment occur
- Most may eventually need insulin
- Beneficial to patients with type 1 DM and hypoglycemia unawareness
- Aim
  - Not insulin independence
  - But reduction of hypoglycemic events
    - Insulin requirements reduction
    - Amelioration of HbA1c

Edmonton Protocol

- Transplanting large number of islets—>10000/kg
- Islet sparing immunosuppression—steroid free, with low dose tacrolimus and IL-2 antibody induction

Preparation

- Pancreas is dissociated during enzymatic digestion with collagenase—islets are separated from acinar tissue during gradient purification—islets are cultured for 72 hours—infused
- Human pancreas contain 1 million islets—half are lost during isolation
- About 10000 islets/kg of weight needed for insulin independence—need many donors

Complications

- Most feared—bleeding (20%) and PV thrombosis (<1%)
- Injection done transhepatic—PV by interventional radiologist
- Mini lap—isolate a small mesenteric vein—guide the catheter into PV—can ligate the vein to reduce bleeding

Future

- Living donor—high morbidity for donor
- Xenografts

Small Intestine

7.1 ANATOMY

- **Largest endocrine organ**

Embryology

- Primitive gut is formed from endodermal lining, the yolk sac. Endodermal layer gives rise to epithelial lining of intestine
- Splanchnic mesoderm surrounding the endoderm form the muscular and all other layers of intestine, and also mesentery
- Nerves and neurons on the wall are derived from neural crest
- All small intestine is derived from midgut except duodenum
- Herniation of midgut occurs through umbilicus—5th week
- Loop divided by vitello intestinal duct into cranial and caudal
- Cranial limb form distal duodenum, jejunum, proximal ileum
- Caudal limb form distal ileum, cecum, ascending colon and proximal two-thirds of transverse colon
- Vitello intestinal duct—obliterates before birth
- In 2%—persist as Meckel's
- Endodermal proliferation causes occlusion of the lumen—5th week
- Mesodermal expansion and apoptosis of endoderm produces recanalization of tube starts at 7th week
- Recanalization—complete by 9th week
- Intestines return to abdominal cavity—by 10th week, undergo 270° rotation
- Jejunum placed in left upper quadrant
- Cecum enters last—initially RUQ and later shift to RLQ
- Primitive SI—lined by cuboidal cells
- Villi begin to form by 9th week—proceed caudally even in colon
- Crypt formation by 10–12th week
- Crypt layer—site of continual cell renewal

- **Crypt cells ascend and differentiate into 4 cell lines**
  - Absorptive enterocyte—95% on int cell population
  - Goblet cells
  - Paneth cells
  - Entero-endocrine

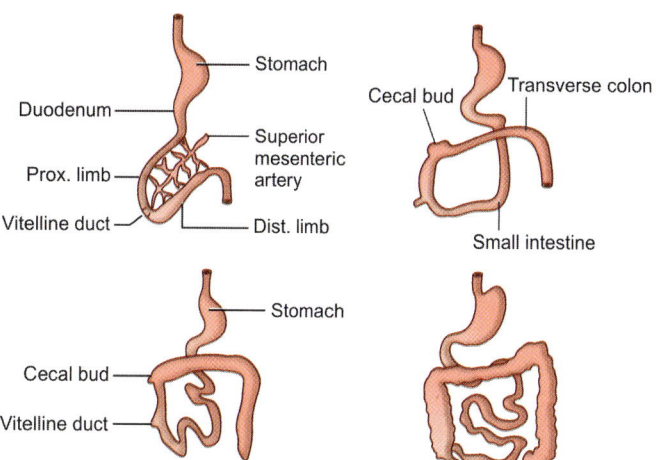

- Paneth cells remain in crypt base-protect intestinal stem cells by maintaining homeostasis
- Other cells ascend the crypt—villous axis and eventually are extruded
- Epithelial cell turns over except for Paneth cells are 3–5 days

Small Intestine—Gross Anatomy

- Length—300–850 cm
- Duodenum—25 cm
- No demarcation between jejunum and ileum
- Proximal two-fifths represent jejunum, distal three-fifths—ileum "Shirt sleeve felt through a coat sleeve"—the feeling on palpating jejunal wall. This is due to the thick wall of jejunum, the mucus membrane can be felt through the muscle wall. The wall of ileum is thin, so feels as single layer.

Duodenum

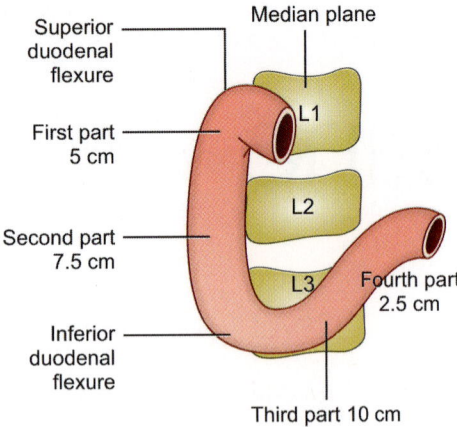

- Root of mesentery attachment—to the posterior abdominal wall to the left of L2 obliquely to the right inferiorly to right SI joint
- Artery: SMA
- Veins follows
- **Nerves**—parasympathetic—through vagus—secretory function
- Sympathetic from plexus around SMA which causes pain

Characteristic	Jejunum	Ileum
Color	Deeper red	Paler pink
Caliber	2–4 cm	2–3 cm
Wall	Thick and heavy	Thin and light
Vascularity	Greater	Less
Vasa recta	Long	Short
Arcades	A few large loops	Many short loops
Fat in mesentery	Less	More
Circular fold (L. plica circulares)	Large, tall and closely packed	Low and sparse; absent in distal part

Microscopic Anatomy

- Serosa—consists of visceral peritoneum—single layer mesothelium
- Muscularis propria—outer longitudinal—thin, inner circular—thick
- Ganglion cells of myenteric plexus of Auerbach between muscle layers
- Submucosa—fibroelastic connective tissue
  - Contain vessels, lymphatics and nerves—Meissner's plexus
  - Strongest layer used for anastomosis
- **Mucosa**

  Muscularis mucosa

  Lamina propria—connective tissue layer
  - Contain plasma cells, macrophages, fibroblasts

- Protective role against microorganisms that penetrate the epithelium—immune function
- Plasma cells secrete—immunoglobulins
- **Epithelium**—continual sheet of cells
  - Crypt—main function is renewal,
  - Also exocrine and endocrine functions and water and ion secretion
  - Villous epithelium helps in digestion and absorption
- 4 cells in mucosa
  - Absorptive enterocytes
  - Goblet cells secrete mucin
  - Paneth cells—secrete lysozyme and cryptidins for defense
  - Entero-endocrine cells secrete GI hormones
- Villi—tallest near distal duodenum and proximal jejunum
  - Shortest—in distal ileum
- Absorptive enterocytes covered by microvilli—increase area by 30-fold
- Microvilli covered by fuzzy coat of glycoprotein—glycocalyx—further increase in absorptive area

Digestion and Absorption

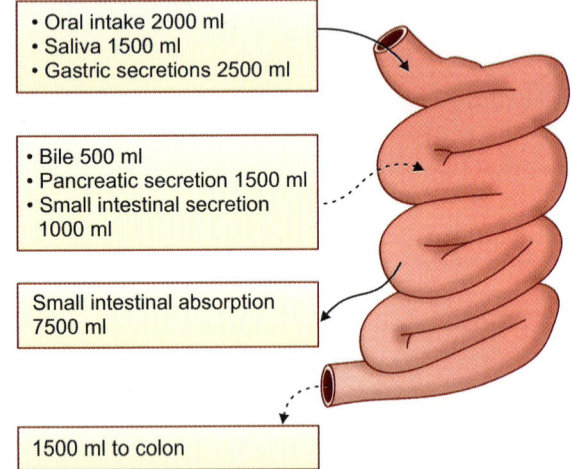

- Liters of fluid and many hundreds of grams of food reach small intestine
- Stomach breaks down particles to 1 mm or smaller
- SI is primarily responsible for absorption of carbohydrates, fat and proteins, ions and water

Carbohydrates

- In Western diet—300–350 gm
- 50% starch, 30% sucrose, 6% lactose. Rest maltose, fructose, sorbitol, etc.

- Starch-polysaccharide with long chains of glucose. Starch contains amylose and amylopectin
  - Amylose—20%—amylase splits it into maltose and maltotriose
  - Amylopectin—80%—amylase splits this into maltose, maltotriose and residual branch saccharides (dextrins)
- Starch—almost totally converted to maltose and other polymers before they pass duodenum and proximal jejunum
- Remaining digestion by brush border enzymes

Carbohydrates: Brush Border Enzymes

- Split disaccharides to monosaccharides
- Glucose—>80% end product of digestion
- Galactose and fructose—10%

3 Transporter Systems

- Sodium-glucose transporter-1 (SGLT-1)
  - Co-transport with Na
  - It is an active transport
  - Glucose and galactose are transported
- Glucose transporter-5 (GLUT-5)
  - Not sodium or energy dependent
  - Fructose is transported
- GLUT-2: Located at basolateral membrane helps in exit of glucose from cytosol into intracellular space
- Transport across intestinal epithelium

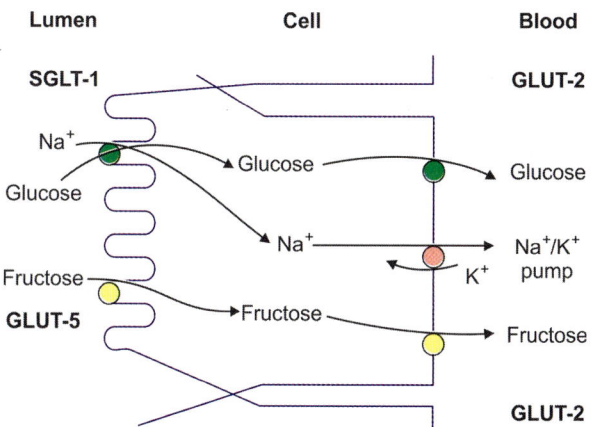

Protein

- Digestion is initiated in stomach—acid denatures protein
- Pancreatic trypsinogen is inactive. Duodenal brush border enzyme enterokinase—activate it to trypsin
- Activated trypsin—activate other enzymes like trypsin, elastase, chymotrypsin
- Produce peptides and smaller proteins which are acted upon upon by carboxy peptidases—split to produce di and tripeptides
- Absorbed by Na mediated active mechanism

- Peptidase enzymes in cells and brush border—further split and generate dipeptides and amino acids and pass into portal system
- 80–90% digestion and absorption completed in jejunum
- 70% absorbed as amino acids

Areas of Absorption

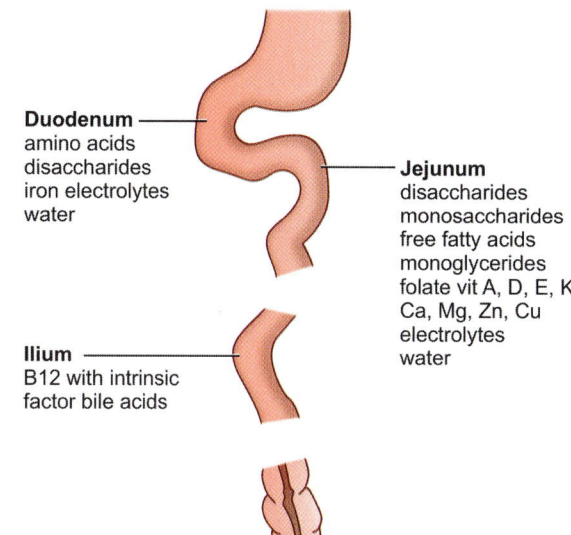

Endocrine Function of SI

- Function as endocrine, autocrine, paracrine and as neurotransmitters
- Signal through G protein—coupled group of receptors found in the body
- Other receptors
  - EGFR, IGFR, Fibroblast GFR, PDGFR
- Some peptides act as neurotransmitters

Immune Function

3 Areas

- Peyer's patches
  - Lamina propria lymphoid cells
- Intraepithelial lymphocytes

Peyer's Patches

- Unencapsulated lymphoid nodules—constitute the afferent limb of gut associated lymphoid tissue—contain microfold (M) cells—recognize antigens—activate B and T cells. Activated lymphocytes then migrate to lymph nodes and then to lamina propria.
- B lymphocytes become IgA
- 60% are T cells
- 40% B cells
- Major immune mechanism—IgA
- SI contains >70% of IgA producing cells in the body

- IgA is produced by plasma cells in lamina propria—secreted into intestine
- IgA—prevents bacterial colonization and adherence to epithelial cells
  - Neutralizes bacterial toxins
  - Neutralizes viral activity
  - Blocks absorption of antigens from gut
- IgA—does not destroy infective organisams or antigens

7.2 SMALL BOWEL NEOPLASMS

- Small bowel—75% of length and 90% surface area of GIT
- Both benign and malignant tumors are rare
- Can arise from epithelium, neural tissues, lymphatics and mesenchymal cells or metastases
- Number of LNs to be examined for optimum staging
  - Nonampullary duodenal ca—5 LNs
  - SI cancer—at least 9 LN

Epidemiology

- <5% of GI tumors are small intestinal
- <2% of malignant GI tumors
- 5-year survival is 80%—with local disease
  - With regional and distal metastasis—survival reduces
- Benign are asymptomatic and most are distally located
- Among symptomatic cases—75% are malignant
- More than 40 histological types are present in malignant, 95% are either adenocarcinoma, carcinoid, lymphoma or GIST.
- Most common benign tumors—stromal tumors and adenoma
- Benign more common in distal SI
- Most common malignant tumor—adenocarcinoma constitute 30–50% of malignant SI tumors
- NET—25 to 30%
- Adenocarcinoma more common in proximal SI
- Other malignant tumors more common—distal SI

Protective factors

- High levels of benzopyrene hydroxylase + folate receptors
- Low bacterial load
- Fast transit time
- High cellular turnover
- Liquid and alkaline medium
- Safe stem cells
- Immune protection—IgA

Risk factors

- FAP
- HNPCC
- Peutz-Jeghers syndrome
- MUTYH associated polyposis
- Other genetic conditions: Gardner syndrome, von Recklinghausen syndromes, cystic fibrosis
- Crohn's disease
- Celiac disease
- Immunosuppression
- Other malignancies
- Smoking
- Alcohol (>80 g/day)
- Red meat
- Salted food

Genetics

- KRAS
- APC gene (5q)
- P53 (17q)
- DCC (18q)
- DPC4 (SMAD4)
- MSI-H—associated with celiac disease—CpG methylation—links celiac disease to cancer

Clinical Features

- Usually vague
- Anorexia, dyspepsia
- Pain abdomen—due to obstruction—most common symptom—intussusception in benign
- Bleeding next common—hematochezia or hematemesis
- Most are asymptomatic

Diagnosis

- Need high index of suspicion
- Correct preop diagnosis made only in 50% of symptomatic
- Upper GI series with follow through—diagnosis in 50–80% of malignant tumors
- CT enteroclysis has 95% accuracy
- MRI enteroclysis has 98% sensitive and 97% specific
- UGI scopy and colonoscopy
- Enteroscopy—push type

– Double balloon enteroscopy can be done. With this, preoperative tattooing can be done and is associated with high rate of perforation
- X-ray abdomen is useful in obstruction
- CT abdomen can detect extraluminal tumors and help in staging
- Angiography useful in vascular tumors

Benign Tumors

- Most common tumors reported in autopsy—adenomas
- Most common benign tumors producing symptoms—stromal tumors
- When a benign tumor is encountered at surgery—resection is warranted—may become symptomatic

Stromal Tumors

- Arise from interstitial cells of Cajal
- 3 histological types: Fusiform (77%), epithelioid (8%) or mixed (15%)
- Express CD 117 (c-kit proto-oncogene)—>95%
  – CD 34 in 70–90%
- Stain +ve for actin, desmin, S100
- Equal in both sexes
- Firm gray white, with whorled appearance on cut section

Treatment

- Surgical resection
- Most common indication or surgery in benign—bleeding

Adenomas

Spigelmann Classification Refer Colorectal Chapter

- 3 types—true adenomas, villous, Brunner gland adenomas
- Adenomas are seen, ileum 50%, jejunum 30%, duodenum 20%
- Mostly single and asymptomatic
- Most common symptom—bleeding/obstruction.
- Villous adenomas—most common site—duodenum—associated with FAP
- Villous and true adenomas are premalignant. Adenoma—carcinoma sequence—related to size >5 cm
- Malignant potential 35–55%

Treatment

- Resection in ileum and jejunum
  – Duodenum—endoscopic resection and can cause more bleeding perforation

– If there are recurrence/invasive features—pancreaticoduodenectomy
- Endoscopic mucosal resection

In FAP

- Duodenal adenomas found in 50–90%
- Increasing age—independent risk factor
- FAP carry 5% lifetime risk of duodenal adenocarcinoma

Brunner Gland Adenoma

- Benign hyperplastic lesions arising from Brunner glands of proximal duodenum
- Symptoms mimic peptic ulcer disease
- Endoscopic diagnosis
- Treatment—excision—endoscopic/surgical
- No malignant potential

Lipoma

- Common in ileum
- Single, intramural lesion in submucosa
- 6th–7th decade
- More common in males
- Only less than one-third are symptomatic
- Most common manifestation—obstruction and bleeding
- No malignant potential
- Treatment—excision only if resection is simple

Peutz-Jeghers Syndrome

- Autosomal dominant inheritance
- Mutation of STK11 gene (LKB1) tumor suppressor gene
- Mucocutaneous melanosis over circumoral, palms, soles, digits, perianal region
- Intestinal hamartomatous polyps—entire jejunum and ileum—most common
- 50% have colorectal and 25% gastric lesions
- Abdominal pain due to intussusception—most common presentation
- Bleeding manifest as anemia—due to autoamputation of polyps
- Extracolonic cancers occur in 50–90% (SI, pancreas, stomach, lung, uterus)
- Resection of only the affected segment—no extensive resection needed
- Not curable

Hemangioma

- Developmental malformation—submucosal proliferation of blood vessels
- Most common—in jejunum
- 3–4% of all benign tumors, 60% are multiple

Associated with

- Osler-Weber-Rendu disease
- Turner syndrome—cavernous haemangiomas of intestine
- Most common symptom—bleeding
- Angiogram and Tc 99m RBC scanning—localise—resection warranted
- Localised also by intraoperative transillumination and palpation

MALIGNANT TUMORS

Tumor type	Cell of origin	Frequency	Predominant site
Adenocarcinoma	Epithelial cell	36–50%	Duodenum
Carcinoid	Enterochro-maffin cell	20–40%	Ileum
Lymphoma GIST	Lymphocyte Interstitial cell of Cajal	12–15% 10–15%	Ileum

Diagnosis

- X-ray, small bowel follow through
- CT
- Double balloon enteroscopy
- Video capsule enteroscopy
- Octreotide scan
- Tc 99 radionucleide scan
- There is an increase in incidence of NETs

Clinical Features

- Almost always produce symptoms—most common pain and weight loss
- Obstruction in 15–35%—due to infiltration and adhesions vs intussusception in benign
- Diarrhea with mucus and tenesmus
- Bleeding with anemia—more in GIST
- Palpable mass in 10–20%
- Perforation in 10%—usually in lymphomas and sarcomas

NET

- Arise from enterochromaffin cells (Kulchitsky) cells from neural crest situated at base of crypts of Lieberkuhn-Argentaffin cells
- Foregut-respiratory tract, thymus-secrete-low serotonin, more 5 HTP (hydroxytryptophan) or ACTH
- Midgut—high serotonin
- Hindgut—serotonin and somatostatin and peptide YY
- Most common site—appendix (most common) and GIT

Carcinoid Syndrome

- In liver metastasis
- Direct secretion into venous system bypassing portal system—lung, ovary

NET-Pathology

- 70–80% asymptomatic
- Appendiceal NET—only 3% metastasis, ileal NET—35% metastasis
- Size <1 cm—associated with 2% metastasis
- Size 1–2 cm—50% metastasis
- >2 cm—80–90% metastasis
- Submucosal lesions—yellow on cut surface
- Seen on antimesenteric border of SI—associated with larger mesenteric mass of LN with desmoplastic reaction—mistaken for primary
- Produce kinking—obstruction
- Multicentric in 20–30% (mostly any GIT malignancy)
- Synchronous adenocarcinoma in colon—in 10–20%
- MEN 1 association in 10%

Clinical Features

- Most common—abdomen pain—due to obstruction-desmoplastic reaction due to humoral agents and intussusception
- Diarrhea—due to partial obstruction and may be secretory and causes weight loss
- Mesenteric nodes cause venous engorgement and ischemia

Malignant Carcinoid Syndrome

- In <10% of NET
- Usually from GIT—SI carcinoid with hepatic metastasis
- Also from bronchus, pancreas, ovary—extra abdominal disease without liver metastasis
- Manifestations—cardiac
  - Vasomotor
  - GIT
- Substances responsible—serotonin, 5HTP, histamine, dopamine, substance P, PG

Clinical Features

- Cutaneous flushing (80%)
- 4 types
  - Diffuse erythematous short lived, on face neck
  - Violaceous associated with longer duration with permanent cyanotic flush, injected conjunctiva
  - Prolonged flushes may last 2–3 days and with lacrimation
  - Bright red patchy flushing—typically seen in gastric NET

- Hepatomegaly (76%)
- Right-sided valvular heart disease (40–70%)
- Asthma—25%—due to serotonin and bradykinin
- Diarrhea
  - Episodic after a meal, watery, explosive
  - Serotonin—responsible
- Cardiac—mainly right side of heart
  - In 15% left side of heart
  - Most common—pulmonary stenosis (90%)
  - Tricuspid insufficiency (47%)
  - TS (42%)
- Malabsorption and pellagra (dermatitis, dementia, diarrhea—3Ds)—due to diversion of dietary tryptophan

Diagnosis: NET

- Elevated humoral factors—basis of diagnosis
- Serotonin—in liver and lung converted into 5 HIAA
  - 24-hour urine 5 HIAA—highly specific—not sensitive
  - CgA-Sp 95%, sensitivity 55%
  - Combined CgA and 2-hour urine 5HIAA
  - Combined CgA and N-terminal probrain natriuretic peptide (NT-proBNP)
- Measurement of serotonin, substance P, neurokinin A—not reliable

Imaging

- Barium studies
- CT—solid mass with surrounding strands, kinking of bowel
- MRI—in liver metastasis
- Indium labelled 111 petetreotide—binds to somatostatin 2 and 5 receptors
- PET CT—only useful in high grade
- Ga-DOTATATE PET/CT is the choice for localizing and in metastasis

NET: Treatment

Surgery

- Based on site, size and metastasis
- <1 cm without regional LN metastasis—segmental resection
- >1 cm, multiple or with LN metastasis, regardless of size—wide excision of bowel and mesentery

- Terminal ileum—right hemicolectomy
- Explore for multicentric lesions
- Anaesthesia can precipitate carcinoid crisis—manifested as hypotension, bronchospasm, flushing, arrhythmias and treated with IV octreotide 50 to 100 µg bolus—infusion 50 µm/hr

In Liver Metastasis

- Surgery
- TACE, TARE
- Liver transplant

Adenocarcinoma

- 50% of malignant tumors of SI
- M>F
- More common in duodenum and jejunum
- Associated with Crohn's disease—more common in ileum
- Vague presentation—pain, weight loss

Treatment

Surgery

- If tumor invasion to adjacent structures present NACT—surgery after 2–3 months
- Radical resection with lymphadenectomy
- Pancreaticoduodenectomy, right hemicolectomy—depending on lesion site

Postop Chemo

- In poorly differentiated
- If <10 LN sampled
- In metastatic—FOLFOX—first line, FOLFIRI—second line
  - **Duodenal adenomas**—<1 cm endoscopic removal
- >2 cm—surgical—pancreaticoduodenectomy (PD) if involving D2
- 1–2 cm—EUS—if in mucosa—endoscopic removal and follow-up
- In FAP—surveillance endoscopy—endoscopic removal—if surgery needed—standard PD

Metastatic Tumors

- More common than primary
- Most common from—cervix, ovary, kidney, stomach, pancreas, colon
- By direct extension or implantation
- Extra-abdominal malignancy—most common—melanoma

Colon and Rectum

8.1 ANATOMY

Dimensions

(Large Intestine: 150 cm)

- Cecum—diameter—7.5 cm, length—10 cm
- Diameter >12 cm—necrosis can happen
- Appendix—from cecum 3 cm below ileocecal valve
  - At the convergence of tenia coli
  - Fold of Treves—only antimesenteric appendage found on small intestine at the ileocecal junction
- Ascending colon: Length—15 cm
- Transverse colon: Length—45 cm
- At hepatic flexure there is nephrocolic ligament
- At splenic flexure there is phrenocolic ligament
- White line of Toldt—fusion of mesentery with posterior peritoneum
- Nephrocolic ligament—overlies right kidney, duodenum, and porta hepatis
- Phrenocolic ligament lies ventral to spleen
- Descending colon—length 25 cm
  - Diameter smaller than ascending colon
  - From splenic flexure to pelvic brim
- Sigmoid—15–50 cm (Avg 38 cm)

Sigmoid Mesocolon

Inverted 'V'

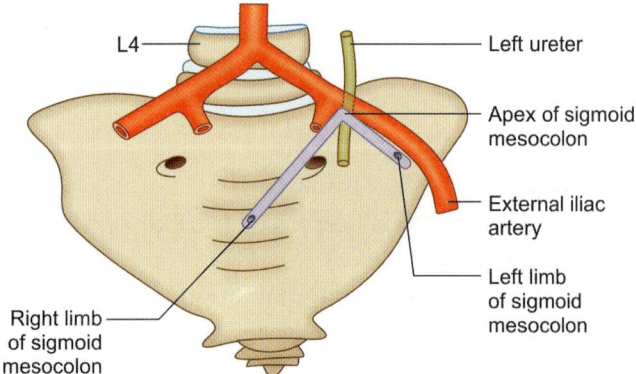

- Apex near division of left common iliac artery
- Left limb medially to left psoas mm
- Right limb in the pelvis ends at the midline at S3
- Ureter lies under sigmoid mesocolon and intersigmoid recess

Rectum

- 12–15 cm—from sacral promontory or from converging of tenia coli
- Distally dentate line-anatomist view
  - Proximal border of anal sphincter—surgeon's view

Anal Canal

- 4 cm

- Variable length of colon depends on transverse colon
  - Longer in older, women and thinner individuals.
  - Transverse colon lies below umbilicus in 10% women.

Bauhin's valve—ileocecal valve

Also known as:
- Tulp's valve
- Tulpius valve
- Valve of varolius
- Colic valve
- Ileocecal eminence

Taeniae

- Condensations of longitudinal muscles
- Colon has a thin layer of longitudinal muscle completely encircling colon

Taeniae of transverse colon

- Taenia mesocolica—connected to mesocolon
- Taenia omentalis—attaches to greater omentum
- Taenia libera—no attachments seen

- Length of taeniae is shorter than colonic length causing puckering which results in haustra—saccular appearance

Appendices Epiploicae

- Peritoneum covered fat pieces
- Most numerous along taeniae
- Absent on appendix, cecum and rectum
- Flat on right colon
- Pedunculated and most prominent on sigmoid

Ileocecal Junction

- Superior ileocecal fold—contains anterior cecal artery
  - Covers superior ileocecal recess
- Inferior ileocecal fold—from antimesenteric aspect of ileum to mesentery of appendix
  - No vessel in this, so called blood less fold of Treves
  - Inferior ileocecal recess lie inferior and posterior to this fold
- Gerlach's valve—mucosal fold at the opening of appendix

Rectum

- Posterior surface is almost completely extraperitoneal—adherent to presacral tissues
- Anterior surface of upper third—covered by visceral peritoneum
- Peritoneal reflection—7–9 cm from anal verge in men –5–7.5 cm in women
- POD, cul-de-sac, rectouterine pouch

Folds/Valves of Houston

- Three of them
- Upper and lower to the left
- Middle to the right
- No specific functions
- Mobilization of them gives extra 5 cm length
- Posterior aspect of rectum—mesorectum is thick
- Thin investing fascia cover mesorectum—fascia propria
- Lies on presacral fascia
- Dissection between fascia propria and presacral fascia during rectal dissection—holy plane of Heald
- Lymphatics are inside mesorectum important in TME

Para Rectal Fascia

- Endopelvic fascia—lines walls and floor of pelvis
- Applied to periosteum of sacrum—presacral fascia

- Presacral fascia—thin condensation of endopelvic fascia—also forms lateral pelvic stalks/ligament—anterolateral structures containing middle rectal artery

Rectosacral Fascia (Waldeyer)

- Thick condensation of endopelvic fascia
- Attachment from presacral fascia to fascia propria
  - From S4 vertebra to anorectal ring
- Division provides entry into deep retro-rectal pelvis
- Dissection should be between presacral fascia and fascia propria

Recto Prostatic Fascia (Denonvilliers)

- Membranous partition at lowest part of rectovesical pouch
- Separates prostate and urinary bladder from rectum
- Single fibromuscular structure—several layers fused
- Covers seminal vesicle
- Rectovaginal fascia—in females
- Prevents spread of prostatic carcinoma to rectum

Pelvic Floor

- Pubococcygeus, iliococcygeus, puborectalis—levator ani
- Between sacrum, obturator fascia, ischial spines and pubis
- Supports pelvic organs and continence
- Levator hiatus—opening in decussating fibers of pubococcygeus
- Passage of anal canal, urethra and dorsal vein in men
  - Anal canal, urethra and vagina in women
- Puborectalis around rectum—in a state of continuous contraction
  - Relaxation happens during defecation
- Pubo coccygeus and iliococcygeus exert lateral pressure on levator hiatus and provide continence

Blood Supply

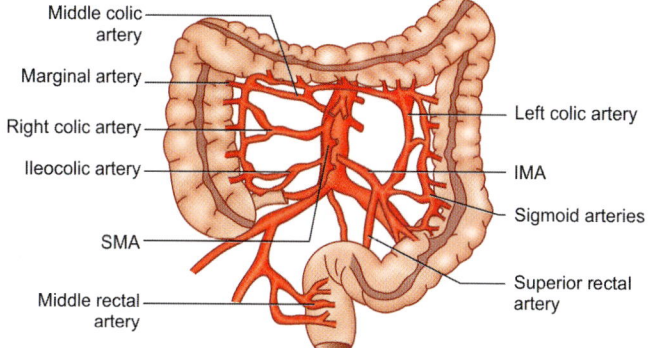

Collaterals—Between Celiac Artery and SMA

Superior pancreatico duodenal artery from celiac and inferior pancreatico duodenal from SMA—they form anastomosis around head of pancreas and duodenum

Arc of Barkow

It is between left and right gastroepiploic and mesocolic vessels.

Arc of Buhler—Between GDA and SMA

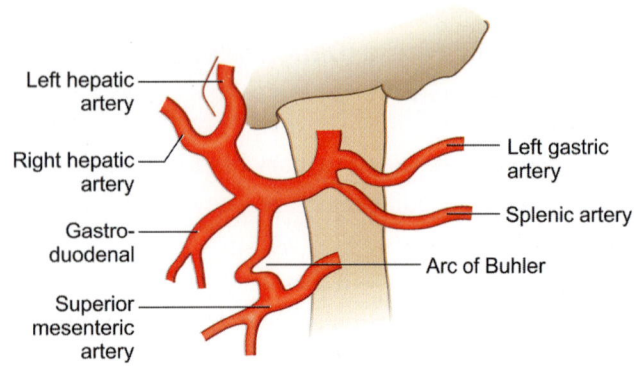

SMA–IMA Collaterals

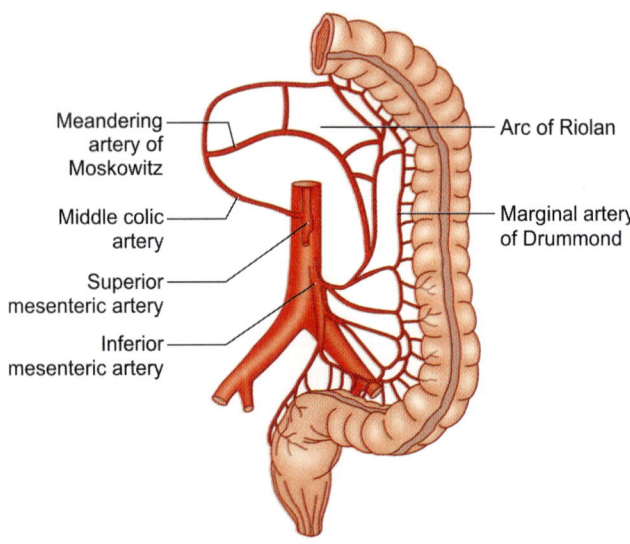

- Arc of Riolan—mid-distal branch of middle colic artery to left colic artery
- Arc of Moskowitz—proximal branches of middle colic artery to ascending branch of left colic artery
- Marginal artery of Drummond

IMA–iliac Artery Collaterals

Between superior rectal and internal iliac artery

SMA

- SMA territory ends at distal transverse colon
- IMA territory starts at splenic flexure
- SMA supplies entire small bowel
- 12–20 jejunal and ileal branches to the left
- Up to 3 main colonic branches to the right
- Most constant branch—ileocolic artery
- RCA is absent in—2–18%
- MCA—complete absence—4–20%
- Accessory MCA—10%
- Splenic flexure—50 % cases lack clearly identified arteries
  - Survive on adjacent vasa recta
  - Known as critical point of Griffith

IMA

- Originates at L2-L3, 3 cm above aortic bifurcation
- Most proximal branch: LCA
- 2–6 sigmoid branches
- Terminates as superior rectal/hemorrhoidal artery
- Middle rectal (hemorrhoidal) artery from internal iliac artery—enters rectum slightly anterior to lateral pelvic ligaments
  - Absent in 40–80%
- Inferior rectal (hemorrhoidal) artery—branch of pudendal artery which is a branch of internal iliac artery

Venous Drainage

- Follows arteries
- Right colon—SMV-PV
- Left colon, rectum—IMV which joins splenic vein to the left of aorta
- Anal canal—middle rectal and inferior rectal vein drains to internal iliac veins and to IVC
  - Also to superior rectal vein, which drains to IMV.
  - Bidirectional

Lymphatics

- Follows arteries
- Most of colon and proximal two-thirds of rectum drains to para-aortic LN and to cisterna chyli
- Distal rectum and anal canal
  - Para-aortic LN or
  - Laterally through internal iliac—superficial inguinal nodes
  - Dentate line roughly marks the watershed line

Nerves

Right Colon and Transverse Colon

- Sympathetic—preganglionic from T6–T12—preaortic ganglia
  - Postganglionic along blood vessels
- Parasympathetic—through right vagus
- Follow branches of SMA—synapse on bowel wall

Left Colon and Rectum

- Sympathetic—preganglionic—L1–L3-preaortic plexus—postganglionic—follow IMA, SRA

Lower Rectum and Anal Canal

- Sympathetics from pelvic plexus—adherent to lateral pelvic wall near lateral pelvic ligaments
- Condense to form hypogastric nerves—responsible for delivery of semen to prostatic urethra
- If injured can develop ejaculation problems.

Pelvic Parasympathetics

- Nervi erigentes
- From S2–S4
- Preganglionic parasympathetic merge with post-ganglionic sympathetics
- Injury near prostatic plexus (mixed sympathetic and parasympathetics) causes impotence and atonic bladder
- High ligation of IMA can cause injury to hypogastric nerves near sacral promontory—sympathetic dysfunction—retrograde ejaculation bladder dysfunction

Physiology

- Colon is involved in recycling of nutrients
- Depends on
  - Metabolic activity of colonic flora
  - Motility, secretion
  - Mucosal absorption
- Rectum—involved in
  - Elimination of stool
  - Dehydration
  - Defecation

Recycling

- SI absorbs most of the nutrients
- Ileal effluent—rich in water, electrolytes
- Colon can absorb many nutrients, electrolytes, nitrogen

- Accomplished by presence of bacterial flora
- Ileal effluent—succus entericus
  - Rich in electrolytes, bile salts

Colonic Flora

- Enormous quantity of autochthonous flora (indigenous)
- >400 species of bacteria
- Large intestine contains 10^{11} to 10^{12} bacterial cells/gram
- Contributes to 50% of fecal mass
- Most are anaerobes
- Bacteroides predominate throughout colon
  - Constitutes two-thirds of total count in proximal colon
  - And 70% of bacteria in rectum
- Escheritia, Klebsiella, proteus, Lactobacillus, Enterococci—facultative anaerobes
- These bacteria feed on protein sloughed from bowel wall and undigested carbohydrates

Functions of Colonic Microflora

- Barrier function—maintain epithelial integrity
- Nutritive—use plant polysaccharides
- Stimulate epithelial cell differentiation and angiogenesis
- Immune—gut associated lymphoid tissue
  - Innate and adoptive immunity
- Short chain FA—produced by fermentation of starch
  - Principal source of nutrition for colonocyte
- Probiotics—dietary supplements containing live cultures of bacteria and yeast
  - Beneficial to colonic and host function
  - Most used—lactobacillus and bifidobacterium
  - Stimulate immunity, anti-inflammatory functions, suppress pathogenic organisms
- Prebiotics—non-digestible oligosaccharides (inulin)
  - Stimulate growth of some bacteria

Fermentation

- Colonic mucosa receives nutrition from luminal contents
- SCFA butyrate—primary energy source
- Symbiotic action between colon and bacteria
- Main source of energy for bacteria—fiber from complex carbohydrates (starch and non-starch polysaccharides)—after fermentation

- Lignin, psyllium—not fermented—hydrophilic causing water absorption and bulking
- Cellulose is fermented and adds to minimal stool bulk but provide nutrition to colonocytes
- Fruit pectins—completely metabolized by bacteria
- End product of fermentation—SCFA and gas
  - CO_2, methane, H_2
- Gases from bacterial fermentation—50–75% of flatus
  - Rest swallowed air
- Protein fermentation—putrefaction—toxic products like phenol, indoles, amines
  - This production is inhibited by bacteria with alternative carbohydrate sources
  - Contribute to carcinogenesis

Short-Chain Fatty Acids

- Primary end products of fermentation
- Only 5–10% of them are lost in feces
- Three primary FA: Acetate, propionate and butyrate in 3:1:1
- SCFA metabolized in three main sites
  - In colonocytes, butyrate as primary energy source
  - In hepatocytes—use all three for gluconeogenesis
  - Muscle cell oxidize acetate to generate energy
- SCFA provides 70% of colonocyte energy needs, reduce glucose oxidation and spare other amino acids
- SCFA influences ileocolonic brake, inhibition of gastric emptying and controls nutrients reaching ileocolonic junction
- Acetate—transported to liver—synthesize cholesterol
- Nonabsorbable, nonfermentable fibers like phyllium—decrease production of acetate—reduce cholesterol levels
- Propionate—glycolytic in liver—inhibits cholesterol synthesis
- Butyrate—inhibits growth of neoplastic cells
  - Regulates cell adhesion molecules

Urea Recycling

- Colonic bacteria contains urease
- In low protein diet—can recycle nitrogen
- An alternate solution for dialysis

Absorption

- Total absorptive area of colon—900 cm^2
- Fluid delivered to cecum—1000–1500 ml

- Total water in stool 100–150 ml/day
- This 10-fold reduction makes colon—most efficient site of absorption per surface area
- Sodium at cecum—200 mEq/L, stool 20–50 mEq/L
- Water is absorbed passively
- Sodium is transported against chemical and electrical gradients—spending energy
- Lack of butyrate—due to lack of bacteria—in antibiotic treatment—less water and Na absorption—diarrhea
- SCFA also maintains blood flow, mucosal cell renewal, and maintain intraluminal pH for homeostasis of luminal bacteria
- Colon also absorbs—so part of enterohepatic circulation
  - Transported passively by nonionic diffusion
  - When colonic absorptive area exceeded—bacteria deconjugate bile acids—interfere with water and Na absorption—secretory or cholecteric diarrhea
  - Seen in right hemicolectomy and ileal resection

Secretion
Secrete and Excrete K

- In renal failure
- Inhibited by spironolactone
- In IBD, cholera, shigellosis
- Requires Na$^+$, K$^+$–ATPase and Na-K 2Cl cotransporter, an apical K channel

Secrete chloride

- In diarrhea

Secrete H$^+$ and bicarbonate

- Involving colonic carbonic anhydrase
- Involved in systemic pH regulation

Motility
Segmental and Propagated Activity
Segmental

- Single or rhythmic bursts of contractions
- Propel fecal matter distally
- Pressure gradient towards rectum
- Mixing and optimal absorption

Propagated Activity
- Low amplitude and high amplitude

Low Amplitude
- Associated with distension of viscus and passage of flatus

High Amplitude
- Mass movements or migratory motor complexes
- Shifts large quantity of contents in colon distally
- In defecation

Formation of Stool
- > 3 loose stools/day—diarrhea
- <3 stools/week—constipation
- Colonic transit time—F>M
  - Premenopausal > postmenopausal
  - Smokers < nonsmokers

Defecation
- Rectum—a reservoir
- Stool in rectum—anorectal reflex—to close sphincter
- Rectocolic reflex—for emptying colon contents into rectum
- Circadian rhythm of colonic activity maximum—immediately after waking up.
- After meals—fatty meal prolonged reflex

8.2 DIVERTICULAR DISEASE
Nomenclature
- Diverticulum = sac-like protrusion of the colonic wall
- Diverticulosis = describes the presence of diverticuli without inflammation
- Diverticular disease—clinical term—presence of symptomatic diverticula
- Diverticulitis = inflammation of diverticuli

Epidemiology
- Before the 20th century, diverticular disease was rare
- Prevalence has increased over time
- 1907 first reported resection of complicated diverticulitis by Mayo
- Increases with age
- Gender prevalence depends on age
  - Younger age—males are more common, older age—females more common.

- Anatomic location of diverticuli varies with the geographic location
- Western nations (North America, Europe, Australia) have predominantly left-sided diverticulosis
- 95% diverticuli are in sigmoid colon
- 35% can also have proximal diverticuli
- 4% have only right-sided diverticuli
- In Asia, diverticula are more common on right side of colon—true diverticula—up to 70%
  - Those who migrate to west—more in distal colon
- Diverticula—one of the most common findings on colonoscopy—in the absence of symptoms—no need to change lifestyle or treatment
- Sigmoid and descending colon—most common sites due to:
  - Hypertrophy of muscle layers
  - Smaller luminal diameter
  - Less fiber in diet—less bulk of stool in colon—decrease in colonic luminal content—requires generation of increased colonic pressures to propel feces forward
- In Asia and Africa diverticulosis in general is rare and usually right-sided
- Prevalence <0.2%
- Colonic pseudodiverticulum more like a local hernia
- Mucosa-submucosa herniates through the muscle layer (muscularis propria) and then is only covered by serosa

Interactions of
- High intraluminal pressure
- Disordered motility
- Alterations on colonic structure
- Low fiber diet

Diverticuli are formed on the mesenteric side of the antimesenteric tenia coli
- At areas of weakness where vasa recta penetrate muscular layers
- Protrusion of mucosa and submucosa—pseudo-diverticulum
- As diverticula become more prevalent—they develop between two antimesenteric taeniae

Pathophysiology
- Diverticuli develop in 'weak' regions of the colon. Specifically, local hernias develop where the vasa recta penetrate the bowel wall
- Law of Laplace: $P = kT/R$
- Pressure = k × Tension/Radius

- Sigmoid colon has small diameter resulting in highest pressure zone
- Segmentation = motility process in which the segmental muscular contractions separate the lumen into chambers
- Segmentation → increased intraluminal pressure—mucosal herniation—diverticulosis—pulsion diverticula
- May explain why high fiber prevents diverticuli by creating a larger diameter colon and less vigorous segmentation

Lifestyle Factors Associated with Diverticular Disease

Low fiber → diverticular disease
- Low fiber—low bulk—need more force to propel the fecal matter
- More risk with red meat—not so with chicken and fish

Colonic Wall

- Increase in elastin deposition in taeniae by >200%—increased collagen cross-linking—stiffening of colon wall—less resistant to stretch on increasing luminal pressure
- Sigmoid with narrowest diameter—more pressure
- Submucosa develop small tears—herniation

Altered Motility

- Segmentation—simultaneous contraction of two neighboring haustra—create temporary closed segment—increase in luminal pressure
- Reduced number of interstitial cells of Cajal and enteric glial cells cause disorganized colonic contraction

Triggers for Inflammation

- Obstruction of diverticula
- Fecal stasis
- Alteration of bacterial flora in colon
- Local ischemia
- Fecal stasis leads to
  - Slow transit through colon
  - Entrapment of feces in diverticula—diverticula are devoid of muscles—so it is difficult to expel fecal matter—alteration in the flora leads to local ischemia—breakdown of colonic wall—trigger inflammation

Bacterial Flora

- Low fiber diet—change in bacterial flora—diminish barrier function—inflammation—also affect enteric nervous system

Lifestyle Factors

- Obesity associated with diverticulosis—particularly in men under the age of 40
- Lack of physical activity
- NSAID—increase diverticulitis and bleeding—alteration in the permeability of colon

Steroids

- Risk of perforation due to reduction in collagen turn over

Smoking

- More chance of perforation/abscess
  - Alcohol—more symptomatic disease
  - Family history—increased risk

Uncomplicated Diverticulosis

- Usually an incidental finding at time of colonoscopy

Symptomatic Un Complicated Diverticular Disease (SUDD)

- Considered 'asymptomatic'
- However, a significant minority of patients will complain of cramping, bloating, irregular bowel habits, narrow caliber stools
- Some consider it is part of IBS
- Treatment: Fiber
- Bulk content reduces colonic pressure preventing underlying pathophysiology that lead to diverticulosis
- 20 to 30 g fiber per day is needed; difficult to get with diet alone.

Segmental Colitis Associated with Diverticulosis (SCAD)

- Overlap with IBD
- Localized inflammation of diverticula—called diverticular colitis

Diverticulitis

- Diverticulitis = inflammation of diverticula
- Results from—food impaction at diverticula—perforation of a diverticulum—pericolonic inflammation
- Most common complication of diverticulosis
- Occurs in 10–25% of patients with diverticulosis

Pathophysiology of Diverticulitis

- Micro or macroscopic perforation of the diverticulum → subclinical inflammation to generalized peritonitis

- Previously thought to be due to fecaliths causing increased diverticular pressure; this is really rare
- Erosion of diverticular wall from increased intraluminal pressure → inflammation—focal necrosis-perforation
- Usually inflammation is mild and micro perforation is walled off by pericolonic fat and mesentery

Diagnosis of Diverticulitis

- **Classic history:** Increasing, constant, LLQ abdominal pain over several days prior to presentation with fever
- Crescendo quality—each day is worse
- Constant—not colicky
- Fever
- Previous episodes of similar pain
- Associated symptoms
  - Nausea/vomiting 20–60%
  - Constipation 50%
  - Diarrhea
  - Urinary symptoms (dysuria, urgency, frequency)
- Right-sided diverticulitis tends to cause RLQ abdominal pain; can be difficult to distinguish from appendicitis

Physical Examination

- Low grade fever
- LLQ abdominal tenderness
- Usually moderate with no peritoneal signs
- Painful mass in 20% of cases
- Rebound tenderness suggests free perforation and peritonitis

Blood routine: Mild leukocytosis
- 50% of patients will have a normal WBC count

Radiology

- Modality of choice—CT
- Information on location, extent, severity and changes outside lumen
- CT enterography
- US/MRI—not as reliable

Colonoscopy—risk of perforation
- 3–5% have other conditions like adenocarcinoma
- Gastrograffin/barium enema—only in diverticulosis

Treatment of Diverticulitis

- **Complicated** diverticulitis = Presence of macro-perforation, obstruction, abscess, or fistula—majority may require surgery

Uncomplicated diverticulitis = Absence of the above complications with only pericolonic inflammation

Uncomplicated Diverticulitis Treatment

- Most recover without surgery
- 50–70% will not have any further episodes
- Bowel rest or restriction
- Clear liquids or NPO for 2–3 days
- Then advance diet
- Majority managed as OP cases
- Admission and IV antibiotics if concern about peritonitis

Antibiotics

- Coverage of fecal flora
- Gram-negative rods, anaerobes
  - Monitoring clinical course
- Pain should gradually improve in several days (decrescendo)
- Normalization of temperature
- Tolerance of oral intake
- If symptoms deteriorate or fail to improve within 3 days, reassessment
- After resolution of attack → high fiber diet with supplemental fiber
- **Follow-up:** Colonoscopy in 4–6 weeks
- Flexible sigmoidoscopy and barium enema reasonable alternative

Aim of Colonoscopy

- Exclude neoplasm, IBD
- Evaluate extent of the diverticulosis

Prognosis After Resolution of Uncomplicated Diverticulitis

- 30–40% of patients will remain asymptomatic
- 10–35% develop subsequent attack
- <5% develop complicated diverticulitis
- Roughly 1% ultimately requires surgery

Recommendation for Further Treatment

- Individualized
- Based on
  - Frequency and severity
  - Overall medical condition
  - Comorbidity

Surgery
Indications in Uncomplicated

- Risk of subsequent attacks of diverticulitis—long >5 cm segment and family history
- Risk of complicated diverticulitis after recovery from diverticulitis—<5% after uncomplicated diverticulitis

- Risk of perforation—immunesuppression, renal failure, collagen disease, severity on CT
- Number and interval between attacks >3 episodes in 2 years
- Multiple attacks of diverticulitis over a short time—due to unresolved ongoing inflammation—'**smoldering diverticulitis**'—may need surgery
- After 4–6 weeks of diverticulitis and colonoscopy
  - Sigmoid colectomy—anastomosis in upper rectum—to minimize recurrence.
  - To remove all diseased colon.

Complicated Diverticulitis
- Acute—abscess, perforation, obstruction
- Chronic—stricture, fistula

Abscess
- Fever, leukocytosis, pain
- Ileus due to inflammation of small bowel
- Large >4 cm abscess—antibiotics and drained by guided aspiration—with or without resection
- Small <4 cm—antibiotics
- Failure to resolve—laparotomy

Perforation

Hinchey classification	
Stage I	Pericolic abscess or phlegmon
Stage II	Pelvic, intra-abdominal, or retroperitoneal abscess
Stage III	Generalised purulent peritonitis
Stage IV	Generalised fecal peritonitis
Modified Hinchey classification	
Stage 0	Mild clinical diverticulitis
Stage Ia	Confined pericolic inflammation—phlegmon
Stage Ib	Confined pericolic abscess
Stage II	Pelvic, distant intra-abdominal or retroperitoneal abscess
Stage III	Generalised purulent peritonitis
Stage IV	Generalised fecal peritonitis

- Hinchey I and II
  - Antibiotics, percutaneous drainage
  - Later colonoscopy—surgery
  - Current recommendation—elective resection after a single episode of complicated diverticulitis

- Hinchey III and IV
  - Surgical emergency
  - May present with sepsis
  - CT/X-ray may show intraperitoneal air

Surgical Options
- Hartmann procedure
- Resection—anastomosis—with colostomy
- Lap irrigation with warm saline and drains—may obviate the need for elective colectomy
  - In Hinchey III
  - Colectomy or colostomy not done
  - Fail to improve—consider colectomy
- Hartmann vs anastomosis with diversion
  - No difference in outcome
  - Stoma reversal was higher (90%) with primary anastomosis,
  - Hartmann—55%
- Hansen classification—includes asymptomatic diverticulosis and diverticulitis
- Was vary modification of Hinchey classification

SCAD
- Present with crampy pain, diarrhea
- Endoscopy—congested, friable granular mucosa with superficial ulcers—most often to crests of colonic folds, sparing diverticular opening, the rectum and areas of unaffected colon
- Rectum—normal

Peritonitis Treatment
- Resuscitation (fluid/electrolyte)
- Antibiotics
- Ampicillin + Gentamycin + Metronidazole
- Imipenem/cilastin
- Emergency exploration
- Mortality 6% in purulent peritonitis and 35% in fecal peritonitis

Abscess
- Occurs in 20% of patients with acute diverticulitis
- Percutaneous drainage followed by single stage surgery in 70–80% of patients

- CT guided drainage
  - Leave in until drain output less than 10 mL in 24 hours
  - May take up to 30 days
  - Catheter sinograms helpful to show persistent communication between abscess and bowel
- Small abscesses too small to drain percutaneously (< 1 cm) can be treated with antibiotics alone
- These patients behave like uncomplicated diverticulitis and may not require surgery

Fistulas

- 5% of complicated diverticulitis—develop fistula
- Occurs in up to 80% of cases requiring surgery
- Major types
  - Colovesical fistula 65%—dome of bladder
  - Colovaginal fistula 26%—exclusively after hysterectomy
  - Coloenteric, colouterine 10%
  - Colocutaneous—at site of drain
- Passage of gas and stool from the affected organ
- Colovesical fistula:
  - pneumaturia, dysuria, fecaluria
  - 50% of patients can have diarrhea and passage of urine per rectum

Diagnosis

- **CT:** Thickened bladder with associated colonic diverticuli adjacent and air in the bladder (not been instrumented). Is the investigation of choice
- **Barium enema:** Direct visualization of fistula track in 50% of cases in colovesical fistula
- Flexible sigmoidoscopy is low yield (0–5%)
- Cystoscopy—reveal cystitis and bullous edema at fistula site
- Sigmoid—vesical fistula—more common in men— uterus protects in women

Colovaginal fistula

- CT scan—if not apparent, do limited gastrograffin enema
- Fistula pinched off—vaginal side and not sutured and left open for drainage or also can be treated with omentum interpose.

Treatment of Fistulas

- Antibiotics
- Colonoscopy—to rule out malignancy/Crohn's disease

Surgery

- Resection of affected colon
- Fistula tract can be "pinched off" most of the time
- Suture closure for larger defects
- Foley left in 7–10 days
- Elective single stage resection is ideal, ~6 weeks after episode
- Two-stage procedure (Hartmann procedure)

Obstruction

- Obstructive symptoms occur in 65% of patients with acute diverticulitis
- Complete obstruction in 10%
- Stricture is rare
- Partial and insidious
- CT enterography/colonoscopy to exclude malignancy

Diverticular Bleeding

- Most common cause of brisk hematochezia (30–50% of cases)
- 5–15% of patients with diverticulosis will bleed
- 70% of diverticular bleeding stops without need for intervention
- Risk of rebleeding 10% in one year, 50% in 10 years
- Right-sided diverticula responsible for more than half of bleeding
- After second episode of bleeding, risk of rebleeding 20–50%

Pathophysiology of Bleeding

- Diverticulum herniates at site of vasa recta
- Over time, the vessel becomes draped over the dome of the diverticulum separated only by mucosa
- Later, there is segmental weakening of the artery → ruptures and bleeds
- Bleeding occur at the neck of the diverticulum

Symptoms

- Most only have symptoms of bloating and diarrhea but no significant abdominal pain
- Painless hematochezia
- Start—stop pattern; "water faucet"
- Diverticulitis rarely causes bleeding

Management

- Resuscitation
- Localization
- Supportive care with blood products

Localization

- Right colon is the source of diverticular bleeding in 50–90% of patients

Possible Reasons

- Right colon diverticula have wider necks and domes exposing vasa recta over a great length of injury
- Thinner wall of the right colon
- Colonoscopy after resuscitation
  - Can localize site of bleeding and offers possible therapeutic intervention (inj. epinephrine, cautery, clip, etc.)
  - Often limited by either brisk bleeding obscuring lumen or no active bleeding with clots in every diverticuli

Tagged Red Blood Cell Scan

- Can localize bleeding source
- 95% sensitivity
- 85% specificity
- Can detect bleeding as slow as 0.1 ml/min
- Often not particularly helpful

Angiography

- Accurate localization
- 30–45% sensitive
- 100% specific
- **Need brisk active bleeding:** 0.5–1 mL/min
- **Offers therapy:** Embolization, vasopressin
  - Success rate >90%
- 5–10% risk of intestinal infarction

Surgery

- Segmental resection
  - If site can be localized
  - Rebleeding rate of 0–14%
- Blind hemicolectomy in rebleeding.
- Surgery based on RBC localization, still incidence of recurrent bleeding in one-third.
- Subtotal colectomy does not completely eliminate chance of rebleeding and causes more morbidity.

Diverticular Associated Colitis

- Pathologic features of Crohn's/ulcerative colitis in the diverticula
- Tenesmus, hematochezia, diarrhea.
- Endoscopy—focal erythema, submucosal ecchymosis, erosions, ulcers
- Segmental colitis
- Medical treatment—25% recurrence rate
- May consider surgery for recurrence/complications

In Immunocompromised

- Diverticulitis—is not more prevalent
- More complications
- Low threshold for colectomy after single episode
- Prophylactic colectomy—in pre-transplant—controversial

Right-sided Diverticulitis

- Rare
- In younger
- CT—choice
- In complicated—right hemicolectomy

In Younger Patients

- May be more virulent
- Young age (<50)—not a routine indication for elective resection

Giant Colonic Diverticula

- Rare
- Most occur—antimesenteric side of sigmoid colon
- Barium enema—diagnostic
- Complications—perforation, obstruction, volvulus
- Treatment—resection of involved colon and diverticulum

8.3 COLORECTAL NEOPLASIA

- Third most common cancer in males
- Fourth among females
- Incidence increasing in Asia and in India
- High incidence in western world; decreased recently.
- Major factors—diet and lifestyle

Modifiable Risk Factors

- Diet
- Red meat and fat
  - Affects distal colon especially
  - Generation of heterocyclic amines
  - Narrow lumen and prolonged contact time
- **Dietary fibers—protective**
  - Dilute carcinogen
  - Speed up transit

– Certain fibers bind mutagens
– Change fecal pH
– Leafy vegetables, folate, calcium—protective
- Alcohol
  – Positive dose response ratio
- Smoking
  – High relationship
  – More chance for affecting rectum
  – Relation with dose and duration
- Exercise and obesity

  Cancer prevention benefits of exercise
  – Reduce inflammation and generation of free radicals
- Central obesity more chance of cancer

Clinical Risk Factors

- Familial syndromes
  – FAP
  – HNPCC
- IBD
  – Crohn's disease
  – Ulcerative colitis
- Polyps
- Familial cancer syndromes
  – 75% sporadic
  – 25% hereditary
- 15–20% familial
- 3% HNPCC
- 1% FAP

FAP

- Autosomal dominant—caused by mutation of APC gene
- > 100 polyps throughout colorectum
- 100% chance of malignancy by age 55
- Average age of cancer—42

HNPCC

- Lynch syndrome
- Cancer developing from adenomatous polyps
- **Lynch I:** only CRC
- **Lynch II:** CRC with endometrial, ovarian and gastric Ca.
- 80% with Lynch syndrome develop CRC in lifetime

IBD

- **UC:** Incidence of malignancy proportional to
  – Extent of colonic involvement
  – Age of onset
  – Severity
  – Duration—after 8–10 years

- **CD:** Also increase risk
  – Inflammation-induced cancer

Sporadic

- Absence of family history
- Common in age group—60–80 years
- Isolated colorectal cancer
- Genetic mutations limited to the tumor
- Genetics of initiation and progression can progress in the same line as hereditary

Familial

- Genetic polymorphism
- Gene modifiers
- Defect in tyrosine kinases

Note

Most common risk factor—age

Following sporadic ca—40% develop metachronous polyps

6%—second CRC

Familial and nonfamilial causes of colorectal cancer
Syndromes with adenomatous polyps
APC gene mutations (1%)
• Familial adenomatous polyposis
• Attenuated APC
• Turcot syndrome (two-thirds of families)
MMR gene mutations (3%)
• Hereditary nonpolyposis colorectal cancer types I and II
• Muir-Torre syndrome
• Turcot syndrome (one-third of families)
Syndromes with hamartomatous polyps (.1%)
• Peutz-Jeghers (LKB-1)
• Juvenile polyposis (SMAD4, PTEN)
• Cowden (PTEN)
• Bannayan-Riley-Ruvalcaba
• Mixed polyposis
Other familial causes
• Familial h/o adenomatous polyps (MYH)
• Familial h/o colon cancer
• Familial colon—breast cancer
Nonfamilial causes
• Personal history of adenomatous polyps
• Personal history of colorectal cancer
• IBD
• Radiation colitis, ureterosigmoidostomy, acromegaly, Cronkhite-Canada syndrome

Concept of Mutagenesis

- Initiation—promotion model
- First step—initiation-DNA damage
- Promotion—cellular proliferation
- Initiating and promotional factors can be modified, thus reducing tumorigenesis.
- Mutagens—ubiquitous on colonic mucosa
- Protective mechanisms in mucosa detoxify them.
- Can prevent interaction between mutagens and mucosa

Mutations in three Distinct Genes

- Chromosomal instability pathway—80%
  - Oncogenes
  - Tumor suppressor genes
- Microsatellite instability pathway—20%
  - DNA mismatch repair genes
- Gene methylation and inactivation of tumor suppressor gene
  - CIMP—CpG Island methylator phenotype
  - Seen in 32% CRC as predominant lesion
- Chromosomal instability—changes in chromosome number and structure, leading to changes in amount, structure and proteins
- Microsatellites are base pairs repeated in chromosomes, any damage to them are repaired by mismatch repair genes.
- Mismatch repair genes (MMR)
  - MSH1, MLH1, MLH2, PMS1, PMS2
- APC mutation seen in two-thirds in adenoma
- K-RAS—more common in larger lesions
- P53 mutation is seen—only in carcinoma
- 70% adenomas and cancers in left side of colon
- Synchronous lesions in 3–5%

Colorectal Cancer Distribution

Distribution of CRC

- Rectum—35–40%
- Sigmoid colon—18–24%
- Caecum—10–15%
- Transverse colon 6–7%

- Ascending colon—6–7%
- Descending colon—3–5%
- Splenic flexure—3%
- Hepatic failure—2%
- Anus 2%
- Appendix 0.5–1%

- Adenoma—carcinoma sequence in sporadic and hereditary colorectal cancer

Genetics

- Tumor suppressor genes
- DNA MMR genes
- Proto oncogenes
- Promoter hypermethylation events

Tumor Suppressor Genes (TSG)

- Inhibitory control deregulation by mutation develop tumor due to
  - Point mutation
  - Loss of heterozygosity
  - Frame shift mutation
  - Promoter hypermethylation
- First gene mutated-gate keeper gene-normally regulate cell cycle
- Failure of regulation of cell cycle by TSG leads to Loss of function
- Both alleles should be mutated-for tumor formation

Wnt Pathway

Wingless Related Integration Pathway

- Closely associated with APC b catenin pathway
- Normally reduced intracytoplasmic b catenin-inhibit Wnt expression
- When APC is mutated, b catenin levels rise—wnt activated
- Wnt leads to activation of target genes like cyclin D1, MYC—cell proliferation and tumorigenesis
- Earliest mutation in adenoma—ca sequence-in APC gene

Fearon -Vogelstein model

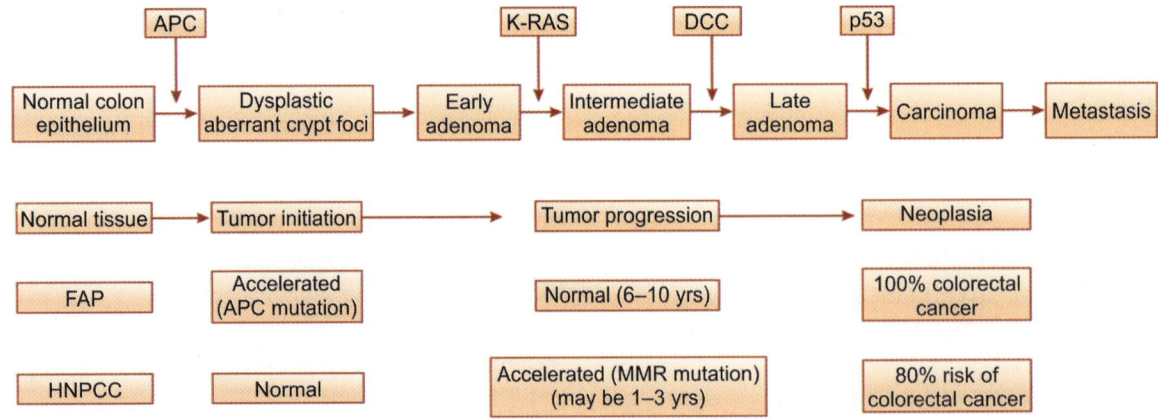

- Earliest phenotypical change—**Aberrant crypt formation**
- Most consistent genetic aberrations leads to abnormally short proteins—known as APC truncations
- Most relevant mutation in APC gene—truncation mutation

APC Gene

- Located on Chr 5q21
- Forms cytoplasmic complex with GSK (glycogen synthase kinase)—3 beta, beta catenin, and axin
- Beta catenin—structural component of cell adherence junctions, also binds in the cytoplasm to Tcf/LEF—nucleus—activates transcription of genes such as *c-myc*-regulate cell growth and proliferation
- APC—cell cycle control by regulating intracytoplasmic pool of beta catenin
- Germline APC truncation—responsible for FAP
- 30% of them have *de novo* germline mutation with no family history
- No gender predilection
- >100 adenomatous polyps in colon and rectum
- Manifest by late second or early third decade of life
- Most patients die of cancers by fifth decade
- APC truncation mutation similar to this occur in 85% sporadic colorectal Ca
- Most APC mutations occur near area responsible for β-catenin binding
- Mutation near 5′ end leads to short truncated protein: Attenuated FAP
  - <100 polyps
  - Tendency to spare rectum
- Classic FAP—mutation in codons from 1250 to 1464
- Mutations along 3′ end leads to much attenuated phenotype or no detectable abnormality
- Another APC mutation at I 1307 location—in Ashkenazi Jews
  - Point mutation
  - Responsible for 25% ca colorectum in Jews—most important cause

MYH Mutations and MAP

Mut Y DNA Glycosylase H

- MYH gene responsible for base excision repair and repair oxidative DNA damage
- Inheritance recessive in nature

- Can promote APC defects—MYH associated polyposis (MAP)
- All with biallelic MYH mutation—increased risk of Ca
- Can have 100–1000 polyps and also duodenal adenomas
- Surgery for polyps similar to AFP—IPAA
- In biallelic carriers upper and lower GI scopy are indicated every 1 to 2 years
- MAP implies more risk for siblings than offspring unless both parents possess recessive gene allele

p53 Mutation

- Most common mutated TSG in human neoplasia
- Chromosome 17p
- P53 mutation in CRC 75%—develop late
- Normally p53—induce apoptosis or cause G1 cell arrest—allowing DNA repair
- Role in apoptosis, called guardian of the genome
- IN CRC, if p53 intact—there is survival advantage

Genes Located in 18q

- SMAD2, SMAD4, DCC
- DPC gene—TSG adjacent to DCC

MMR Genes

- hMLH1, hMSH2, hMSH3, hPMS1, hPMS2, hPMS6
- Result in HNPCC
- 3% CRC—caused by HNPCC
- MMR gene mutation leads to errors in S phase when DNA is newly synthesized and copied
- MMR mutation exists in 10–15% of sporadic CRC
  - 95% tumors in HNPCC

Oncogenes

- Proto oncogenes—produce proteins—promote cellular growth and proliferation
- Mutation to proto oncogene—gain in function
- Mutation in one of the two allele is enough
- Leads to uncontrolled proliferation—cancer

Products of Oncogenes

- Growth factors
  - TGF-α, EGF, IGF
- Growth factor receptors
  - erdB2
- Signal transducers
  - src, abl, ras
- Nuclear proto-oncogenes transcription factors
  - myc

Adenoma–Carcinoma Sequence

- Most CRC develop through this
- Larger polyps—more risk
- FAP adenomas are histologically same as sporadic adenomas
- Peak incidence of discovery of benign CR polyp—50 years
- Peak incidence of CRC—60 years

Polyps

Histologic classification of colorectal polyps	
Neoplastic	*Non-neoplastic*
Adenomatous	**Hyperplastic**
• Tubular	**Hamartomas**
• Villous	• Juvenile
• Tubulovillous	• Peutz-Jeghers
Serrated	**Inflammatory**
• Traditional serrated	**Submucosal lesions**
• Mixed	• Lymphoid
• Sessile serrated adenoma	• Lipoma
Rare malignant lesions	• Leiomyoma
• Carcinoid	• Neuroma
• Melanoma	• Angioma
• Lymphoma	
• Mesenchymal tumors	

- Neoplastic—adenoma; potential for CRC
- Multiple polyps—more chance.
- Polyps mean—"Many feet"
- Most common type of colorectal polyp—adenoma—seen in 25–55% of adults
- Most common neoplastic—adenoma
- Most common non-neoplastic—hyperplastic polyp
- Most polyps originate as sessile lesions later traction cause pedunculation

Adenomatous Polyps

- Tubular
  - Branched tubular glands
  - 60–85% of adenomas
  - Pedunculated
  - Less atypia (on size)
- Tubulovillous
  - Mixed
  - 10–25% of adenomas
- Villous
  - Long finger-like projections
  - 5–10% of adenomas

- More of sessile
- More atypia and dysplasia

Risk of cancer
Tubular <1 cm—risk <5%
>2 cm— risk 35%
Villous >2 cm risk 50%

- **Polyp**— size and malignancy
  - <5 mm diameter—0–0.05% chance of malignancy
- Tubular adenoma—80% dysplastic tubules packed tightly and extend to normal lamina propria
- Villous adenoma—80% villous fronds made of core lamina propria surrounded by adenomatous epithelium—these fronds are crypts which have elongated at least twice the normal length
- Tubulovillous—have >20% tubular components, <80% villous

Adenomas

- Most common site sigmoid colon—40%
- Least common—rectum—3%
- Most are asymptomatic
- Usually redder in color than normal mucosa

Treatment

- Complete colonoscopy
- Removal—by snare

Surgery is Indicated

- Tumor extended through muscularis mucosa—invasive ca
- Invasive—more LN metastasis

Haggitt Classification

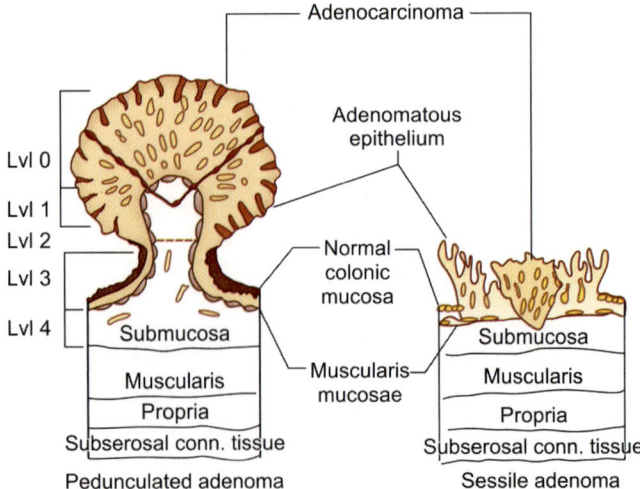

- Level 0—Carcinoma *in situ* muscularis mucosa not invaded
- 1—Invaded muscularis mucosa into submucosa limited to head
- 2—Invaded the neck, between head stalk
- 3—Ca invaded any part of stalk
- 4—Invaded submucosa below the stalk, but above musc propria
- All sessile polyps with invasive carcinoma are level 4

Sessile Type with Invasive Cancer

Chance of Mets-10%

- Poorly differentiated
- Cancer cells in lymphovascular spaces
- So treated aggressively
- Pedunculated levels 1, 2 and 3—low risk of metastasis so local excision with clear margin
- If well differentiated, no LV invasion and completely excised—depth of invasion guides further treatment

Hyperplastic Polyps

- Most common colonic polyps
- Benign—no malignant potential
- Serrated appearance
- 90% <3 mm
- Contain adenomatous elements which can turn malignant
- So better excised
- In serrated adenoma higher incidence of Ca right colon in women and smokers
- Associated with microsatellite instability
- They are pale, flat
- Most common site rectosigmoid
- Arise from faulty epithelial maturation and failure of apoptosis
- Main component—mature goblet cells

Serrated Adenomas (Polyps)

- Traditional
  - Contain low/high grade dysplasia of crypt surface
- Mixed
  - Combination of serrated architecture of hyperplastic polyps and dysplasia of adenomatous polyps
- Sessile
  - Morphology of both hyperplastic polyps and traditional serrated polyps
- Show dilatation of crypts with extension parallel to muscularis mucosa or herniation through it
- All serrated adenomas—secrete focal mucin

Hamartomatous Polyps

- Localized outgrowth of mature, normal intestinal epithelial cells
- Endoscopy—round, pink, pedunculated
- Lined by epithelium—core made of submucosa which does not involve muscularis mucosa

- Pathogenesis
  - Mucosal ulceration/inflammation—blocks colonic glands—proliferation and dilatation of glands—growth of granulation tissue and connective tissue
- When > 3 polyps—suspect polyposis syndrome

Inflammatory Polyps

- Pseudopolyps
- Arise from mucosal ulceration and repair
- Uniform in width from base to head
- In UC, CD
- Treat the cause
- There is malignant potential

Polyposis Syndromes

Gastrointestinal polyposis syndromes			
Polyp histology	*Syndrome*	*Genetics*	*Gene(s) lost*
Adenomatous	FAP	Germline APC mutation	5q21
	AFAP	Germline APC mutation	5q21
	MAP	Biallelic germline MUTYH mutation	1p32.1–34.3 MLH1: 3p21
	Lynch syndrome	Germline MMR mutation	MSH2: 2p16 MSH6: 2p16 PMS2: 7p22
Hyperplastic/ serrated hamartomas	Familial CRC type X	Unknown	Unknown
	Juvenile polyposis syndrome	Germline SMAD 4 mutation	18q21.1
		Germline BMPR1A mutation	10q21–122
	Serrated polyposis syndrome	Unknown	Unknown
	Peutz-Jeghers syndrome	Germline LKB/ STK 11 mutation	19p13.3
	PTEN hamartoma tumor syndrome	Germline PTEN mutation	10q23.3
	Cronkhite-Canada syndrome	Unknown	N/A
Mixed	Hereditary mixed polyposis syndrome	Unknown	15q 14–22
		Possibly CRAC1	

Hamartomatous Polyposis Syndromes

- JPS (Juvenile polyposis syndrome)
- PJS (Peutz-Jeghers syndrome)
- PTEN hamartoma syndrome (Cowden, Bannayan-Riley-Ruvalcaba)
- Cronkhite-Canada syndrome

Polyposis Syndromes

FAP

- APC gene—Chr 5q21
- Cockayne—1927—described the hereditary transmission—autosomal dominant
- Lemuel Herrera—in 1986—mutation of APC gene
- Multiple colonic polyps
- Gastric, duodenal, periampullary polyps—in 50%
- Extraintestinal manifestations
  - Epidermoid cysts
  - Desmoid tumors of abdomen
  - Osteomas
  - Brain tumors
- Gastric polyps are fundic gland hyperplasia—not adenomatous—limited malignant potential
- Duodenal polyps are adenomatous have malignant potential
- Can develop ampullary ca
- Adenomatous polyps can develop cancer in jejunum and ileum
- Rarely cancer of extrahepatic biliary tree, pancreas, adrenal, thyroid, Liver

CHRPE

Congenital Hypertrophic Retinal Pigment Epithelium

- Most common extracolonic manifestation—CHRPE-in 75%
- Mutations between codons 543 and 1309 of APC gene—associated with high risk of CHRPE
- Bilateral lesions suggestive of FAP
- Can find isolated lesions without FAP
- Can be used to identify FAP family

FAP

Gene is expressed in 100% patients with mutation
- Autosomal dominant—so expression in 50% of offspring
- 10–20%—no family history—spontaneous germline mutation
- For testing, DNA from peripheral blood leucocyte used
- All patients develop cancer if untreated
- Average age of discovery of new patient—29 years
- Median age of adenoma development—17 years
- Average age of new cancer—39–40 years
- Death by 44 years

Gardner Syndrome

- Polyps, osteoma, epidermal cysts
- Osteomas over skull, mandible—most common sites—benign
- Supernumerary teeth, dentigerous cyst

Turcot

- With brain tumor

Thyroid Cancer in FAP

- Incidence 1–2% in FAP
- Most common—papillary Ca
- Females more
- Average age 27 years
- More multifocal and with LN metastasis
- In one-third may present before FAP, one-third concurrent, one-third has FAP at the time of diagnosis of TC
- May be associated with CHRPE gene location
- Commonest pathological type—cribriform morular type—if this pathology is detected—screen for FAP

Desmoid Tumor in FAP

- One-third in FAP develops desmoid
- Locally aggressive—no metastasis, fatal due to local infiltration
- Second most common cause of death in FAP, after CRC
- 80% intra-abdominal
- Early lesion—flat—desmoid precursor lesions
- Mutation towards 3' end of APC gene

  Risk factors
  - History of prior surgery—2 years after
  - Females
  - Family history
- Seen on first surgery—in 2%

  Staging
  - Stage I—<10 cm, asymptomatic—not growing
  - Stage II—symptomatic, not growing <10 cm
  - Stage III—symptomatic 11–20 cm
  - Stage IV—rapid growth, symptoms, >20 cm

Treatment

- First line: NSAID—Sulindac and Indomethacin
- Antiestrogens—Tamoxifen, Raloxifen
  - Combination
- Most commonly used—agents Vinblastine, MTX
  - Doxorubicin

- Tyrosine kinase inhibitors: Imatinib
- Role RT—in postop or inoperable

Surgery

- Reserved for selected cases—not first line
- Postop RT
- High chance of recurrence and short bowel syndrome
- Abdominal wall desmoids excised with 2 cm margin
- Cytotoxic drugs reserved for severe tumors

Upper GI Neoplasia in FAP

- Gastric fundal polyps—very low risk
- Antral polyps more risk—seen in 10% of FAP

Duodenal Adenomas

- Duodenal adenomas—found in >90% of FAP
- Duodenal polyps progress similar to colorectal polyps
- Duodenal cancer risk—4%—second most common malignancy
  – Spigelman type IV—36%
- Associated with less colorectal polyps
- No known gene mutation position

Spigelman Classification

Modified Spigelman classification for staging duodenal polyposis in FAP patients			
	Points		
Variable	**1**	**2**	**3**
Number of polyps	1–4	5–20	>20
Polyp size (mm)	1–4	5–10	>10
Histology	Tubular	Tubulovillous	Villous
Dysplasia	Low grade		High grade
Stage 0 (no polyps) 0 points, Stage I 1–4 points; Stage II 5–6 points, Stage III 7–8 points, Stage IV 9–12 points			

- Low risk stage 0, I, II—screening endoscopy—2 to 3 years
- High risk stage III, IV—endoscopy every 6 to 12 months
- Surgical intervention in Stage IV and some stage III
- **Duodenal adenomas**
  – **Surgical therapy**
- Reserved for high risk
  – Extensive polyposis
  – Rapid growth
  – Villous lesion with high grade dysplasia
  – Spigelman IV
- Pancreaticoduodenectomy in
  – Cancer, large, rapidly enlarging with dysplasia
- Others
  – Local excision, ampullectomy

Pancreatic Tumor in FAP

- Increased incidence of adenocarcinoma, cystic tumors, acinar cell and islet cell tumors

Hepatoblastoma in FAP

- Absolute risk <2%
- No specific genotype

Adrenal Adenoma in FAP

- Present in 7–13% in FAP
- Clinical features and management similar to nonFAP tumors

Brain Tumors in FAP

Turcot Syndrome, Brain Tumor Polyposis Syndrome

- Most common medulloblastoma—80%
- Absolute lifetime risk 7 times that of normal population
- Overall lifetime risk of brain tumor in FAP is only 1–2%
- Codons 697 to 1224—more risk
- More in cerebellum
- More in females

FAP—Medical Treatment

- Sulindac, celecoxib, omega 3 FA
- Do not prevent occurring
- Suppress formation of polyps
- Cause regression of polyps

Surgery

Timing of prophylactic colectomy		
Urgency	*Timing*	*Indication*
Immediate	Next available list	Cancer Symptoms Complications of colonoscopy
Soon	Within 3 months	Profuse polyposis (>1000 adenomas) Multiple are >1 cm adenoma High grade dysplasia in an adenoma
Sometime	Annual	Mild polyposis (100–1000 adenomas) Asymptomatic Social factors
Defer	Delay as much as possible	High risk of desmoid disease High comorbidity

- Abdominal colectomy + Ileorectal anastomosis
- 6–12 monthly proctoscope
- If mutation occurs after codon 1250—3 times more risk of rectal cancer than before this codon
- If there are no polyps in rectum and if mutation is before codon 1250—ileorectal anastomosis may be considered.

Surgical Procedures

- Total colectomy, ileorectal anastomosis, ileostomy
- Total proctocolectomy, ileostomy
- Total proctocolectomy, IPAA
  – One stage, two stage
- Total PC with end ileostomy
  – Mainly in older patients
  – Poor sphincter function
  – Carcinoma distal rectum
- **Restorative proctocolectomy and IPAA**
  – Total proctocolectomy
  – Pouch created using 30 cm of ileum
  – Anastomosed to anus
  – By stapling or
  – Hand sewn—after stripping distal rectal mucosa
- IPAA: Anastomosis

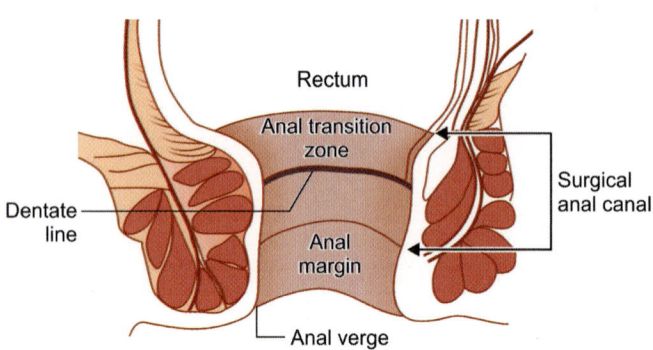

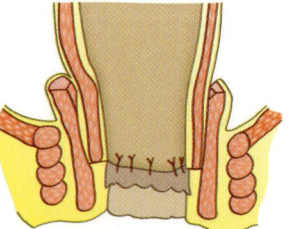

Trans anal mucosal resection and hand anastomosis

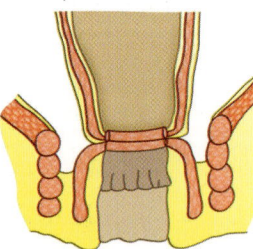

Stapled anastomosis

Trans anal Mucosal Resection or Stapled

Risk of Cancer after Ileorectal Anastomosis

- 5 years—4%
- 10 years—6%
- 15 years—8%
- 20 years—25%
- One-third (30–40%)—develop florid polyposis of rectum—may need proctectomy in 20 years

Risk Higher

- >20 rectal polyps,
- >1000 total polyps,
- Mutation between 1250 and 1464,
- Towards 3′ end of codon 1250 of APC gene

IPAA Risk of Neoplasia

- Following double stapling—30%
- Mucosectomy and handsewn—15%

Attenuated AFP

- Fewer <100 polyps
- More proximal
- Average age of CRC—55 years
- Lifetime risk of CRC—69%

Mutations

- Near 5′
- Exon 6 and exon 9
- After codon 1580 Near 3′ end
- Higher risk of gastric, ampullary cancers
- CHRPE, Desmoids—rare
- Needs colonoscopy for evaluation
- Tendency for rectal sparing
- Treatment
  – Similar to FAP
  – Small no. of polyps—polypectomy—surveillance
  – Colectomy and IRA

MUTYH Associated Polyps

MAP

- Autosomal recessive
- No role in sporadic CRC
- Fewer polyps
- More proximal distribution
- Average age of diagnosis—45
- Risk of CRC—100% in 4–7 decades
- Duodenal polyps 18–26%
- There will be fundic gland polyps
- Extraintestinal cancers
  – Breast, endometrium, bladder, skin
- Desmoid and osteomas: Do not occur
- Most are microsatellite stable

Treatment

- Endoscopic polypectomy and surveillance
- Some say prophylactic surgery
- Colectomy and IRA
- If rectum involved Total proctocolectomy and IPAA

Lynch Syndrome

- First described by Alfred Warthin in 1913:
  – 'Family G'
- Later in 1966 Henry Lynch—'Cancer Family syndrome'
- Most frequent hereditary colorectal cancer syndrome

- Accounts for 3–4% of all CRC
- Autosomal dominant
- Mean age 44 years
- 80% with Lynch syndrome develop CRC in lifetime
- 70% of cancers on right colon
- 20–30% Rectal ca, 16–24% as initial px
- Predominantly mucinous/poorly differentiated/signet ring
- More synchronous/metachronous cancers
- Good outcome after surgery
- 60% occur before the age 50

Clinical criteria for hereditary non-polyposis CRC

Amsterdam criteria

At least 3 relatives with colon cancer +
- 1 affected is a 1st degree relative of other 2
- 2 successive generations affected
- At least one case diagnosed <50 yrs of age
- FAP excluded

Modified Amsterdam criteria

Same as Amsterdam, except that cancer must be associated with HNPCC instead of specifically colon cancer

Bethesda criteria
Amsterdam criteria or any one of the following:
- 2 HNPCC associated cancers in one patient including synchronous/metachronous cancer
- Colon cancer and a 1st degree relative with HNPCC associated cancer and/or colonic adenoma
- Colon or endometrial cancer diagnosed <45 years
- Undifferentiated or signet cell type right sided colon cancer diagnosed <45 yrs
- Adenomas diagnosed <40 years

Genes Responsible for Lynch

- Germline mutation of MMR genes
- hMLH1 (3p21)
- hMSH6 (2p16–21)
- hPMS2 (7p21)
- hPMS1 (2q)
- hMSH2 (2p21)

- hMSH2 or hMLH1—responsible for >90% mutations
- hMSH6—increased endometrial cancer
- In sporadic cancers
  - Defective function is due to methylation that silences the gene—rather than mutation—CpG island methylator phenotype (CIMP)
- Most commonly affected gene in sporadic cancer-MLH1
- Microsatellite instability
  - Microsatellite stable (MSS)
  - MSI-L-low instability
  - MSI-H-high
  - MSI-H have better prognosis for same stage than MSS
- Absence of MMR protein—decreased responsiveness to 5FU
- 20% have spontaneous germ line mutation so, family history may not reflect
- In CRC <50 years do genetic testing and if MMR is positive—other family members should be tested
- Absence of MMR mutation with suggestive history of Lynch—does not exclude Lynch
- In 50% with clear history—DNA testing may be negative

Testing

- IHC for MMR mutation on tumor tissue
  - Good sensitivity and specificity on cancer tissue
  - Low on adenomas—70%
- MSI testing-compare the length of microsatellites in tumor DNA to normal DNA in blood
  - Only 60% adenomatous tissue show accuracy
- So in adenomatous polyps with suspicion of Lynch syndrome—gene sequencing is done

Extracolonic Manifestations
Urogenital

- Ca endometrium
  - Risk 45%
  - Higher in MSH2 and MSH6
- Upper urothelial cancer
  - 6% lifetime risk
  - High risk in MSH2 mutation
- Gastric cancer
  - Incidence 30–70%
  - MSH6—low risk
  - MSH2—higher risk
  - More intestinal type

Screening

Colonoscopy starting at 20 years
- Every 2 years till age 35—then annually
- Endometrial vacuum curettage, USG, CA-125-at age 25
- Urine occult blood—renal ca
- Needs frequent surveillance

Treatment
- Adenomas—managed by colonoscopy
- Abdominal colectomy with ileorectal anastomosis
- TAH + BSO
- Annual proctoscopy for rectum
- Role of prophylactic colectomy—not clear

- Lynch associated CRC have better prognosis than other CRC for same stage
- Lynch with rectal cancer—role of TPC with IPAA—role to prevent metachronous ca
- Proximal cancer colon after proctectomy alone—16–55% in 10–15 years

Variations of Lynch

Muir-Torre Syndrome

- Lynch syndrome with
  – Sebaceous adenomas and cancer
  – Hair follicle tumor—keratoacanthoma
  – Sebaceous adenomas of trunk and extremities—most common presentation
- Most common mutation MSH2

Turcot Syndrome

- CRC and brain tumor
  – Associated with MMR mutation in Lynch—Glioblastoma
- Associated with APC mutation: Anaplastic
  – Astrocytoma, ependymoma, medulloblastoma

Constitutional Mismatch Repair Deficiency (CMMRD)

- Biallelic inheritance of MMR variations
- CRC before age 20, adenomatous polyps 10–100
- Café au lait skin lesions
- Brain tumors
- Mean age of first cancer 16 years

Familial CRC Type X

- Similar to Lynch
- Family history similar to Amsterdam criteria
- But no MMR mutation
- More of left-sided cancer
- Slightly older 60 years vs 40—between Lynch and sporadic
- More well differentiated, aneuploid, less often mucinous
- Have twofold risk for CRC than general population
- But lesser than Lynch patients
- Colonoscopic surveillance—similar to Lynch
- Treatment based on phenotype
- Polyps managed by scopy
- No extra colonic malignancy—no screening needed
- Segmental colectomy preferred over total—synchronous lesions less
- Screening colonoscopy at 45

Mutation Negative Lynch or Tumor Lynch or Lynch Like

- No MMR mutation
- Tumor profile is like Lynch syndrome but no germline mutation

Serrated Polyposis Syndrome
(Hyperplastic Polyposis Syndrome)

- Multiple hyperplastic polyps in colon and rectum
- May have serrated adenomas and adenomas
- Polyps—6 to 40 in numbers
- Age 4–6th decade
- WHO criteria for diagnosis
  1. Presence of 5 or more hyperplastic or serrated polyps proximal to sigmoid colon, with two or more measuring at least 1 cm
  2. Any number of polyps proximal to sigmoid, with a first degree relative with SPS
  3. >20 hyperplastic or serrated polyps, any size, anywhere in colon
- Risk of CRC—40–50%
- Family history of CRC
- CRC develops at early age, multiple
- BRAF mutation and methylation of CpG islands—the neoplastic pathway
- Polyps are treated by endoscopic removal
- Surgery depending on polyps/CRC
- Colectomy with IRA, preferred surgery

Hamartomatous Polyposis Syndromes

- Juvenile polyposis syndrome
- Peutz-Jeghers syndrome
- PTEN hematoma tumor syndrome
  – **Cowden**
  – **Bannayan-Riley-Ruvalcaba**

JPS

- Most common polyps in pediatric population
- Solitary hamartomas present in Rectosigmoid-separate from JPS
  – Age 4–5 years
- Average age of presentation—19 years
- Criteria for diagnosis—one of the three
  1. 3 to 10 hamartomatous polyps on colonoscopy
  2. Hamartomatous polyps outside colon
  3. Any number of hamartomatous polyps in a patient with family history of juvenile polyps

3 Types

- Juvenile polyposis coli—hamartomatous polyps only in colon
- Generalised juvenile polyposis—hamartomatous polyps in colon, stomach, SI
- Juvenile polyposis of infancy—diarrhea, protein losing enteropathy, bleeding, rectal prolapse—often fatal

Clinical Features

- Spherical/lobular polyps
- Pedunculated
- Size up to 3 cm
- Vascular
- May be ulcerated
- Present with—diarrhea, intussusception, prolapse
- Extraintestinal manifestations—seen in 10–20%
  - Heart defects
  - Polydactyly
  - Clubbing
  - Malrotation
  - Hydrocephalus, macrocephalus
  - Undescended testis
- Family history in 25–50%
- Autosomal dominant
- Genes associated
  - SMAD4
  - BMPR1A
  - ENG
- SMAD4—associated with hereditary hemorrhagic telangiectasia also
- Sporadic hamartomatous polyps—no risk of cancer
- JPS risk of adenoma—carcinoma
- CRC risk—40%
  - Mean age 35–45
- Risk of pancreatic, gastric and intestinal cancer present

Screening:

- Colonoscopy at age 15–18
- UGI scopy started at 25
- If clinical and genetic study negative—1–2 yearly screening till age 35
  - If mutation seen—until the age of 70

Treatment

- Polyps—managed endoscopically
- **Surgery**—For complications
  - Large number, bleeding, hypoproteinemia
- Following surgery—endoscopic surveillance needed

PJS

- Characterized by
  - GI hamartomatous polyps <100
  - Mucocutaneous melanin pigmentation

- Caused by mutation of
  - TSG-STK11 gene known as LKB1
  - Located on chromosome 19p13.3
  - 25%-*de novo* STK11 mutation—no family history
- Diagnosed when any of the following:
  1. Two or more of histologically confirmed hamartomatous polyps
  2. Any number of hamartomatous polyps with family history of PJS
  3. Mucocutaneous pigmentation with family history of PJS
- Polyps size 1 mm to 4 cm
- Most common location jejunum and other SI—60%
- Colon in 50%
- Stomach also
- Polyps in nose, bronchus, biliary tract
- Melanotic macules
  - Most common site vermillion border of lips—95%
  - Then buccal mucosa
  - Other sites—digits of hand and feet, perianal, genital regions
  - Appear in infancy and early years—maximal level in adolescence—fade away after puberty
- Most common presentation—abdominal pain due to intussusception
- Others
  - Bleeding
  - Anemia
  - Biliary obstruction
  - GOO
- One-third present in—first decade
- Two-thirds by third decade
- Colorectal cancer risk—nearly 40%
- Average age of first malignancy—45 years
- Ca esophagus, stomach, Ca SI, and colon
  Extraintestinal cancer
  Thyroid, lung, pancreas, GB cancer
- In women, cancer of ovary, uterus
- Men—Sertoli cell tumor
- In PJS—major cause of death—cancer
- Cancer in PJS due to mucosal instability

Mallorca guidelines for screening and surveillance of PJS is used

PJS: Treatment

- Aggressive endoscopic polypectomy

Surgery in

Adenomatous change
Complications
- No role for prophylactic colectomy

PTEN Hamartoma Tumor Syndrome

Phosphatase and Tensin Homolog Protein-encoded by PTEN Gene

Cowden and Bannayan-Riley-Ruvalcaba, syndromes

- Gene mutation mutation—10q23.3
- PTEN is a tumor suppressor gene
- Intestinal polyps and extraintestinal manifestations
- There is evidence of increased CRC
- Colon can have hamartomatous polyps

Cowden Syndrome

- Autosomal dominant

  Features
  - Benign hamartomas
  - Malignant tumors of breast, thyroid, uterus, brain, mucocutaneous tissue
- 85% will have germline mutation of PTEN gene
- Breast cancer risk 30–50% in men also
- Thyroid—benign and cancer (10%)
- Renal cell carcinoma

Bannayan-Riley-Ruvalcaba

- Features
  - Macrocephaly
  - Developmental delays
  - Pigmented speckling of penis
  - Lipoma and hamartomas of intestines
  - Incidence of GI polyps—45%
  - >60%—PTEN mutation

Screening and Surveillanace for PTEN Mutation

- Breast cancer screening starting at 18 years mammogram at 30
- Thyroid cancer screening starting at 18 years
- Endometrial cancer screening at 35 years
- RCC screening also
- Colonoscopy at 20—1–2 yearly
- OGD at 30 years

Manifestations of PTEN mutations—treated similar to sporadic counterparts

Gorlin syndrome—Nevoid basal cell carcinoma syndrome

Proteus syndrome—Elephant man syndrome
- No obvious colonic involvement
- But may require evaluation of Colon-subepithelial polyps

Cronkhite-Canada Syndrome

- Acquired GI polyposis syndrome
- Not an inherited disorder

- Infection, toxins, nutritional deficiency, stress—all suspected
- Features
  - Hamartomatous polyps
  - Dystrophy of nails, alopecia
  - Cutaneous pigmentation
- Arise from tissues of ectodermal in origin

Manifestations

- Present in 6th decade with cutaneous and GI manifestations
- Watery diarrhea, dysgeusia (altered taste)
- Anemia, hypoproteinemia
- Electrolyte disturbance
- Polyps found throughout GIT—sparing esophagus
- Most common site in GIT—stomach

Complications

- Mucosal ulceration,
- GI bleeding
- Rectal prolapse, intussusception
- Increased risk for CRC and carcinoma stomach

Management

- Screening for CRC and stomach—yearly
- Supportive care, fluid—electrolyte management
- Steroids, antibiotics
- Anabolic steroids
- H2 blocker, PPI
- Medical treatment for 6–12 months
- Steroid for recurrence
- Surgery for bleeding, cancer—more morbidity

Hereditary Mixed Polyposis Syndrome

- Autosomal dominant
- Colon polyps of varied histology
- Increased risk of CRC
- No extraintestinal manifestations
- Polyps—hamartomas, adenomas, serrated, hyperplastic
- Can develop early age CRC
- No risk for any other cancer
- Spread throughout colon <15 in number
- Colon only organ involved

Genes

- CRAC1 gene on chromosome 15q14-22
- THBS1 on chromosome 15q21.1

Differential Diagnosis

- FAP and PJS—they have extraintestinal manifestations
- Lynch and MAP—they do not have hamartomatous polyps
- Juvenile polyposis is more difficult to differentiate.
- Colonoscopy started at 18–20 years—1–2 yearly
- Total abdominal colectomy and IRA—in selected patients
  - Choice if CRC develops
- Rectal stump surveillance needed

Risk Stratification for CRC Screening

Average Risk For CRC (must fulfil all)

- Age 50 years or older
- No personal history of polyps or CRC
- No first degree relative with polyps or CRC
- Fewer than 2 second degree relatives with CRC

Moderate risk for CRC (any criteria)
- First degree relative with CRC or polyp at age younger than 60 years.
- First degree relative with CRC or polyp at age 60 years or older
- Two or more second degree relatives with CRC

Increased risk for CRC (any criteria)
- Gene carrier or at risk for FAP
- Gene carrier or at risk for HNPCC
- After genetic testing of a family member—by venipuncture—noninheritance is seen—he can be avoided from further screening

---

Recommendations for colorectal cancer screening

Patients with average risk:

1. **FOBT:** Yearly screening. 2 samples from each of 3 consecutive stools without rehydration. Positive test—colonoscopy follow-up.
2. Flexible sigmoidoscopy: Every 5 yrs
3. FOBT plus flexible sigmoidoscopy: FOBT annually and sigmoidoscopy every 5 yrs.
4. Colonoscopy every 10 yrs
5. Barium enema every 5 yrs

Patients with increased risk:

1. **Family history of colorectal cancer or polyps:** 1st degree relative with colon cancer or adenomatous polyp diagnosed by less than 60 yrs of age or two 1st degree relatives with the same diagnosed at any age—screening colonoscopy starting at 40 yrs of age or 10 yrs younger than age of earliest diagnosis in family(whichever first), repeated every 5 yrs
2. **HNPCC:** Colonoscopy every 1–2 yrs starting at ages 20–25 yrs or 10 yrs younger than earliest diagnosis in family (whichever first). Genetic testing.

---

3. **FAP:** Flexible sigmoidoscopy start at ages of 10–12. Genetic testing (upper endoscopy with side viewing scope) done every 1–3 yrs
4. **Personal history of adenomatous polyps:**
   - If one or more polyps that are malignant or large and sessile or incomplete colonoscopy, then follow-up colonoscopy must be in short-term basis.
   - If 3 or more polyps, follow-up colonoscopy in 3 yrs
   - If one or two polyps alone, which are less than 1 cm, follow-up scopy in 5 yrs
5. **Personal history of colorectal cancer:**
   - Colonoscopy incomplete at the time of diagnosis, then repeat colonoscopy in 6 months after surgical resection
   - Complete colonoscopy done at diagnosis, repeat colonoscopy in 3 yrs, if normal, repeat every 5 yrs
   - IBD, surveillance colonoscopy recommended.

Colorectal Cancer

- Right-sided cancer has increased in incidence
- 40% of CRC proximal to the area of sigmoidoscopy
- Bleeding from right-sided Ca—can produce melena
- In one-third of colonic cancer—Hb normal stool no occult blood
- Colonoscopy—gold standard
- Lifetime risk—6%
- In other GI solid tumors—Invasion of lamina propria into muscularis mucosa is T1
  - In CRC—T1—is involvement of submucosa
- Longitudinal intramural lymphatic spread is limited to 2 cm. So, 5 cm clearance is advisable
- Paracolic LN along marginal artery—most abundant and most important
- Lymphatic spread—stepwise paracolic—intermediate—principal nodes
- Rarely skip metastasis can occur due to retrograde spread due to tumor blockage of main efferent channels—gastrocolic omentum
- 7–8 cm above anal verge, at the level of middle rectal valve—lymphatic watershed line
- High ligation of IMA—no advantage—may increase autonomic nerve injury
- Mesorectal excision 5 cm distally in high rectal growth
- **TME** is done in middle and low rectal growth only
- **CRM** (Circumferential Resection Margin)—Is the distance in mm from the deepest point of tumor invasion in the primary cancer and the margin of resection in the retroperitoneum or mesentery
- Achieved by resection of pericolic/rectal fatty and fibrous tissue and pelvis
- The term does not apply to the anatomic serosa of the colon or rectum that is peritonealised

Tumor Regression Score: By Ryan

Description	TRS
No viable cancer cell (complete response)	0
Single or small groups of cancer cells (near complete)	1
More than single cells with residual cancer, which shows tumor regression (partial response)	2
No tumor regression, with extensive risk of cancer (poor or no response)	3

Prognostic Factors in Colorectal Cancer—CRM

- Surgically dissected nonperitonealised surface
- Colon—the area of retroperitoneum
- Mid and lower rectum—entire surface
- In rectum all mesorectal tissue and LN removed and the margin is mesorectal fascia
- CRM is positive if less or equal to 1 mm clearance
  - >2 mm can predict local recurrence

Prognostic Factors

- CEA
- Tumor deposits
  - Number of satellite tumor deposits discontinuous from tumor edge, not associated with LN mets
  - Tumor regression grade after NACT/RT
- Circumferential margin
- Resected margin
- Microsatellite instability
- Perineural invasion
- KRAS mutation status, if mutated cause lack of response to EGFR monoclonal antibodies

Staging Investigations

- CXR
- CT chest abdomen, pelvis
- EUS
- MRI
- PET-CT

Surgery

- Mechanical preparation not favoured for colonic cancer—mainly done for low rectal cancers
- Risk of anastomotic leak in ileocolic and colocolic—4 to 8%
- Omentum attached to the removed colon—resected

Colonic Resections

- Right hemicolectomy
- Extended right hemicolectomy
- Left hemicolectomy
- Sigmoidectomy
- Segmental resection

Follow-up Therapy

Stage 0—(Tis, N0, M0)

- Very low risk of LN metastasis
- Excision of polyp
- Follow-up colonoscopy
- If cannot be excised—segmental resection

Stage I

- Observe with colonoscopy—after one year
- If polyps detected—scopy annually—until scopy reveals no polyps
- Then colonoscopy 5 yearly
- If family history or syndromes—more frequent scopy
- CEA every 3 months for 2 years—even if preop value normal
  - Rising value suggestive of metastasis

Stage I: Malignant Polyp (T1N0M0)

- Malignant polyp with carcinoma in the head with no stalk involvement—<1% chance of LN involvement—resected endoscopically
- LV invasion, tumor budding, PD tumors, tumor within 1 mm of resection—segmental colectomy
- Sm 1—low risk
- Sm 2—intermediate risk
- Sm 3—high risk
- Sessile polyp with invasive carcinoma extending to submucosa—segmental colectomy

Stage II (T2, 3N0, M0)

- Surgical resection
- Postop chemo role not clear
- 5-FU based chemo or Oxaliplatin in—young patients with high risk in
  - Insufficient LN sampling (<12)
  - T4 lesions
  - Poorly differentiated
  - Perforation
- Oxaliplatin not indicated in good risk stage II
- Follow-up with 3 monthly CEA—2 years

- Then 6 monthly for 5 years
- Annual CT for 3 years
- In stage II with MSI—single agent FU/LV—not beneficial
- So in stage II MMR testing may be important

Stage III (Any T, N1, M0)

- Postoperative chemotherapy with FOLFOX
- MSI-H will not benefit from 5-FU based Chemo

Stage IV-M1

- If Asymptomatic—Chemotherapy
- Isolated metastasis—surgery
  - Survival 15–24%—5 years
- 5FU regimens
- Cetuximab-chimeric monoclonal antibody to EGFR
- Panituzumab-human-monoclonal antibody to EGFR
  - Indicated only in KRAS mutation negative
- Bevacizumab-vascular endothelial GR inhibitor
- With FOLFOX

Stage IV—Metastasis

- Most common site-liver
- 15% will be limited to liver—of these 20% resectable for cure
- Second commonest site—lung-in 20%—1 to 2% will be resectable
- HIPEC
- Stenting
- Radiotherapy

Prognosis

- Stage I—90%—5 years
- IIA—85%
- IIB—70%
- III—50%
- IV—<5%

Oxaliplatin

- Oxaliplatin by itself having only minimal antitumor action—but when combined with leucovorin/FU active
- **MOSAIC trial**—Multicenter International Study of Oxaliplatin/FU/Leucovorin in the adjuvant treatment of colon cancer—FOLFOX

- Only effective in Stage III—no advantage of Oxaliplatin in stage II
- Platinum based
- No nephrotoxicity—have neurotoxicity and myelosuppression
- **MOSAIC**—Postop FU/LV by 48-hour infusion every other week plus or minus a two-hour infusion of Oxaliplatin—FOLFOX
- NSABP—National Surgical Adjuvant Breast Bowel Project
- C-07 trial—addition of Oxaliplatin to weekly schedule of FU/LV by IV injection—FLOX regimen
  - Oxaliplatin on weeks 1, 3, 5 and 8
  - Substantial amount of diarrhea
- **CapeOx regimen**
- Capecitabine oral + IV Oxaloplatin
- Showing better results than Ox + FU/LV- IV

FOLFIRI

- Irinotecan plus 48-hour infusion of FU/LV
- Demonstrated limited benefit
- Irinotecan, Bevacizumab, Cetuximab—all have limited role in adjuvant treatment
- Main role is in the metastatic set up

Summary

- Stage III and high risk Stage II—FOLFOX preferred
- Cape Ox and FLOX—alternatives
- Irinotecan, Bevacizumab and Cetuximab only in metastasis
- If to be treated with fluoropyrimidines alone—FU/LV or Oral Capecitabine plus Leucovorin—good option
- Stage II role of adjuvant chemo—unsettled

Treatment of stage IV CRC

- IFL (Irinotecan infusion plus bolus 5FU/LV) vs FOLFOX—FOLFOX preferred-
- Advantage due to infusional 5FU
- FOLFIRI (infusional FU/FV plus Irinotecan vs FOLFOX—same response
- FOLFOX vs CapeOx—same response
- So the frontline Chemo regimens in metastasis—FOLFOX, FOLFIRI, CapeOx

- Bevacizumab (anti-VEGF) monoclonal antibody
  – More effective with chemo
  – Delay wound healing
  – Half life 21 days
  – Discontinued 6 weeks prior to surgery

Cetuximab and Panitumumab-anti-EGFR Monoclonal

- Effective only if KRAS nonmutated—wild type
- Both show 10% single agent response
- Most common side effect—acne-like skin rash—a sign and measure of antitumor activity
- Combination of anti-VEGF plus anti-EGFR—not recommended
- To make stage IV disease operable—Irinotecan regimen with Bevacizumab is better

Postresection followup

- 80% postsurgery recurrence occur in 3 years
- CEA 3–6 monthly for 2 years and every 6 months for 5 years
- CECT chest abdomen pelvis—annually for 3 years
- Colonoscopy—at 1 year or after 6 months, if there is no colonoscopy done prior to surgery—then 3 years later—then every 5 years
- PET—not routine
- Clinical—3–6 monthly—for 3 years—then annually for 2 years
- After 5 years—symptomatic evaluation
- Colonoscopy continued indefinitely—look for synchronous/metachronous lesions

CEA

Normal value <5 ng/ml

- Half life 7–14 days—measured several weeks after surgery
- Serial values parallel progression/regression
- Preop value should fall in 2–3 weeks postop
- Newly elevated CEA—repeat to see lab error—Full body CT—if negative—colonoscopy
- CEA shows steep rise—if liver or lung the first or only site of metastasis
- Value of PET in evaluation of elevated CEA—questionable

Rectal Cancer

Denonvilliers fascia, Waldeyers fascia, investing fascia (fascia propria)

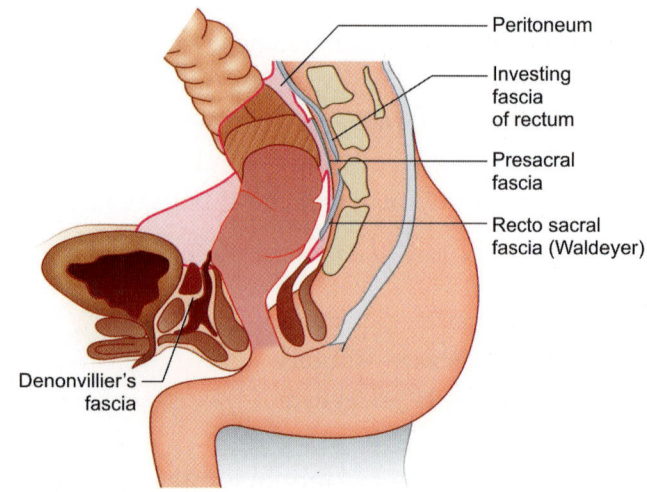

- Most common symptom—hematochezia
- Internal intussusception—mucosal trauma—polypoid lesion—benign columnar epithelium residing deep to muscularis mucosae—Colitis Cystica Profunda
- Above peritoneal reflection—covered by peritoneum anteriorly and on sides—posteriorly mesorectum
  – Below completely extra peritoneal
- Mesorectum tapers towards anorectal ring—almost absent 2 cm proximal to levator ani, where longitudinal muscle becomes the internal sphincter

Evaluation

- Assessment of relation of lesion with sphincter, invasion, depth and LNs
- Precise location best seen by rigid proctosigmoidoscopy/flexible sigmoidoscopy
- Depth by
  – Digital examination
  – EUS—most useful in T1—for local excision
  – MRI—most accurate in local staging
  – CT—for metastasis

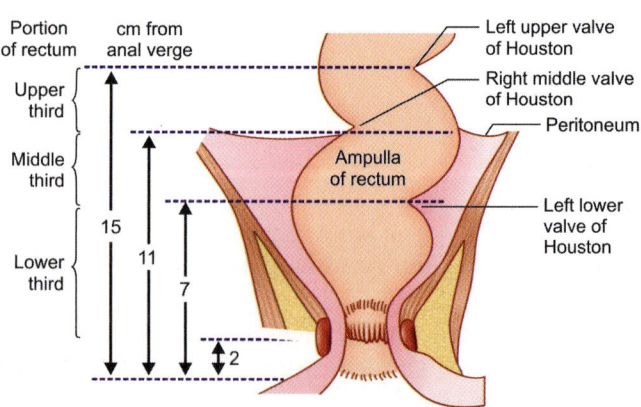

Upfront Surgery
Low Rectal Cancer

- cT3a/b-levator free, MRF (mesorectal fascia) free, N0
- No other invasion

MRI Based T Staging of Rectal Cancer

T1	Invades submucosa
T2	Invades muscularis propria
T3	Invades subserosa
T3a	Tumor extends less than 1 mm, beyond muscularis propria
T3b	1–5 mm beyond MP
T3c	5–15 mm beyond MP
T3d	>15 mm beyond MP
T4a	Invades peritoneal reflection
T4b	Invades other organs

Surgical Treatment—Rectal Cancer
- Total mesorectal excision (TME)
- Circumferential clearance
- Longitudinal clearance

Treatment—Rectal Tumors
- Anterior resection—resection of rectum if done above peritoneal reflection—high AR
- Low anterior resection—resection below peritoneal reflection
- Ultra low anterior resection—resection and anastomosis at the level of levator ani
- Intersphincteric resection—rectum resected along with internal sphincter and colo-anal anastomosis done—continence is dependent on external sphincter only
- Abdomino perineal resection
- Extra Levator Abdomino Perineal Excision (ELAPE)—in very low tumors involving levator muscle or close to them—wide resection of levator muscles, with possible flap cover of the defect

Correct Technique of TME
- Improved survival from 50 to 75%
- Decreased local recurrence from 30 to 5%
- Decreased incidence of impotence and bladder dysfunction from 85 to <15%

- Ligation of lymph vascular pedicle at the origin of superior rectal artery, distal to origin of LCA—low tie
- Ligation of IMA at its origin—high tie
- Meso-rectal spread of tumor is usually 3 to 4 cm distal to tumor—so lower end of resection of mesorectum—5 cm distal to lower end of tumor. So, TME is not done in upper rectal cancer and it is called tumor-specific TME.
- Some mesorectum is left attached to distal rectal stump
- TME is done in middle and lower rectal cancers.

LAR Anastomosis
- LAR syndrome-frequency of stools
  - **To increase capacity of the colonic end (neo-rectum)**
- J colonic pouch using 6 cm pouch
- Coloplasty
  - 8–10 cm long incision, 4–6 cm from divided end and closed transversely

Neoadjuvant CRT
- Upper third rectal ca—treated as rectosigmoid—no NACRT

For Mid and Lower Third Rectum
Indications-after MRI
- cT3b-d-tumor within 1 mm from mesorectal fascia
- cT4, N1
- Extramural vascular invasion
- Infiltration of internal and external sphincter and intersphincteric space
- Stage II or higher (T3c or higher)

Long Course: CRT
- Preop 4500–5040 cGy with infusion of 5FU—Leucovrin, 5FU alone or Capecitabine—5 to 6 weeks—surgery 6–10 weeks later—diverting ileostomy—closed 10 weeks later
- Complete response in 20%

Short Course
- 25 Gy—1 week—1 week rest—surgery—no chemo
- Goal of RT—better local control

- Even if a pathologically complete response to CRT—postop chemo should be given—FOLFOX
- Concurrent CRT—5FU preferred
- Total neoadjuvant therapy (TNT)—systemic chemotherapy followed by chemoradiation only with no surgery

Rectal Cancer-Local Excision Indications

- Within 10 cm from dentate line
- <3 cm in size
- <30% of circumference
- T1N0 lesions-LN metastasis 8%
- Well/Mod differentiated
- No lymphovenous spread
- For evaluation MRI preferred over EUS
- CT mainly for metastasis

Kikuchi Classification for Nonpedunculated T1 Lesions

Sm1—invasion <1 mm

Sm2—between sm1 and sm3

Sm3—invasion near to muscularis propria

Rectal Cancer-Local Treatment

- Trans anal excision
- Trans coccygeal excision
- Trans sphincteric excision
- Trans anal microscopic endosurgery (TEM)
- Fulgeration
- Radiotherapy

T1 N0, T2N0 Lesions

- Radical procedure better with TME for T2 N0
- Small good risk T2N0—can offer local excision with CRT
- Criteria
  – T1 N0, sm1
  – <3 cm, <30% circumference
  – Distal, accessible
  – No poor histopathology features like poor differentiation, LN invasion, perineural invasion

Local Recurrence After Local Excision

- T1N0—8%
- T2N0—20%

Trans anal Excision

- Tumors <10 cm from anal verge—amenable for
- <3 cm—hybrid approach—distal lesion dissected with TAE-parks retractor-the TAMIS
- Not preferred these days

Trans Coccygeal—Kraske

- Lesions in middle or distal third of rectum
- Especially for lesions of posterior wall of rectum.

Trans Sphincteric—Mason and York

- Similar to trans coccygeal
- Divide levator ani muscles and external sphincters in midline
- Later closed
- More incontinence
- Not done these days

TEM (Transanal Endoscopic Microsurgery)

- For more proximal lesions
- LN metastasis
  – T1sm1—0–3%
  – T1sm2—3–15%
  – T2—25%
  – T3/T4—58%

TAMIS

Atallah—2010
- Port—37 to 44 mm length

Trans Anal-Trans Abdominal TME

TATA-Marks—1984

- Abdominal dissection is done
- Distal dissection trans anally—rectum divided distal to tumor proximal end closed—TME completed—specimen removed—anastomosis
- Can decide where to divide rectum under vision

TA-TME (Trans anal TME)

- Entirely trans anally
- Rectal resection and TME
- Usually done as a hybrid procedure—TATA
- Mobilization of splenic flexure may be difficult
- Abdominal mobilization—up to peritoneal reflection and sacral promontory—anal dissection to proceed and peritoneum opened from anal side

Summary

- Patient-Mobile tumor, <3 cm, 30% circumference
  - T1, T2 with no signs of locoregional/LN metastasis, mobile
- Preop-ERUS, MRI
  - CT for metastasis
- Follow-up
  - Clinical, CEA 3 monthly—for 2 years, 6 monthly–5 years
  - CT yearly for 3 years along with change in CEA
  - Colonoscopy after 1 year—every 3–5 yearly
- Radical surgery—for salvage

Trials Evaluating CRT and TEM in T2 Lesions

- **CARTS trial**—TEM after long course CRT
- **TREC**—TEM and RT in early rectal cancer—following short course RT
- Combined—**STAR-TREC trial**

Lap vs Open

- Lap—inflammatory mediators released less—less immunosuppression—less chance of recurrence
- Long term oncologic function—comparable

To Assess the Vascularity of Colon

- Indocyanine clearance
- Inj 5–10 mg of indocyanine—visualized with near infra-red light—it absorbs infra-red and emits fluorescence

Recurrent CRC

- Incidence of local recurrence 5–15%
- 50% of them will be resectable
- 30–50%—luminal
- 90% relapse within 5 years
- Post NACRT 30% after 5 years
- 90% distant metastasis—within 5 years

Role of PET

- Not routine
- To confirm—distant metastasis before liver resection
- In raising CEA
- In equivocal imaging

Recurrence

- Best assessed by MRI
- As recurrence may be extra luminal
- CRC recurrence—treatment
  - Trimodal

- Preop CRT—surgery with IORT—Chemo
- If previously radiated—10–30 Gy
- Otherwise 50.4 Gy

Contraindications to resection in locally recurrent rectal cancer

- Extensive pelvic wall involvement
- Tumour extension through sciatic notch
- Encasement of iliac vessels
- Sciatic pain
- Predicted R2 resection
- Morbid patient
- Bilateral ureteral obstruction except bladder trigone

Pulmonary Mets

- Second commonest site after liver
- <10% metastasis isolated to lung
- Only 2% resectable
- Indications for resection
  - <3 lesions
  - Each <3 cm
  - Good lung function
  - No extra pulmonary metastasis except liver and primary is controlled

Evidence-Based Recommendations

- Category 1—definitely proven based on published trials and used in management
- Category 2—an extensively studied biologically or clinically—has prognostic value—but not validated by robust studies
- Category 2B—shown promise in multiple studies but data insufficient to be included as 1 or 2A
- Category 3—not yet sufficiently studied
- Category 4—Well-studied and proven no prognostic significance

Prognostic Factors in Colorectal Cancer

- Cat 1—TNM staging, LVI, residual tumor following sx, elevated CEA
- Cat2A—histologic grade, CRM
- Cat2B—MSI, histologic type, loss of heterozygosity of chr 18q (DCC allelic loss), tumor border
- Cat3—microvessel density, molecular markers
- Cat4—tumor size, and morphology

Important Prognostic Factors in CRC

- TNM stage
- CEA

- Resected margins
- **Nodes**
  - Minimum 12 nodes to be examined
  - No. of nodes is considered
- LVI

  Identification of tumor cells within an endothelial lined channel or elastic lamina
  - e.g. L0 L1, V0 V1
  - Tumor contained within afferent vessels and not in lymph nodes is considered L1N0

CRM

Tumor regression grading after NACRT

- 0—No regression
- 1—Minor-Dominant tumor mass, Fibrosis <25% tumor mass
- 2—Moderate—Fibrosis 25–50%
- 3—Good regression—Fibrosis >50%
- 4—Total regression

Histologic Type

- Signet ring cell—worst type (1% of all CRC)
- Mucinous also (10% of CRC)

Infiltrating Border: Adverse vs Expansile Border

- Microvessel density—tumor-induced angiogenesis cause more recurrence and poor survival
- Presenting with obstruction and perforation—poor prognosis

MSI

- MSI-H—poorly differentiated, peritumoral lymphocytic infiltration, medullary type, larger, right sided
  - Longer survival
- MSI-L/MSS—left sided tumor—negative prognostic factors

Loss of Heterozygosity of 18q

- Loss of DCC gene—impairs apoptosis—resistance to chemotherapy
- Poor prognosis
- MSI stable/BRAF mutated—poor prgnosis
- MSI stable/BRAF-wild type—intermediate prognosis
- MSI high/BRAF-wild type—favourable

Perineural Invasion

KRAS mutation status—lack of response to EGFR monoclonal antibodies

Gene Expression Profiling

- ColoPrint—18 gene signature on fresh tissue
- Oncotype DX—utilizes reverse PCR on formalin fixed tissue
- ColDx—634 gene signature using formalin fixed paraffin embedded tissue—for stage II
- ColoGuideEx—13 gene signature for stage II
- ColoGuidePro—7 gene signature for stage III tumors

NET of Colon and Rectum

- Accounts for 0.90% of colonic and 0.5% of rectal tumors
- Argentaffin staining—reducing silver
- Argyraffilic—lack of ability to reduce silver in the absence of a reducing agent
- Midgut—argentaffin positive
- 85 to 95% of hindgut tumors contain argentaffin positive cells
- Carcinoid syndrome seen in 10–18%
  - Episodic flushing
  - Non-bloody watery diarrhea
  - Abdomen pain
  - Right-sided heart failure
- Serotonin—hypermotility
- Kalleikrein—wheezing, flushing
- No primary GI tumor produce carcinoid syndrome—hormones metabolised in liver—otherwise in liver metastasis—or alternate systemic venous drainage
- Colonic—more common in females
- Rectum—equal in both sexes
- Colonic NET—worst prognosis among GINET—5 years 65%
- Rectal NET—best prognosis 5 years 95%
- Rectum more common than colon

Rectum

- Most are asymptomatic
- Usually <1 cm with no LN or metastasis
- 4% present with distant metastasis

Colon

Symptomatic—pain, bleeding, obstruction, altered bowel habit
- Typically >2 cm
- Two-thirds have regional or distant metastasis
- Colorectal—arise from
  - Serotonin producing EC cells
  - Glucagon like peptide producing cells
  - PP producing L cells

Rectum

- Mainly from L cells
- Most are polypoid or submucosal

Diagnosis

- EUS to assess depth and size
- MRI/CT for metastasis—in >2 cm and high grade
- Not necessary to estimate tumor burden in liver for staging
  - But important for treatment
- Gallium labelled octreotide scan
- Markers
  - CgA—tumor load, poor prognosis, monitor response to treatment
  - 5-HIAA
  - Pancreostatin
  - Neurokinin A
- Colonic NET—positive for both CgA and synaptophysin
- Rectal NET—Do not express CgA—but only synaptophysin

Treatment
Colonic

- Surgical resection—choice
- <1 cm tumor—endoscopic submucosal resection, chance of high non R0 resection

Rectal

- <2 cm, with no high risk features
  - EMR, ESD, TAMIS, TEM
- High risk features—oncologic resection and TME indicated
- >2 cm—high chance of metastasis
- Adjuvant RT, chemo—not considered

Follow-up

- Low risk tumors—routine follow with radiology not required
- High risk—CgA 6 monthly—guide CT evaluation

Metastatic Disease

- Somatostatin analogues (CLARINET trial)—choice
- Interferon alfa
- HA embolization

NE Carcinoma

- Very aggressive—NORDIC NEC trial
- 5-year survival—5% with mets, 18% without
- Multimodal therapy

8.4 ANAL NEOPLASMS

- Anal trigger zones—1to 12 mm
- Anal canal in men 3–6 cm
- Anal canal in women 2–4 cm
- ATZ contain—transitional urothelium like epithelium-contain cloacogenic, transitional and basaloid—variants of squamous epithelium—instead of columnar
- Transformation zone—squamous metaplasia above Dentate line-usually lined with columnar epithelium

- Anal verge—junction of mucous membrane of anal canal and skin
- Perianus or anal margin—area of 5 cm radius around anal verge
- Skin lesions—area >5 cm away from perianus

Anal Canal Cancer

- Most common cancer—SCC (epidermoid—70%)
- Second most common—adenocarcinoma
- <2% of large bowel cancer
- Below dentate line—SCC
- Above—basaloid, cloacogenic, transitional— together known as—epidermoid—70%

Anal Margin Tumors
Condyloma Acuminatum (Anal Wart)

- Caused by HPV
- Most common virally transmitted STD
- HPV-6 and HPV-11 cause benign warts
- HPV-16 and HPV-18—dysplasia and cancer
- Pinkish warts
- In anal canal also
- High resolution anoscopy with 5% acetic acid for diagnosis
- Look for immunosuppression—HIV, drugs

Treatment

- Chemical
  - Podophyllin,
    - Cytotoxic, irritants to skin
  - For only minimal extra anal disease
- Trichloro acetic acid,
  - Less irritant
  - Can be used peri and intraanally
- 5 FU
- Imiquimob 5%—3 times weekly (for 6–10 hours)
  - Not suitable for intra-anal use
- Cautery
- Laser
- Surgery
- All associated with high recurrence 30–70%

Anal Intraepithelial Neoplasia

- Low grade squamous anal intraepithelial lesion (LSIL) includes
  - Anal intraepithelial neoplasia I (AIN I) (low grade), anal and perianal condylomas
- High grade squamous anal intraepithelial lesions (HSIL) include Bowen's disease
  - AIN II and III, SCC *in situ*
- AIN grades are determined according to lack of keratinocyte maturation, and extension of proliferative zone
- Proliferative zone lower third of epithelium—AIN I
  - Lower two-thirds or entire epithelium—AIN II or AIN III
- AIN I and II—may regress—but rarely only AIN III
- AIN III is seen in 80% anal cancer biopsies
- Intraepithelial lesions
  - Prevalence—<1%

HSIL

- More common in
  - Immunosuppression
  - HIV
  - Vulvar *in situ* cancer
  - Cervical carcinoma *in situ*
- Progression to malignancy
  - 10% in 5 years
  - HIV positive MSM (men sex with men)—1 in 600 in per year
  - HIV negative MSM 1 in 4000 in per year

Clinical Features

- Present as condyloma
- Itching
- Scaly lesion

HSIL-Treatment

- *In situ*, localized (if <30% of circumference of anus)
- Local excision with margins—more morbidity
- High resolution anoscopy with acetic acid—aid in localizing—area infected with HPV turn white—show the typical vascular patterns—Lugols iodine paint applied—HSIL appears yellow, normal mucosa or LSIL turn brown—biopsied from HSIL—then electrocautery, infrared treatment
- Local 5% Imiquimob
- Local 5% 5 FU cream
- Multifocal
  - Focally ablated
  - Follow-up—for recurrence and invasive cancer

Verrucous Carcinoma

- Giant condyloma acuminatum or Buschke-Lowentein lesion
- Can cause—fistula, infection, malignant transformation
- Treated with wide excision/APR
- SCC can develop—poor prognosis
- Associated with HPV-6 and HPV-11
- Shows exophytic and endophytic growth unlike normal condyloma

Paget's Disease

- They are intraepithelial adenocarcinoma—arise from apocrine glands or pleuripotent keratinocyte stem cells
- Occur in older—7th decade
- Seen in areas of high density apocrine sweat glands
- Can develop into invasive cancer of underlying apocrine glands
- Commonest symptom—pruritus
- Eczematous plaque with ulcer
- Paget cell—PAS positive, due to mucin, large vacuolated cytoplasm with eccentric nucleus—diagnostic
- Extramammary Paget's disease—associated with underlying invasive cancer—in 30–45%
- Visceral malignancy seen in 50%

Treatment

- Limited noninvasive disease—
  - Wide local excision closure or V-Y plasty
- Recurrent noninvasive lesion—re-excision
- Medically unfit, noninvasive lesions-
  - Topical Imiquimob, 5-FU, Cryo, Argon laser
- Invasive disease—radical resection—APR
- 5-year disease-specific survival of extra mammary Paget—50–70%
- Others—Moh's surgery, systemic chemo, photo-dynamic therapy

SCC of Anal Canal
Etiology

- HPV, HIV
- Most common HPV strain—HPV 16-mediated through oncoproteins E6 and E7—inactivation of p53 and pRB—cancer
- Anal receptive intercourse
- Men sex with men (MSM)—20 times more

- No association with chronic inflammatory conditions, hemorrhoids or diet
- Present as mass, bleeding, pruritus

Staging

- CT chest, abdomen, pelvis—for metastasis
- ERUS—for anal canal wall involvement
- MRI pelvis—for mesorectal and inguinal LNE (local staging)
- PET if >T2 lesion—for LN assessment—not palpable or by CT (<8 mm)
- HIV checking and CD4 count

LN Involvement

- <3 cm lesion—<5%
- T3 and T4—(>5 cm)—20%

Regional LN of Anal Canal

- Superficial and deep inguinal
- Mesorectal
- Superior rectal
- External iliac
- Internal iliac

Treatment

- Chemo RT—concurrent
- Infusional 5FU with Mitomicin C and ERT to pelvis—45 Gy
- Inguinal LN, pelvis, anus, perineum included in the field
- T2 lesion and residual disease after 45 Gy, T3, T4 or with positive lymph nodes—additional 9–14 Gy (total RT 54 to 59 Gy)
- RT should include inguinal LN
- Recurrent/persistent disease—APR
- 15–30%—fail to respond to CRT
- Local recurrence (in 20–25%)—APR
- Excision of postvaginal wall may be required in 70%
- Isolated inguinal LN metastasis—groin dissection. RT may be considered if no prior RT given
- Salvage APR—5-year survival—50% vs 27% after salvage CRT
- HIV patients—same protocol is followed along with ART treatment
  – 2-year survival reported same
- IMRT—better to avoid collateral damage and toxicity
- Nigro protocol—30 Gy RT with 5 FU and Mitomycin

Prognosis

- LN involvement and size—major factors
- Male gender, African Americans, age >65—adverse factors
- HIV—negative prognostic factor
- HPV—favorable factor

Follow-up

- DRE, anoscopy, LN evaluation—for 5 years
- Most of the recurrence occurs in 3 years
- CT only for advanced disease

Perianal Cancer

- Account for 3–4% of all anorectal lesions
- Involves 5 cm around anus-perianus—anal margin
- Having stratified squamous epithelium
- Common cancers—SCC, Verrucous ca, Paget's disease, BCC

Perianal SCC

- Similar to skin SCC
- If anal canal SCC extending to skin—treated like anal canal ca
- Differentiated from anal canal SCC by looking for presence of skin appendages, keratinisation, and location
- Mets to inguinal LN
- CT chest abdomen and pelvis

Treatment

- Based on size and location
- Small T1, N0—wide local excision—1 cm margin
- Involving anal sphincter—APR or CRT
- Larger lesions with inguinal LNE—needs CRT
- >2 cm lesion—RT of inguinal region
- >5 cm—RT of pelvic nodes also

Anorectal Melanoma

- 1% of all melanoma
- <4% of all anal/perianal cancers
- Most common site of melanoma in GIT—65% in anus and perianus
- Nonspecific presentation
- 50% have metastasis at presentation
- 25%—amelanotic—diagnostic difficulty

5-year survival

- R0 resection 20%
- Involved margins—5%
- Local disease—30%
- Regional—17%
- Mets—0%
- APR vs wide excision—R0 resection is important
- First line—wide excision
- Radio and chemoresistant—surgery is the mainstay
- Tyrosine kinase inhibitor—imatinib
- Anti-CTLA-4 antibody—ipilimumab
- Mucosal melanoma has different genetics than cutaneous

Adeno ca Anal Canal

- From columnar epithelium of canal ducts—also from mucosa
- Second most common ca of anal canal
- 10–20% of anal canal cancers
- More aggressive than SCC
- Differentiating from Ca rectum difficult—not important—same treatment
- CRT with APR—choice

Risk Factors

- Chronic inflammation
- Crohn's disease
- Chronic fistula
- Crohn's disease associated cancer—0.3–.7%, Most common type adenocarcinoma, then the SCC
- Neoadjuvant CRT, then surgery—preferred

BCC Anal Canal

- <1% of all BCCs
- Pearly borders with central depression
- Treated with wide excision
- APR for extensive tumors involving sphincters
- Not aggressive—100% cancer-specific survival

Appendix

9.1 APPENDIX ANATOMY AND APPENDICITIS

- Vestigial organ
- Presents only in human, certain anthropoid apes and the wombat
- At birth short and broad
- Later due to differential growth of cecum, appendix develops into a tubular structure by 2 years
- Growth of cecum in children rotates appendix into retrocecal position, in 30% rotation does not occur, thus assuming other positions

Embryology and Anatomy

- Derived from midgut
- First appears at 8 weeks of gestation as an outpouching of cecum
- Later rotates to a more medial location
- Appendicular artery is a branch of ileocolic artery, this is an end artery, thrombosis leads to gangrene of appendix
- Accessory appendicular artery may be seen
- Lymphatics drain to anterior ileocolic nodes
- In adults appendix has no known function

Histology

- Mucosa is of colonic type with columnar epithelium, neuro endocrine cells, goblet cells
- Lymphoid tissue is found in the submucosa
- Length varies 5 to 35 cm (avg 9 cm)
- Base is located at the convergence of taeniae
- Tip may vary in location
- Position of appendix:
  - Most common—retrocecal within peritoneal cavity: 60%
  - Pelvic in 30%, retroperitoneal in 7–10%

Duplication of Appendix

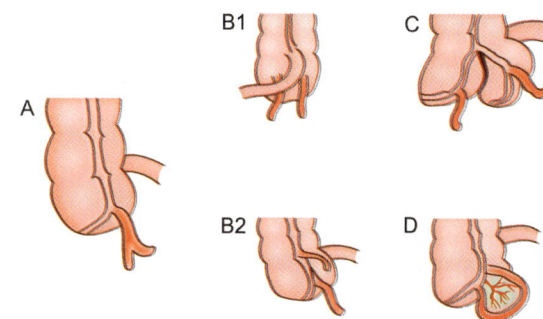

Modified Cave-Wallbridge classification	
Classification appendix duplication	Features
A	Single caecum with various degrees of incomplete duplication
B1 (bird type or avian type)	Two appendices symmetrically placed on either side of the ileocecal valve
B2 (taeniae coli type)	One appendix arises from the cecum at the usual site, and the second appendix branches from the cecum along the lines of the tenia at various distances from the first
B3	One appendix arises from the usual site, and the second appendix arises from the hepatic flexure
B4	One appendix arises from the usual site, and the second appendix arises from the splenic flexure
C	Double cecum, each with an appendix
D (Horseshoe appendix)	One appendix has two openings into a common cecum
Triple appendix	**One appendix arises from the cecum at the usual site, and two additional appendices arise from the colon**

Appendicitis

- Appendicectomy has protective effect on ulcerative colitis due to
  - Release of dimeric forms of IgA from plasma cells and
  - Th2 response by IL-13 producing natural killer T cells

History

- In 1886 Reginald Fitz identified appendix as the primary cause of RIF pain
- First appendicectomy by Claudius Amyand in an inguinal hernia: 1735
- He coined the term appendicitis and recommended surgery
- In 1889 Chester McBurney described migratory pain and the point
- 1894: McBurney incision
- 1982: First lap appendectomy-Kurt Semm
- 8% of western population have appendicitis some time in life
- Peak incidence 10–30 years
- Most common general surgical emergency
- Worldwide perforated appendix—the leading general surgical cause of death
- Rare in infants
- Incidence increases up to early adult life, peak by teens and early 20s
- After middle age risk is small

Etiology

- Decreased fiber and high intake of refined carbohydrates

Pathophysiology

- Obstruction of lumen—major cause due to
  - Inspissated stool,
  - Fecalith,
  - Lymphoid hyperplasia,
  - Parasites,
  - Tumor.
- Lumen is small compared to length, develops closed loop obstruction
- Obstruction leads to bacterial overgrowth, continued secretion of mucus and gas by bacteria and intraluminal distension and increase in pressure
- Luminal distension causes visceral pain in periumbilical area
- Later when tip gets inflamed—parietal peritoneum is involved—pain shifts to RIF
- Luminal distension—impairment in lymphatic and venous flow—mucosal ischemia—gangrene—perforation

- Local perforation or generalised
  - Local abscess
  - General peritonitis—septic shock
- Fecalith or appendicolith is composed of inspissated fecal material, calcium phosphate, bacteria and epithelial debris. Rarely some foreign body may be also there in the mass
- Finding a fecalith is an indication for prophylactic and interval appendicectomy

Most common anaerobic bacteria—*Bacteroides fragilis*
Most common aerobic bacteria—*E. coli*

Diagnosis

- 'Cope's early diagnosis of the acute abdomen'
- Never place appendicitis lower than second in DD of acute abdomen pain in a previously healthy person

Types of Appendicitis

- Acute nonobstructive catarrhal appendicitis
- Acute obstructive appendicitis
- Recurrent appendicitis
- Subacute appendicitis
- Stump appendicitis
- Early diagnosis—important goal

Clinical Features

- Starts with periumbilical pain—due to the midgut visceral discomfort associated with anorexia, nausea
- Later localizes to RIF as inflammation of parietal peritoneum over appendix causing somatic pain
- Usually single bout of vomiting
- Urinary symptoms, microscopic hematuria
- Can cause constipation or diarrhea
- May present with small bowel obstruction
- Retroperitoneal appendix can cause—back or flank pain
- Pelvic appendix—suprapubic pain

Murphy's Triad

- Pain
- Vomiting
- Fever

Physical Examination

- Look ill, lying still on bed
- Low grade fever
- Tender RIF, guarding
- Absent BS, McBurney point tenderness
- Involuntary guarding, rebound tenderness due to peritoneal irritation
- Pain on movement like coughing—**Dunphy's sign** seen in retrocecal appendix

- **Rovsing's sign**—palpation of left lower quadrant—produce pain on right lower quadrant
- Obturator sign—pain in RIF on internal rotation of hip—in pelvic appendix
- Psoas sign: Patient lies with right hip flexed for pain relief. Pain on extension of ipsilateral hip—in retrocecal appendix
- PR tenderness anteriorly in pelvic appendix
- A pelvic appendix may not produce somatic pain involving anterior abdominal wall but may produce suprapubic discomfort and tenesmus
- PV tenderness in pelvic appendix
- If perforated
  - Rigidity
  - High fever, tachycardia,
- **Blumberg sign**—is rebound tenderness
- Sherren's triangle hyperesthesia
  - Boundaries—umbilicus, pubic symphysis and anterior superior iliac spine.
- **Pointing sign**—patient can tell where the pain started and where it has moved
- In postilealappendix—appendix lies behind terminal ileum

  Greatest difficulty in diagnosis as:
  - The pain may not shift
  - May cause diarrhea
  - May cause marked retching
  - Tenderness is ill defined, may be to the right of umbilicus

Differential diagnosis of acute appendicitis		
Children	*Adult*	*Adult female*
Gastroenteritis	Regional enteritis	Mittelschmerz
Mesenteric adenitis	Ureteric colic	Pelvic inflammatory disease
Meckel's diverticulitis	Perforated peptic ulcer	Torsion/rupture of ovarian cyst
Intussusception	Torsion of testis	Ectopic pregnancy
Henoch-Schönlein purpura	Pancreatitis	
Lobar pneumonia		

Lab Tests

- Leucocytosis with shift to left—in 90%
- Normal TC and DC found in 10%
- Very high WBC seen in gangrene and perforation
- Urine—may show minimal pyuria
- Microscopic hematuria
- Other blood tests are not very useful

The Alvarado (MANTRELS) score	
	Score
Symptoms	
Migratory RIF pain	1
Anorexia	1
Nausea and vomiting	1
Signs	
Tenderness	2
Rebound tenderness	1
Elevated temperature	1
Laboratory	
Leukocytosis	2
Shift to left	1
Total	**10**
Score >7 appendicitis strongly predictive	
Score 5–6 equivocal need radiological studies	

- Helpful in diagnosis and predicting perforated appendix
  - CRP
  - Bilirubin
  - IL-6
  - Procalcitonin

Radiological Studies

- X-ray abdomen
  - Not very useful
  - Mainly to rule out other conditions like obstruction, perforation, stones, etc.
  - Appendicolith is visible in 5% on X-ray
  - Pneumoperitoneum—is not typically seen in appendix perforation
- Barium enema:
  - Nonvisualization of appendix
- USG
  - Noninvasive and easily available
  - Sensitivity 85%, specificity 90%
  - Diameter >7 mm (>6 mm)
  - Target sign
  - Enlarged, immobile noncompressible structure appendicolith
  - Ring of fire appearance

CT scan with only IV contrast. No oral or rectal contrasts
- 90% specificity and sensitivity
- >7 mm appendix (>6 mm)
- Wall thickening >2 mm—halo or target sign
- Periappendiceal fat stranding, edema, free fluid
- Mass, abscess, appendicolith
- But not routinely done
- Mainly in older patients where diagnosis is in doubt
- Not so in younger

MRI
- Best in pregnant lady
- Without contrast
- Appendicitis
  - >7 mm enlargement
  - >2 mm thickenng
  - Inflammation
- 100% sensitive and 98% specific

Diagnostic Laparoscopy
- Not routine
- When diagnosis is in doubt
- Especially in women

Treatment
- Choice—prompt appendicectomy
- Methods—incisions
  - Grid iron: McArthur-McBurney
  - Rutherford Morison
  - Rockey-Davis transverse
  - Lanz
  - Midline
  - Right paramedian
  - Laparoscopic
- Rockey-Davis incision—transverse incision centered at McBurney's point
- Rutherford Morison—in para and retrocecal appendix. Oblique muscle cutting incision, lower end over McBurney's point and extends obliquely upwards and laterally as necessary. All layers are divided in the line of incision

Postoperative Complications
- Wound infection
- Intra-abdominal abscess
  - CECT diagnostic and guided drainage
- Ileus
- Respiratory complications
- Venous thrombosis/embolism
- Portal pyemia
- Fecal fistula
- Adhesive intestinal obstruction

Antibiotics
- In uncomplicated appendicitis only single postoperative dose is indicated
- In perforated appendix—continued for 4–7 days (STOP-IT trial)

Oral Alimentation
- Started immediately in uncomplicated appendicitis
- In perforated appendix—started when bowel sounds appear and passage of flatus

Novel Techniques
- Natural orifice transluminal endoscopic surgery (NOTES)
  - Transgastric, transvaginal
- Single incision laparoscopic surgery (SILS)
- Robotic surgery

Appendicular Mass (Periappendicular Phlegmon)
- Body's defense mechanism
- Infection localized to RIF
- Mass constituted by—appendix, ileum, cecum, omentum, peritoneum
- Tender, smooth, not mobile

DD
- Ca cecum
- Crohn's disease
- Ovarian cyst
- Actinomycosis
- Mesenteric adenitis, ruptured ectopic pregnancy
- Ileocecal TB

Investigations
- CBC
- USG
- CECT

Management
Ochsner-Sherren Regimen
- Conservative treatment
- Temp, pulse, BP chart
- Mark the mass and monitor the progress
- CECT abdomen
- IV fluids
- Analgesics
- NG aspiration
- Oral fluids

- Discharged when patient improves
- Interval appendicectomy after 6 weeks
- Interval appendicectomy is indicated in only if presented with recurrent appendicitis
  - Also if CT shows appendicolith
- Recurrence—80% occur in 6 months

Contraindications for OS regimen

- Diagnosis in doubt
- Children and elderly
- Burst gangrenous appendix
- Diffuse peritonitis

Criteria to Discontinue Conservative Treatment

- Patients become toxic
- Tachycardia, high fever
- Persistent vomiting
- Signs of diffuse peritonitis
- Increasing size of mass

Appendicular abscess

- Due to suppuration of acute appendicitis
- Usually retrocecal can be subcecal
- Can lead on to pelvic abscess

Clinical Features

- High fever
- Toxicity
- Tender soft mass RIF
- USG, CT—for diagnosis

Treatment

- Antibiotics
- CT-guided drainage

Surgery

- Extraperitoneal drainage of abscess
- Appendicectomy
- Interval appendicectomy
- PR/PV drainage of abscess
- Incidental appendicectomy means appendicectomy done on normal appendix when surgery is performed for some other disease—not advisable

Appendicitis in Pregnant

- Most common nonobstetric emergency in pregnancy and most common reason for general surgical intervention
- Round ligament pain—in second trimester—lower quadrant pain due to traction on suspensory ligaments of uterus
- Appendix is pushed upwards
- Physiological leukocytosis seen in pregnancy so diagnosis is difficult
- Negative appendicectomy 25–50%

Investigations

- USG—done in left lateral decubitus or left posterior oblique
  - Low accuracy
- MRI without contrast—the choice
  - Very accurate
- CT without IV contrast limited study can be done—if US and MRI are not available
  - Radiation is below the dose for fetal malformation
- Impact of appendicitis on pregnancy
  - Preterm labor—11%
  - Fetal loss 6%, if perforated—36%
- So there should be a low threshold for surgery
- Laparoscopic approach has more fetal loss than open—7% and 3%
- Should use low intra-abdominal pressure, in laparoscopic surgery

Chronic or Recurrent Appendicitis

- Patients with recurrent right lower abdomen pain
- Not associated with fever
- Imaging showing appendicolith or dilated appendix
- Appendicectomy relieves the pain, but only indicated if there is radiological evidence

Stump Appendicitis

- Appendicitis developing in a excised appendix stump of >0.5 cm long
- Surgery is indicated
- During laparoscopic surgery critical view of appendix help identification of appendix
  - Appendix is placed at 10 O'clock, taeniae coli libera at 3 O'clock and terminal ileum at 6 O'clock.
  - Identify where the taeniae coli merge to identify the base of appendix

In Infants

- Delayed presentation
- Perforation is higher
- Omentum is underdeveloped, so can develop diffuse peritonitis

Children

- More incidence of vomiting
- Complete aversion to food
- **In Crohn's disease**—appendicectomy can be done if cecum wall is healthy at the appendix base

9.2 NEOPLASMS OF APPENDIX

- 50% present as appendicitis and diagnosed on HPR
- Seen in 0.7 to 1.7% of specimens
- Account for 0.4% to 1% of all malignant GIT tumors
- Most common—carcinoid tumor—seen in 0.3 to 0.9% of appendicectomies

Carr, et al. Classification

Adenoma (tubular, tubulovillous, villous)	
Serrated polyp	
Non-mucinous adenocarcinoma	
Mucinous neoplasm	Low-grade appendiceal mucinous neoplasm (LAMN), high-grade appendiceal mucinous neoplasm (HAMN) Mucinous adenocarcinoma
Adenocarcinoma with signet ring cells (<50%)	

Carcinoids (NET)

- 75% of them <1 cm in size
- 5–10% >2 cm
- Well-circumscribed mucosal
- More towards distal aspect of appendix
- Size—best predictor of malignancy
- If size is <1 cm, usually benign, appendicectomy is enough
- >2 cm—involving base, mesoappendix—right hemicolectomy
- 1–2 cm—depends on factors
- 1–2 cm—right hemicolectomy is indicated if
  - Positive margins
  - Deep mesoappendiceal invasion
  - Higher proliferation rate
  - Angio invasion
- Right hemicolectomy also in—young, appendix base tumor, LVI, LN involvement, high mitotic index and positive margins.
- Carcinoid syndrome—due to liver metastasis—in 3%
- Serum chromogranin A measurement is tumor marker

Goblet Cell Carcinoma

- Have both adeno ca and carcinoid features
- Worse prognosis than carcinoid—better than adeno ca
- High risk of peritoneal recurrence
- Treatment—right hemicolectomy and surveillance for pseudomyxoma peritonei (PMP)

Lymphoma Appendix

- 1 to 3% of all lymphoma
- NHL
- Difficult preop diagnosis
- Appendix diameter could be >2.5 cm
- Treatment—appendicectomy

Adenocarcinoma—types

- Mucinous adenocarcinoma
- Colonic adenocarcinoma
  - Least common
  - Least likely to secrete mucin
  - Most likely to present with acute appendicitis
  - Prognosis—less favorable than mucinous
- Signet ring type—poorest prognosis
- Adenocarcinoid

Adenocarcinoma

- Most common presentation—appendicitis
- May perforate early, still not associated with worse prognosis
- Treatment—right hemicolectomy
- May have other tumors in GIT
- 5-year survival—55%

Mucinous Tumors/Mucocele
Includes

- Mucosal hyperplasia
- Retention cysts
- Mucinous cystadenoma/carcinoma
- Most common presentation is incidental
  - As appendicitis in one-third of cases
- Careful inspection of peritoneum and liver done
- If there is discordance between HPR of appendix and peritoneum—peritoneal histology is given priority
- High-grade dysplasia—neoplastic cells confined to the crypts—do not invade lamina propria
- Intramucosal carcinoma (IMC)—invades lamina propria—may be into but not through muscularis mucosa—Tis
- LAMN—may extend and sometimes through the wall but do not show features of invasion
  - May show desmoplasia
  - But LN enlargement is rare
- LAMN confined to mucosa with intact muscularis mucosa is appendiceal adenoma
- LAMN once confined to wall—depth of involvement not significant
- Involvement of subserosa and beyond—T_3 and T_4

- LAMN with areas of high grade features—HAMN
- Cystic neoplasm—X-ray/CT—calcification seen

Risk of PMP
- Overall in epithelial tumors—9%
- Nonmucinous neoplasm—3%
- Mucinous adenocarcinoma—30–50%

Treatment
- Low grade tumor with no PMP—appendicectomy-colonoscopy—follow-up
  – CT, CEA, CA 19–9, CA125
- High grade tumor—no PMP—high risk of PMP—prophylactic peritonectomy, right hemicolectomy, omentectomy, intraperitoneal chemo, bilateral salphyngoophorectomy

AJCC 8th edition and the PSOGI 2016 classification consensus of mucinous neoplasia of the appendix

Lesion	Peritoneal disease at diagnosis	Treatment
Low-grade appendiceal mucinous neoplasm (LAMN)	Confined to the appendix	Appendectomy with negative margin, sometimes need ileocecectomy
LAMN	Peri-appendiceal Acellular mucin dissecting through the wall or adjacent organs T4a and T4b respectively	Appendectomy with negative margin, resection of acellular mucin
LAMN	Peri-appendiceal Epithelial cells dissecting through the wall or adjacent organs T4a and T4b respectively	Appendectomy with negative margin, peritoneal surveillance with second look laparoscopy vs. HIPEC
LAMN	Distant epithelial cells or acellular mucin (M1a). Low-grade mucinous carcinoma peritonei	Appendectomy with negative margin, omentectomy, HIPEC
High-grade appendiceal mucinous neoplasm (HAMN—rare)	Management is as shown above	With risk stratification prognosis
Mucinous adenocarcinoma	Confined to the appendix	Right hemicolectomy
Mucinous adenocarcinoma	Peritoneal Dissemination High-grade mucinous carcinoma peritonei with or without signet ring cells	Cytoreductive surgery and HIPEC, with systemic chemotherapy for high-grade histologies
Adenocarcinoma (nonmucinous, including goblet cell histology)	Management with more extensive	Mucinous histologies, chemotherapy
Serrated adenoma	Confined to the appendix	Appendectomy

Inflammatory Bowel Diseases

10.1 CROHN'S DISEASE

- In 1932 Crohn described
- Most common primary surgical disease of small bowel
- Affects young 2nd–3rd decade, second peak in 6th decade
- Both genders equally affected
- Smoking—risk double
- Family history—30 fold risk in siblings
  - 14–15 fold in first degree relatives

Crohn's Disease (CD)

- Transmural granulomatous inflammation
- Involve any part of GIT—most common SI and colon
- Segmental
- Mesenteric fat creeping on to bowel
- Lymphadenopathy
- Strictures
- Fistulas

Causes

- Infection
- Genetic
- Immunologic
- Environmental
- Dietary
- Smoking
- Psychological

Infectious Agents Associated

- *Mycobacterium paratuberculosis* (atypical TB)
  - By Dalziel in 1913
- Enteroadherent *E. coli*

Immunologic

- Both humoral and cell mediated immunity
- Role of IL-1, IL-2, IL-8 and TNF-alfa
- Controversial role

Genetic

- Single strongest risk factor—having a first degree relative with CD
- >70 genes associated
- Strongest association: NOD2, IL23R, ATG16L1
- CARD15 gene expressed in CD—can differentiate from UC

Pathology

- Ileal involvement shown with mutations of IL10, CRP, NOD2, ZNF365 and STAT3
- Ileocolonic involvement—with—ATG16L1, TCF4, TCF7L2
- Colonic involvement—HLA, TLR4, TLR1, TLR6
- Small and large bowel disease in 55%
- Small bowel alone in 30%
- Limited to large bowel—in 15%
- Perirectal and perianal involvement seen in one-third especially with colonic disease
- Rectal sparing can occur
- Bowel dull purple red loops
- Fibrosis of serosa
- Skip areas
- Fat wrapping, presence of circumferential mesenteric fat
- Rubbery and not compressible
- Mesentery thickened, shortened
- Fistula can develop
- On opening bowel earliest lesion—aphthous ulcer of mucosa—later transmural linear ulcers—with normal mucosa in between—cobblestone appearance
- Noncaseating granulomas—characteristic seen in 50% resected specimens.
  - Seen on bowel and lymph node—in 60–70%—most common in anorectal disease.
- Mucosa—deep linear ulcers—**railroad track or bear claw ulcers**
- Skip areas seen

Montreal Classification

Crohn's disease	
Age at diagnosis (A)	
A1	16 years or younger
A2	17–40 years
A3	Over 40 years

Location (L)	Upper Gastrointestinal (GI) modifier (L4)
L1 terminal ileum	L1 + L4 terminal ileum and upper GI
L2 colon	L2 + L4 colon and upper GI
L3 ileum and colon	L3 + L4 ileocolic and upper GI
L4 upper GI	–

Behaviour (B)	Perianal disease modifier (p)
B1 nonstricturing, nonpenetrating	B1p (nonstricturing, nonpenetrating and perianal)
B2 stricturing	B2p (stricturing and perianal)
B3 penetrating	B3p (penetrating and perianal)

Clinical Features

- Abdominal pain, diarrhea, weight loss—triad
- Most common symptom—colicky abdomen pain lower abdomen
- Next diarrhea—in 85%
- UC—diarrhea fewer bowel movements rarely contain mucus, blood or pus
- Low grade fever, malaise

Vienna Classification

Vienna classification of Crohn's disease	
Age at diagnosis (years)	A1: <40 A2: ≥40
Behavior	B1: Nonstricturing/nonpenetrating B2: Stricturing B3: Penetrating
Location	L1: Terminal ileum L2: Colon L3: Ileocolic L4: Upper gastrointestinal tract

Complications

- Obstruction
- Perforation
- Fistula
- Bleeding—usually indolent
  - Can bleed massively in duodenal disease
- Malignancy

Malignancy

- Predispose to cancer of SI and colon
- At the site of chronic disease—more so in ileum
- Most are detected late—poor prognosis
- Relative risk of SI cancer >100 times—but absolute risk is still small
- CRC can develop—greater concern
- Can develop dysplasia and cancer
- Ileal adenocarcinoma in CD—has predominence of extracellular mucin
- So, in cases of fistula with mucin, look for cancer
- Extraintestinal cancer
  - SCC of vulva and anal canal
  - Hodgkin's lymphoma and NHL

Perianal Disease

- Occurs in 25% in limited to SI
  - 41% with ileocolitis
  - About 50% with colonic involvement alone (75%—Bailey)
- In 5%—sole presentation

Extraintestinal Manifestations

- Erythema nodosum
- Pyodermal gangrenosum
- Arthritis, arthralgia
- Uveitis, iritis
- Hepatitis, pericholangitis
- Aphthous stomatitis
- Amyloidosis, pancreatitis
- Nephrotic syndrome

All these may precede, accompany or appear independently

Diagnosis

- **Clinical**
- **Barium**
  - Cobblestone (linear ulcers, transverse sinuses and clefts)
  - Long length of narrow terminal ileum (string sign of Kantor)
  - Irregular pattern of bowel movement
  - **Fistulas**
- **CECT**
  - Transmural thickening and extramural
  - Limit repeated CT use due to risk of radiation
- **MRI** may be superior to detect strictures and ileal wall enhancement
- **MR** enteroclysis
  - In stricture, fistulas
- **Capsule endoscopy:** Criteria for abnormal finding—3 or more ulcers in the absence of NSAID intake
  - Concern of capsule retention Capsule in GIT for >2 weeks (13%)

- **Colonoscopy**—in colon and terminal ileum can visualize 50–80 cm ileum
- Single balloon enteroscopy
- Double balloon enteroscopy
  - Most well established—enteral intubation can be achieved for 240 to 360 cm
- Push enteroscopy visualize for 90–150 cm
- Spiral enteroscopy
- Complications—1%

Serology

- Anti-saccharomyces cerevisiae antibody (ASCA)—positive in 60–70%
  - In ulcerative colitis 10–15%
- Perinuclear antineutrophil cytoplasmic antibody (pANCA) positive in 10–15%
  - Positive in ulcerative colitis: 70-80%
- Outer membrane porin of flagellin (anti-CBir1)
- Outer membrane porin of E. coli (OmpC-IgG)

  Noninvasive inflammatory markers
  - CRP, ESR—nonspecific
  - Stool lactoferin—iron binding protein in secretary granules of neutrophils
  - Fecal calprotectin—protein with antimicrobial properties, released by squamous cells in response to inflammation

Management

- There is no cure for CD
- Essentially—medical management
- Surgery only for complications
- Surgery would not cure CD
- Conservation of intestine—the aim
- 70% require surgery within 15 years of diagnosis
- 50% require another surgery in next 10 years

Medical Therapy

- Induction of remission
  - Steroids, 5—ASA, Methotrexate, Infliximab
- Maintenance
  - Azathioprine,
  - 6MP
  - Methotrexate
  - Infliximab
- Biologic therapy
  TNF-alfa inhibitor—Infliximab
  - In steroid dependent, resistant
  - In fistulizing disease
- Adalimumab
- Certolizumab
- Natalizumab

- Aminosalicylates
  - Mesalamine—slow release of 5-ASA—first line therapy
  - 4 g/day

Corticosteroids

- Not ideal for maintenance therapy due to complications
- Budesonide has high first pass liver metabolism—release in ileum and right colon

  Preferred to mesalamine in localised ileal disease as a primary treatment

Antibiotics

- Adjunctive role
- Useful in perianal disease, enterocutaneous fistula, active colonic disease
- Ciprofloxacin, Rifaximine, Clofazimine, Ethambutol
- Should not be used in maintenance therapy or to induce remission

Immunosuppressive Agents

- AZT, MTX, 6-MP—for maintenance therapy
- Adverse effects
  - Pancreatitis, hepatitis, CLD, BM suppression
- Thiopurine methyl transferase (TPMT)—metabolises AZT and 6-MP regulates the therapy
- Reduced TPMT activity cause fatal BM suppression
- Cyclosporine
- FK-506—inhibits IL-2 production—effective in perianal fistula improvement

Anticytokine and Cytokine Therapy

- TNF-alfa—chimeric monoclonal antibody: Infliximab
  - In severe Crohn's disease
  - As monotherapy for maintenance therapy and steroid-induced remission
- Effective in perianal fistula closure
- Adverse effects—opportunistic infections—TB, fungal, demyelination, CCF
- Adalimumab—humanized IgG1 monoclonal antibody—effective in maintenance
- Certolizumab (humanized antibody fragment Fab)—ideal for pregnant and lactating patients—does not cross placenta, not expressed in milk
- Natalizumab—recombinant humanized monoclonal antibody against alfa-4 integrin
  - Adverse effect—progressive multifocal leuko-encephalopathy

- Vedolizumab—humanized monoclonal antibody binds to $\alpha_4\beta_7$ integrin and blocks its interaction with mucosal addressin cell adhesion molecule 1 (MadCAM-1)
  - MadCAM-1—is specifically expressed on blood vessels in GIT—more gut specific—less neuro side effects
- Ustekinumab—human IgG1 MCA—inhibits IL 12/23

Surgical Therapy

Indications for Surgery

- Obstructing stenosis
- Intractable disease
- Suppurative complications
- Neoplastic/preneoplastic lesions
- Failure to thrive
- Toxic megacolon
- Massive bleeding
- Most common indication for surgery—obstruction due to stricture
- In obstruction due to exacerbation of inflammation—stool lactoferin and calprotectin elevated
- In stricture—surgery
- Treatment of choice in obstruction—resection of segment and primary anastomosis
- Approximately 70% will require surgery within 15 years after diagnosis
- 80% require surgery—at some point in life
- Mortality increased in disease onset before age 20 and >13 years of disease
- CD—death rate 2–3 times higher—most commonly related to wound complications and sepsis

Preop Preparation

- Evaluate the GIT
- Nutrition
- Plan ileostomy
- Mechanical bowel preparation—debatable role

Operative Strategies

- Resect only grossly involved segment

Stricturoplasty

Indications

- Multiple strictures
- Previous extensive (>100 cm) resections
- Risk of short bowel syndrome
- Duodenal CD

Contraindications for Stricturoplasty

- Perforation
- Phlegmon

- Peritonitis
- Abscess, fistula
- Fear of cancer
- Malnutrition

Resection is an Important Option

- Stricturoplasty—short segments types
  - **Heineke-Mikulicz** type
  - **Judd**—done when there is an area of perforation on a stricture segment elliptical area is excised and stricturoplasty is done.

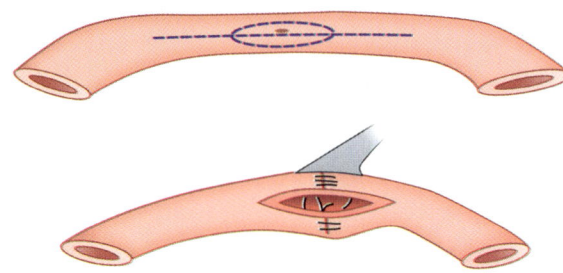

- **Moskel-Walske-Neumayer**—when there is big disparity between stricturous and non-stricturous segments, Y-shaped incision is made and stricturoplasty done.

Long Segment Stricturoplasty

- **Finney's**
- **Jaboulay**—is a side to side anastomosis between non-stricturous bowel loops
- **Michelassi**—long segment side to side anastomosis

Resection

- Resection of only pathologic segment
- Margin—not important—2 cm desirable
- Hand sewn vs stapler anastomosis—subjective
- No difference in end to end and side to side anastomosis

Bypass Procedures

- Exclusion bypass

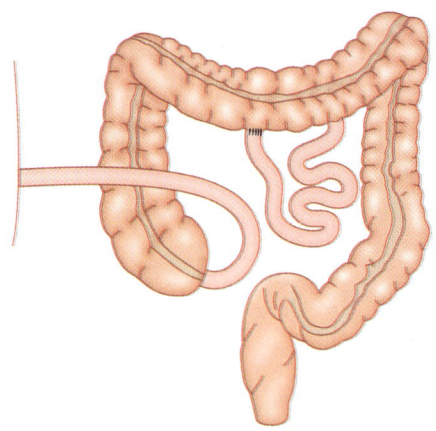

- In ileocecal adherent mass—ileum divided—ileo-transverse end to side anastomosis with or without mucus fistula of ileum
- **Simple continuity bypass**—ileotransverse side to side—continuity bypass

Indications

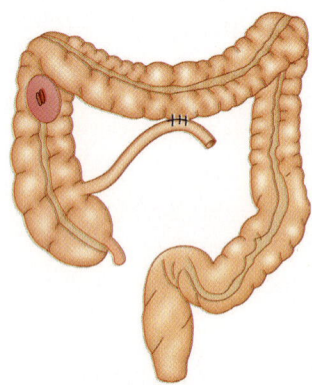

- In gastroduodenal disease
- Poor risk patients
- Had several prior resections

Complicated CD

- Fistulas
- Entero-enteric
- Ileosigmoid
- Enterovesical
- Enterocutaneous
- Enterogenital
- Intensive medical management
- Resection of pathologic segment—closure of the other

Radiologically demonstrated uncomplicated entero-enteral fistula—not an indication for surgery, Infliximab is the option for treatment

Duodenal Disease

- Occurs in 1–5% in CD
- Most commonly in duodenal bulb
- Surgery done only rarely
- Primary indication for surgery—duodenal obstruction—not responding to medical treatment
- Intensive medical management
- Nutrition
- Stricturoplasty
- Balloon dilatation
- **GJ**
- DJ

Perianal Disease
Fistulas and Fissures

- Managed conservatively
- Medical therapy—Infliximab,
  – FK-506, cyclosporin
- Avoid large incisions
- Consider setons
- Advancement flaps
- Fissures are usually lateral,
  – Relatively painless,
  – Large and indolent
- Respond to conservative treatment

Colonic CD

- *Only colon in—10%*
- *Ileocolonic—40%*
- *Small bowel—30%*

Surgical Treatment

- Segmental resection
- Subtotal colectomy
- Proctocolectomy with ileostomy
- Stricturoplasty has only limited role
- IPAA—in limited disease to colon. Role is controversial
  – If ileal and perianal disease—contraindication

Risk of Malignancy

- 100 fold increase
- Still absolute risk is less
- More of mucinous type
- More aggressive
- Poor prognosis

Acute Ileitis

- If diagnosed as acute appendicits, at surgery if ileum is inflammed and appendix normal
  – Appendicectomy done if base of appendix is normal
  – No resection of ileum

10.2 ULCERATIVE COLITIS (UC)
Epidemiology

- More common in developed countries
- All ages are susceptible, more in < 30.
- M:F = 1:1
- More common in Jews, Whites

Causes

- Environmental
- Dietary
  – Inadequate fiber
  – Chemical food additives
  – Refined sugar
  – Cow's milk

- Infectious
  - *Clostridium difficile*
  - *Campylobacter jejuni*
- Smoking—protective effect
- OCP
- Appendicectomy-protective
- Family history of UC

Genetic

- Variations in DNA repair genes
- Variations in major HLA complex genes
- DR 1501—benign course
- DR 1502—more virulent course

  Immunologic response to
  - External and host antigens
  - Anti-colon antibodies seen
  - Defective CMI
  - Leucocyte chemotactic impairment
  - Abnormalities in antigen-specific helper and suppressor T cells

Pathology—Gross

- Major pathology is in mucosa and submucosa
- Spares muscularis
- Typical feature is hyperemic mucosa—ulcer not always present
- Friable granular mucosa
- Later ulcer develops—vary—small erosions to full thickness of mucosa
- Rectum invariably involved—proctitis—hallmark
- Inflammation from rectum—continuous
- Pseudopolyps due to regeneration of inflamed mucosa
  - Composed of nonneoplastic colonic mucosa and inflamed lamina propria
- Continuous uninterrupted inflammation from rectum to variable distance unlike CD
- Entire colon may be involved
- Usually does not involve terminal ileum unlike CD
- Backwash ileitis—inflammation of terminal ileum
  - Inflamed ileum is dilated.
  - In CD terminal ileum will be contracted and narrowed
- Colonic stricture
  - Mostly benign
  - Cancer has to be excluded
- Cancerous stricture suspected when
  - Appearance later in the course of UC
  - Location proximal to splenic flexure
  - Colon obstruction due to stricture.

Montreal Classification

Ulcerative colitis	
Disease Extent (E) (defined as maximal endoscopic extent during follow-up)	
E1	Ulcerative proctitis (limited to the rectum)
E2	Left-sided (limited to colon distal to the splenic flexure)
E3	Extensive ulcerative colitis (disease proximal to the splenic flexure)
Disease severity	
S0	Clinical remission (no symptoms)
S1	Mild (passage of four or fewer stool/day (with/without blood)), absence of any systemic illness, and normal inflammatory markers (ESR)
S2	Moderate (passage of more than 4 stools/day but with minimal signs of systemic toxicity)
S3	Severe (passage of at least 6 bloody stools daily, pulse rate of at least 90 beats/min, temperature of at least 37.5°C hemoglobin of <10.5 g/dl and ESR of at least 30 mm/h)

Histology

- Inflammation of mucosa and submucosa
- Crypt abscess—most characteristic—neutrophils fill crypts of Lieberkuhn
- Crypt branching
- Number of goblet cells and mucin reduced
- Vascular congestion.
- In toxic megacolon all layers of colon involved
- Antineutrophil cytoplasmic antibodies with perinuclear staining pattern (pANCA)—seen in 70–80%—help to differentiate from CD
- Usually muscle layer not involved—in severe inflammation, can involve—toxic megacolon

Clinical Presentation

- UC and CD similar features
- Diarrhea with mucus
- Urgency to defecate more due to proctitis
- Bleeding PR
- Abdominal discomfort—pain is not severe unlike CD
- Perianal finding—rare unlike CD—rectal sparing is seen in CD
- Anal involvement rare in spite of 100% rectal involvement vs CD

Disease Severity

- Mild—rectal bleeding or diarrhea with less than 4 motions, absent systemic signs
- Moderate—more than 4 motions, absent systemic signs
- Severe—more than 4 motions, with one or more signs. Fever>37.5, tachycardia >90, hypoalbunemia <30 g/dl, weight loss >3 kg

Comparison of ulcerative colitis and Crohn's colitis

	Ulcerative colitis	Crohn's colitis
Gross appearance		
Thickened wall	Not seen	++++
Thickened mesentry	Not seen	+++
Serosal fat wrapping	Not seen	++++
Segmental disease	Not seen	++++
Microscopic appearance		
Transmural	Not seen	++++
Lymphoid aggregates	Not seen	++++
Granulomas	Not seen	+++
Clinical features		
Bleeding per rectum	3+	+
Diarrhoea	3+	+++
Obstructive symptoms	1+	+++
Anal or perianal disease	Rare	++++
Risk for cancer	2+	+++
Small bowel disease	Not seen	++++

Colonoscopic features

Distribution	Continuous	Discontinuous
Rectal disease	++++	+
Friability	++++	+
Aphthous ulcers	Not seen	++++
Deep longitudinal ulcers	Not seen	++++
Cobblestoning	Not seen	++++
Pseudopolyps	++	++
Operative treatment		
Total proctocolectomy	Curative	Combined disease: Colon and rectum
Segmental resection	Rare	Absence of anorectal disease
Ileal pouch	Preferred by most patients	Contraindicated
Complications		
Postoperative recurrence	Not seen	++++
Fistulas	Rare	++++
Sclerosing cholangitis	+	Rare
Cholelithiasis	Not seen	++
Nephrolithiasis	Not seen	++

Extraintestinal Manifestations

- Arthritis—knee, ankle, hips—in 20%
- Ankylosing spondylitis—in 3–5%
  - Most prevalent in HLA B27 positive
  - And with f/h/o ankylosing spondylitis
- Erythema nodosum
  - In 10–15%
  - Occur in conjunction with peripheral arthropathy
- Pyoderma gangrenosum—pretibial—ulcerated painful wound
- All improve after colectomy
- Primary sclerosing cholangitis
  - In 5–8% of UC
  - More in young <40 and men
  - HLA—B8 and HLA-DR3—>10 times chance of PSC
  - Quiescent course
  - More chance of colon cancer—5 times—proximal to splenic flexure
  - Colectomy has no effect on PSC

Diagnosis

- X-ray abdomen—Loss of mucosal pattern
  - Lack of fecal matter
  - Dilatation
- Barium enema
  - Loss of haustrations—lead pipe
  - Mucosal changes caused by granularity
  - Pseudopolyps
  - Narrow contracted colon
- Endoscopy of colon and rectum
- Proctosigmoidoscopy in acute phase
  - Confluent, diffuse, symmetrical disease from dentate line proximally
  - Mucosal edema—loss of vascular pattern

Colonoscopy is done after disease is under control and biopsy
- To establish extend of disease
- To distinguish between UC and CD
- To monitor response to treatment
- To evaluate possible cancer

Colonoscopy Features

- Granular mucosa
- Superficial/deep mucosal ulcers
- Pseudopolyps
- Stricture
- Cancer
- Multiple biopsies taken

Differential Diagnosis

- Crohn's disease
- Collagenous colitis
  - Mucosa spared
- Infective colitis
  - *C. difficile, E. histolytica, C. jejuni, Salmonella enteritidis*

Risk of Carcinoma

- Prolonged disease
- Pancolonic disease
- Continuously active disease
- Severe inflammation
- Cumulative risk increases with duration
- 25% at 25 years to 65% at 40 years
- Left side colon involvement has lesser risk than entire colon involvement.
- Develop poorly differentiated and aggressive tumors.
- Stricture in UC—cancer to be rule out
- If cancer cannot be ruled out on endoscopy—surgery is indicated

Surveillance Colonoscopy

- Every 1 to 2 years beginning 8 years after onset of pancolitis and 12–15 years after left-sided colitis
- Traditionally 10 specimens are obtained for biopsy can be up to 30
- Colonoscopic surveillance—debatable value
- Flow cytometry of colonoscopy biopsy
  - Aneuploidy and polyploidy correlate with dysplasia

Dysplasia and Risk of Cancer

- Low grade—risk of Ca—10%
- High grade—30–40%
  - 50% in dysplasia associated with a lesion or mass (DALM).
- 25% cancer in UC—not associated with dysplasia

  Risk of malignancy in stricture
  - Proximal
  - Pancolitis
  - >20 years history
  - Obstruction
- Endoscopic healing—associated with improved long-term outcomes

Treatment: Medical Therapy

Induction of remission and maintenance of remission

- Aminosalicylates
- Corticosteroids
- Immunomodulatory
- Biologics
- Steroid dependent UC—maintained with thiopurines
- Steroid resistant—use cyclosporine or Infliximab

  Aminosalicylates—first line to induce and maintain remission
  - In mild to moderate disease
  - Sulfasalazine (5 ASA with sulfapyridin with diazo bond)
    - Active ingredient 5 ASA
    - Block arachidonic acid metabolism
    - Toxicity related to sulfapyridine
    - Newer—Mesalazine without sulfapyridine— lesser side effects
    - Can be used in active disease and in maintaining remission

Corticosteroids to Induce Remission if 5-ASA not Effective

- **Not as long-term therapy**
- Effective in active UC
- Orally, IV, enema
- Act by blocking phospholipid A2-decrease PG and leukotrienes
- Can cause HTN, DM, infections, osteoporosis
- Hydrocortisone enemas—2–3 times/day in left-sided disease
  - Lesser absorption, side effects
- Newer—Budesonide—water soluble analogue of hydrocortisone—as effective and lesser side effects

Immunomodulatory

Thiopurines—most commonly used

- Used in long-term management
- 6 mercaptopurine, azathioprine
- Act by causing chromosome breaks and inhibiting proliferation of rapidly dividing cells like T cells T> B.
- Useful in induction of remission
- Side effects—BM suppression, pancreatitis

Cyclosporine

- Second line in steroid refractory
- Act by inhibition of IL-2 gene transcription
- Can cause nephro, hepatotoxicity, seizures

- May get infection with *Pneumocystis jirovecii*—prophylaxis with co-trimoxazole or dapsone
- Methotrexate
  – Not preferred
- Tacrolimus
  – Second line therapy in severe active UC unresponsive to steroids

Biologics

TNF-alfa monoclonal antibody—Infliximab (chimeric—human and murine)

- In refractory to steroids
- Before starting rule out infection with *C. difficile*, CMV and TB
- Initial 3 doses followed by 6 weekly dose—IV
- Used in induction of remission

  Adalimumab
  – Humanised monoclonal antibody
- **Golimumab, Certolizumab**—fully human anti-TNF

Surgical Therapy

Indications: For Elective Surgery

- Failure of medical therapy
- Cancer
- Dysplasia:
  – Low grade
  – High grade
  – DALM

Indications—Emergency Surgery

- Fulminant colitis
- Toxic megacolon
- Hemorrhage
- Perforation
- Obstruction
- **20% of CUC require surgery at some point**

Toxic Megacolon and Fulminant Colitis

- High fever
- Severe pain, tenderness abdomen
- Tachycardia, leucocytosis
- Dehydration
- Colonic diameter >5.5 cm on X-ray
- Due to bacterial infiltration of the wall—paralysis of myenteric plexus—dilatation and perforation

Treatment

- IV hydration
- NGT aspiration
- High dose steroids

- Broad spectrum antibiotics
- IV hyperalimentation
- Closely monitored with clinical examination and WBC count
- No improvement/deterioration in 48–72 hours—intervention

Acute Severe Colitis: Definition

Truelove and Witts Criteria

Modified Truelove and Witts criteria for classification of severity of ulcerative colitis			
	Mild	*Moderate*	*Severe*
Bloody stools per day	<4	4–6	>6
Pulse	<90 bpm	≤90 bpm	>90 bpm
Temperature	<37.5°C	≤37.8°C	>37.8°C
Hemoglobin	>11.5 gm/dl	≥10.5 gm/dl	<10.5 gm/dl
ESR	<20 mm/h	≤30 mm/h	>30 mm/h
CRP	Normal	≤30 mg/dl	>30 mg/dl

Fulminant Colitis

- Diarrhea >10 times/day
- Severe anemia
- Need for blood transfusion
- Surgery may be indicated

Predictors of Colectomy

- >8 Stools/day
- Or a combination of
  – CRP >4.5 mg/dl and stool >3 times/day on the third hospital day

Toxic Megacolon and Fulminant Colitis

Treatment—Surgery

- Total colectomy with ileostomy
- Mucus fistula
- Hartmann procedure
- Blow hole colostomy with loop ileostomy
  – Later definitive surgery
- Subtotal colectomy and, closure of rectal stump with ileostomy is preferred. The advantages are
  – Avoiding anastomosis
  – Avoiding pelvic dissection

Massive Bleeding

- Uncommon
- <5% require surgery
- Resuscitation

- Subtotal colectomy may suffice
- If bleeding continues—total proctectomy

Intractability

- Colitis with debilitating symptoms refractory to medical treatment—most common indication for surgery
- They have
  - Persistent abdominal pain, diarrhea, stool urgency, anemia
  - Deterioration of social and professional life.
  - Complications of steroid therapy
  - Extracolonic manifestations
- QOL improves
- Complications of medical therapy avoided
- In extracolonic manifestations

Dysplasia/Carcinoma

- Influence the type of procedure
- Does not exclude the possibility of ileo anal pouch
- Dysplasia or carcinoma
  Proctocolectomy is considered in
  - High grade dysplasia
  - DALM
  - Multiple areas of dysplasia
  - Carcinoma
- Low grade dysplasia also consider proctocolectomy

Total PC with End Ileostomy done in

- Mainly in older patients
- Poor sphincter function
- Carcinoma distal rectum

Surgical Procedures

- Total proctocolectomy with ileostomy
- Restorative proctocolectomy with ileo anal anastomosis
- Total proctocolectomy with continent ileal reservoir (Kock pouch)
- Segmental colectomy—inadequate.
- Total colectomy with ileo rectal anastomosis in rectal sparing—rarely done, can cause intractable disease and diarrhea
- Total proctocolectomy, IPAA can be done in one stage, two stages or three stages
  - One stage—proctocolectomy with IPAA with no ileostomy
  - Two-stage: PC with IPAA and covering ileostomy and later ileostomy closure
  - Three-stage
  - Subtotal colectomy with ileostomy
  - PC with IPAA and covering ileostomy
  - Closure of ileostomy

Total Proctocolectomy with End Ileostomy

- Removes all diseased mucosa.
- But requires permanent ileostomy
- High morbidity due to
  - Perineal wound healing
  - Adhesions
  - Ileostomy
  - Pelvic dissection
- Done in old patients with poor sphincter function and in malignancy

Total Proctocolectomy with Continent Ileostomy

- Kock in 1969
- Ileal pouch created and a valve created by intussuscepting ileal limb
- Continent
- Complications
- Loss of valve, pouchitis, fistula, stricture
- Not done these days
- Not indicated in obese, old, mentally disordered and in CD

Restorative Proctocolectomy and IPAA

- Total proctocolectomy
- Pouch created using 30 cm of ileum
- Anastomosed to anus by
  - Stapling or
  - Handsewn—after stripping distal rectal mucosa
- Stripping of the mucosa and hand sewn anastomosis. Does not eliminate cancer risk completely

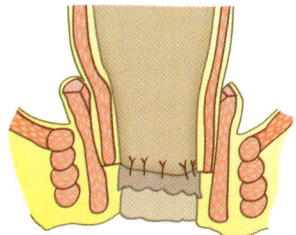 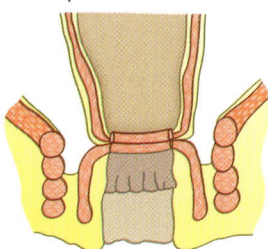

Trans anal mucosal resection and hand anastomosis

Stapled anastomosis

Double Stapling

- Retains anal trigger zone
- Can cause 'cuffitis'
- And dysplasia and cancer

Surgery in Dysplasia

- Influence the type of procedure
- Does not exclude the possibility of ileo anal pouch
- Dysplasia rectum—mucosectomy preferred

IPAA in Malignancy

- No contraindication in
  - Colonic cancer
  - Upper and middle third rectal cancer stage I and II with no neoadjuvant treatment

  Better avoided
  - Lower third rectal cancer
  - Stage III—after CRT

Pouch Comparison

- W pouch has more capacity and compliance
- But long-term no major difference
- Most popular—J pouch

Contraindications for IPAA

- Crohn's disease
- Anal cancer requiring RT
- Fecal incontinence

Early Surgery

- Avoid toxicity of drugs
- Dependence on drugs
- Cost can be reduced
- Potentially curable intestinal disease
- Avoid chance of malignancy

Variations of IPAA

- Mesorectal sparing—reduces leak and sepsis

  Pouch lengthening is achieved by:
  - Pouch length 6 cm below pubic symphysis—reach dentate line almost 100%
  - Ligation of ileocolic artery—add 3 cm
  - Ligation of distal SMA can add another 6.5 cm
  - Mobilization of mesentery
  - Relaxing incisions on mesentery

Early Complications of IPAA

- Sepsis
- PV thrombosis
- Int obstruction
- Bleeding

Late Complications

- Stricture
- Int obstruction
- Pouchitis

- Fistula
- Dysplasia/malignancy
- Cuffitis
- **Anastomotic leak 6–18%—more in**
  - Technical reasons
  - Obesity
  - Anti-TNF treatment
  - Steroid treatment

Leak Treatment

- CECT/Gastrograffin study
- Stable patient—transgluteal drain
- Peritonitis—Laparotomy-lavage-diversion

Pouchitis

- Nonspecific inflammation of pouch
- Causes pain, bloody stools
- Friable mucosa with bleeding

Pathogenesis

- Mucosal ischemia
- Immune deficiency
- Stasis
- Infection
- Recurrence of UC
- CMV, *C. difficile*

Treatment

- Metronidazole oral/topical
- Steroids, antibiotics
- Probiotics

Pouch Revision

- In complications
- Careful laparotomy
- Abdomino perineal mobilization
- Assess the problem
- Redo the pouch/anastomosis

Risk of Malignancy

- Need close follow-up
- If dysplasia—biopsy done every 6 months to 1 year
- No dysplasia—biopsy done every 1–2 years
- More in stapled anastomosis as the rectal mucosa is retained
- Pouch advancement or excision may be needed

Benign Diseases of Anal Canal

11.1 ANAL FISSURE

- Linear ulcer found in midline, distal to dentate line up to anal verge
- Occurs distal to the dentate line
- Most common—posterior midline (90%) > anterior fissures (10%) > lateral fissures (<1%)
- Acute fissure—laceration in anoderm
- Chronic fissure—ulceration with scarred edges
  - Sentinel tag distally
  - Hypertrophied anal papilla proximally
  - Visible muscle fibres at depth
  - Sentinal tag and papilla—consequences of healing and breakdown
- Lateral fissures—rule out Crohn's disease, tuberculosis, syphilis, HIV/AIDS, or carcinoma.

Pathogenesis

- Passage of large and hard stools
- Low-fiber diet
- Previous anal surgery
- Trauma
- Infection—syphilis, TB, herpes, CMV, chancroid
- Increased resting anal canal pressures—sawtooth pattern on manometry
- Vascular-anal resting pressure hypothesis
  - Reduced anal blood flow in the posterior midline
- Also due to frequent defecation and diarrhea
- Previous anal surgery—stricture predispose
- Posterior midline most common reasons
  - Reduced mucosal perfusion
  - Supplied by end arterioles
  - Sphincteric arterioles branch at right angles which transverse internal sphincter
  - Exaggerated shearing forces acting there during defecation
  - Less elastic anoderm—due to increased density of longitudinal muscles in that region
- Increased sphincter tone further reduce blood supply
- Normal sphincter resting pressure is 60–100 cm H_2O, it is raised in acute fissure characterized by saw-toothed pattern in manometry

- In herpes simplex virus infection—multiple superficial ulcers with vesicles
- Anterior fissure—more common in women following delivery

Clinical Features

In AAF

- Cutting or tearing type pain
- Minimal bleeding on tissue paper on wiping
- Constipation—pain—fear to defecate

In CAF

- C/o Lump-sentinel pile, discharge
- Pain will be mild and bleeding may be absent

Diagnosis

- Very painful
- Simple spreading of the buttocks
- Endoscopy postponed
- Examination under anesthesia—cultures, biopsies, therapeutic interventions

Atypical: Appearing Fissures

- Symptoms of inflammatory bowel disease
- Sexual activity and drug history
  - HIV screening.
  - Syphilitic ulcers—dark-field, wet microscopy.
  - Tuberculous ulcer—will show acid-fast bacilli on staining

Treatment

Goals

- Relaxation of the anal sphincter without causing fecal incontinence
- Passage of soft and formed stools
- Relief of pain

Medical

- Warm water sitz bath, stool bulking agents
- Warmth reduce pain and relax sphincters
- Mineral oil not advisable-detrimental on colonic mucosa, and difficult to clean

Acute anal fissures (those presenting within 6 weeks of symptom onset)
- Topical nitric oxide (e.g. nitroglycerin 0.2% to .4%)
  - Relax sphincter, increase blood flow
  - But can cause headache
  - Relief in 5 minutes, lasts up to 12 hours
- Healing in 4–6 weeks

Chemical Sphincterotomy
- Calcium channel blockers (e.g. diltiazem 2%, nifedipine 0.2%)—first line
  - Better healing rate and safer
  - Oral medication not effective
- Botulinum toxin injections—temporary chemo-denervation—relaxation of internal sphincter—promote blood flow—healing
  - Injected 50 units on either side of fissure into internal sphincter
  - 10% develop temporary flatus incontinence
- Topical arginine—NO donor
- Topical bethenecol—muscarinic agonist
- Conservative methods—heal 90% of acute anal fissure, 40% of chronic anal fissure

Surgical Management
Indications
- Severe or chronic fissures
- Failed to respond to medical therapy.

Lateral Internal anal Partial Sphincterotomy (LIS)—Operation of Choice
- Open or closed (stab incision)
- Lateral approach better than midline. Midline approach is through the fissure which can produce keyhole deformity of anus.
- Sphincterotomy to the level of the dentate line produce higher rate of healing

Posterior midline sphincterotomy may produce key hole deformity

Closed Lateral Sphincterotomy-Notaras
- Sphincter divided in full length of fissure may be up to dentate line
- Incontinence in lateral sphincterotomy
  - Total incontinence—14%
  - Flatus in 9%
  - Liquid or solid stool in 2%

Fissurectomy—curettage of base of anal fissure and excision of rolled out edge and excision of sentinel pile/skin tag

- Defect created is covered by advancement flaps
- Anal four finger dilatation causes uncontrolled stretching and so it is discouraged

Chronic or recurrent fissure with hypotensive anal sphincter:
- Fissurectomy with endoanal advancement flap—alternative surgical approach
- Pneumatic balloon dilatation—good healing rate
- Anal dilatation by finger insertion technique discouraged

Hypertrophied papilla—causes bleeding and itching
- It is called cryptitis
- It is treated by laying open/excision

11.2 HEMORRHOIDS
- Haima = blood (greek)
- Rhoos = flowing
- Pila = a ball (latin)
- Normal, vascular tissue within the submucosa located in the anal canal suspended by longitudinal connective tissue and muscle fibers
- Aids in anal continence by providing bulk to the anal canal.
- Located in the left lateral, right anterior, and right posterior quadrants—3, 7 and 11 O' clock anal cushions

Anal Cushions
- Give a washer effect—allows complete closure of anal canal
- Involved in a recto anal inhibitory reflex—small amounts of rectal distension—produce contraction of external sphincter and relaxation of internal sphincter—allows sampling—allows anorectal junction to distinguish between solid, gas and liquid and adjust continence
- Contribute 15–20% of anal resting pressure
- Anal canal—with advancing age ratio of connective tissue increases—leads to loss of elasticity which fragment the anchoring muscle fibers supporting anal cushions leads to prolapse of hemorrhoidal tissue

Blood Supply
- Superior rectal artery from IMA
- Middle rectal artery from internal iliac
- Inferior rectal artery from pudendal artery internal iliac artery
- Venous watershed—dentate line

Etiology
- Portal hypertension
- Hemangiomas
- Infection
- Constipation—straining

- Anal hypertonia
- Ageing

All these are old concepts

Etiology: Current concept

- Abnormalities with weakening of the connective tissue of vascular cushions
- Excessive straining
  - Chronic constipation
  - Low-fiber dietary intake
- Internal anal sphincter dysfunction

External hemorrhoids—distal to the dentate line, covered with anoderm

- They are from inferior hemorrhoidal plexus and are not true hemorrhoids. They are usually recognized after a complication-like thrombosis
- Thrombosis can produce severe pain

Internal hemorrhoids—bright red, painless bleeding or prolapse.

- Dripping or squirting of blood in the toilet.
- Mucus and fecal leakage
- Pruritus.

Secondary Internal Hemorrhoids

- Most important cause—carcinoma anorectum, other causes
  - Hypotonic anal sphincter, pelvic mass
  - Neurological—paraplegia, multiple sclerosis
- Anorectal varices in PHT—are not hemorrhoids—surgical intervention may be dangerous

GRADE SYMPTOMS AND SIGNS

Haemorrhoids: Clinical features

- Haemorrhoids or piles are symptomatic anal cushions.
- They are more common when intra-abdominal pressure is raised, e.g. in obesity, constipation and pregnancy.
- Classically, they occur in the 3, 7 and 11 o'clock positions with the patient in the lithotomy position.
- Symptoms of haemorrhoids:
  - Bright—red, painless bleeding mucus discharge
  - Prolapse
  - Pain only on prolapsed

Goligher's Grading

- First degree bleeding—no prolapse
- Second degree—prolapse with spontaneous reduction
- Third degree—prolapse requiring manual reduction
- Fourth degree—prolapsed, cannot be reduced

Examination

- Left lateral position
- Digital per rectal examination
- Anoscopy: Assess location, grade of prolapse, ask patient to strain
- Rigid proctoscopy
- To rule out proximal source of bleeding consider-colonoscopy

Treatment

Nonoperative Management

- Dietary modifications—fiber supplementation and increasing fluid intake

In grades 1, 2 and some 3

- Anal ointments—reduce trauma to hemorrhoidal cushions
- Rubber band ligation Barron's can produce rare complication of postbanding sepsis

Sclerotherapy

- Injection of a low volume (3 to 5 ml) of sclerosant (e.g. 3% normal saline) into submucosa
  - Sodium morruate, sodium tetradecyl sulphate
  - Phenol in arachis oil or almond oil
  - Injected to apex of pile pedicle
  - Pain means wrong location
- Infrared and laser coagulation, bipolar coagulation
- Ultroid therapy uses direct current

All these are based on principle of local tissue destruction, fibrosis and fixation of anal cushions.

- Infrared which has penetration of 3 mm applied to apex of hemorrhoid, all three hemorrhoid can be treated in one sitting

Rubber Band

- First described by Blaisdell in 1958
- Devices with suction and nonsuction—forceps
- Contraindications for banding-immunosuppression (HIV, on chemo), coagulopathy, on antiplatelet medication
- If severe pain occurs after banding, band may have been placed above dentate line, hence band removed
- Sclerotherapy—not contraindicated in anticoagulation

Surgical Management

Indications

- Grade III or grade IV
- Complicated by strangulation, ulceration, fissure, or fistula
- Symptomatic external hemorrhoids

Thrombosed External Hemorrhoids

- Excision of the mass is advised if they present within 72 hrs. incision of this masses not advised because can produce rethrombosis

- If they present late—conservative management

- Untreated—may resolve, suppurate, fibrose and can burst and bleed

- Majority of cases resolve which is called **'a 5-day, painful, self-curing lesion'** (Milligan)

HEMORRHOIDECTOMY IN

- Prolapsed hemorrhoids

- Coagulopathic patients

- Acutely thrombosed gangrenous internal hemorrhoids—debatable

---

Hemorrhoidectomy

- Closed (Ferguson or Parks) hemorrhoidectomy
- Open (Milligan-Morgan) hemorrhoidectomy

- Whitehead hemorrhoidectomy—relocate the prolapsed dentate line

- Stappler hemorrhoidopexy

- Doppler guided trans anal devascularisation

Parks' Ligament (Treitz's muscle)

Three taeniae of colon broaden over sigmoid—and rectum in an outer layer of longitudinal muscle—this gives off anchoring muscle extensions to the internal anal sphincter and to the anal cushions called the Treitz's muscle. They keep anal cushions in position—allowing them to function normally.

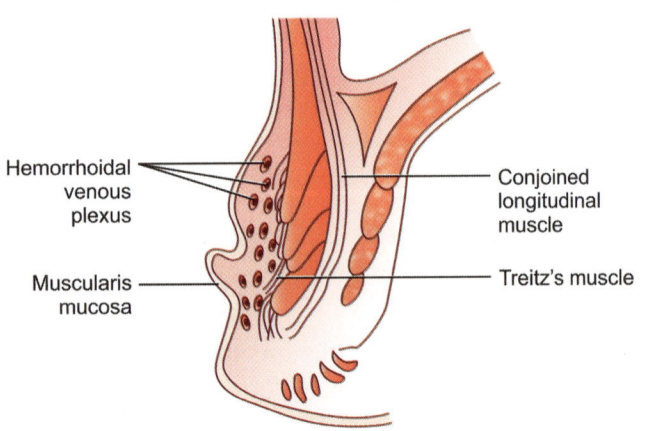

- It fixes conjoined longitudinal muscle to submucosal tissues, passing through internal sphincter.

- Consist of muscular fibroblastic tissue located around anal glands and support hemorrhoidal plexus.

- When submucosal cushions prolapse, they get stretched and fragmented

- Divided in hemorrhoidectomy

- Use of various energy sources like diathermy, harmonic, LigaSure—no advantages

Whitehead Hemorrhoidectomy

- Circumferential excision of hemorrhoidal cushions just proximal to dentate line, then rectal mucosa is advanced and sutured to dentate line

- Produce rectal ectropion called Whitehead's deformity, so this procedure is not popular

Nonexcisional Hemorrhoidectomy or Pexy Procedure—Procedure for Prolapsing Hemorrhoids (PPHS)

Stapled Hemorrhoiodopexy (SH)

- Purse string 3–4 cm above dentate line incorporating only mucosa and submucosa

  – Less pain and reduced operative time and hospital stay

  – Recurrence rate higher

Hemorrhoidal Arterial Ligation Operation (HALO)

- Doppler guided hemorrhoidal artery ligation, or

- Transanal hemorrhoidal dearterialization (THD)+/– mucosopexy

- By Morigana—1995—based on closure of blood flow to hemorrhoids via terminal branches of superior rectal artery—with Doppler with a specially designed proctoscope

- Mucosopexy corrects prolapse

Complications

- Pain—most common

- Urinary retention (in up to 30% of patients)

- Fecal incontinence (2%)

- Infection (1%)

- Delayed hemorrhage (1%) in 5 to 10 days—due to early separation of ligated pedicle
- Stricture (1%)
- Postop metronidazole—reduces pain

11.3 ANORECTAL SUPPURATION

- There are about 8–10 crypt glands at the level of dentate line—arranged circumferentially—penetrate internal sphincter—lumen terminates at intersphincteric plane
- They are the path for infection
- Infection begins in anal glands
- Abscess is acute and fistula is the chronic sequela

Etiology

- Most common—nonspecific cryptoglandular infection.
- Fecal bacterial plugging of the ducts—obstruction and subsequent abscess formation
- Cryptoglandular theory of anal sepsis—Parks theory
- Later pus travel via pathway of least resistance

Other Causes

- Foreign bodies
- Malignancy
- Trauma
- Tuberculosis
- Actinomycosis
- Leukemia
- Postoperative infection, inflammatory bowel disease
- Simple skin infections
- Cigarette smoking

Anorectal Abscesses

- Originate in the intersphincteric space.
- May extend vertically upward or downward, horizontally, or circumferentially.

Classified Into

- Perianal, ischiorectal
- Intersphincteric, supralevator
- Submucosal, deep postanal.

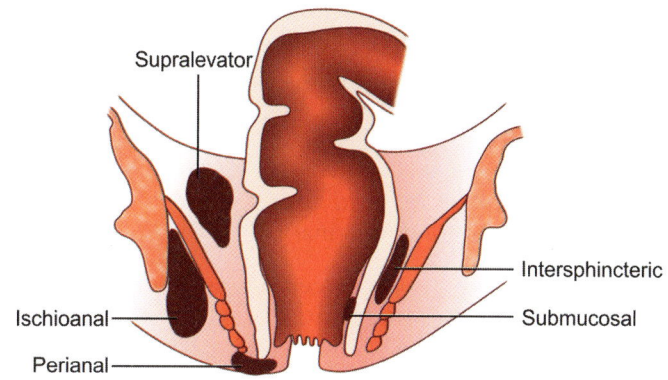

- Multiple perirectal spaces produce classic "horseshoe" abscess
- **"Floating anus":**
  - Circumanal spread of intersphincteric, supralevator, or ischiorectal collections.

Clinical Features

- Perianal—localized swelling, hyperemia, induration, tenderness, discharge
- Pain out of proportion to findings
- Intersphincteric abscess—pain, tender swelling
- Upward extension—supralevator abscess—vague pelvic/anorectal discomfort
- May be also due to pelvic infections
  - Diverticulitis, PID, appendicitis, ruptured viscus
- Horizontal spread—internally to anal canal can produce submucous abscess
  - Externally into ischiorectal abscess produce large erythematous area and can extend to supralevator space
- Transphincteric extension in posterior midline produce postanal abscess
- Circumferential extension cause horseshoe abscess

Treatment

- Incision and drainage
- Depending on site—LA/regional anesthesia
- Intersphincteric abscess—into canal by dividing internal sphincter at the level of abscess

Recurrent Abscesses

- Examination under anesthesia—after imaging of the abdomen or pelvis

Horseshoe Abscesses: Modified Hanley Procedure

- Posterior midline incision (partial distal sphincterotomy + fistulotomy)

- All the muscles attached to coccyx, superficial external sphincter and lower edge of internal sphincter—divided (original Hanley)

- Modified Hanley procedure—partial distal internal sphincterotomy, external sphincters splayed and coccyx musculature need not be divided. Along with this counter incisions over ishiorectal fossae and connecting drains are placed

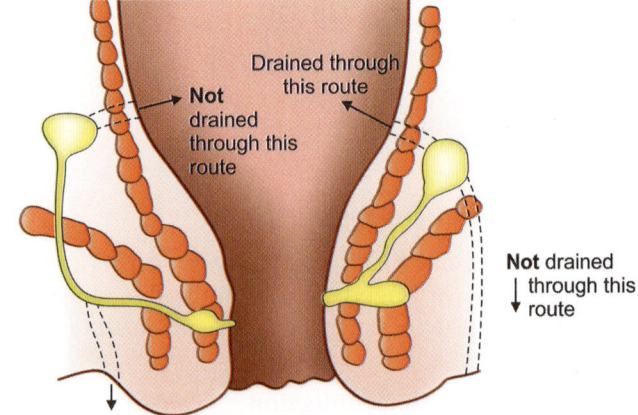

- **Ischiorectal fossa abscess drainage can injure inferior rectal branch of internal pudendal nerve**

Primary Fistulotomy is Considered in

- History of previous anorectal sepsis
- Ischiorectal abscess with an internal opening readily apparent
- Horseshoe abscess and intersphincteric abscess

Fistula in Ano

Clinical Features

- Pain, slight fever
- Passage of flatus or feces through external opening from rectal internal opening
- Pain on defecation
- Mucopurulent drainage
- Pruritic symptoms

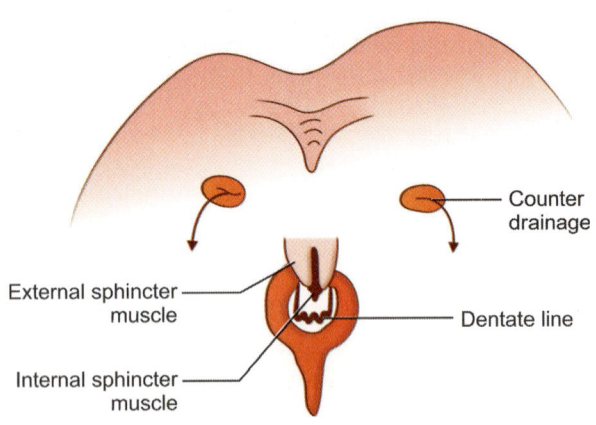

- Posterior incision up to tip of coccyx
- Intersphincteric abscess—drained by laying open internal sphincter and fistulotomy is done by incising anal gland
- Submucosal abscess drained internally
- Supralevator collections that result from

  – An upward extension of an intersphincteric abscess should be drained transrectally as transperineal drainage through IR fossa can result in suprasphincteric fistula

- Supralevator collections that result from the cephalad extension of a transsphincteric fistula or an ischiorectal collection, should be drained transperineally—through ischioanal fossae. If drained trans rectally may result in extrasphincteric fistula

- Supralevator collection if arises from abdominal source—drained trans abdominally

Parks Classification

Intersphincteric

- Confined to the intersphincteric plane. Most common type

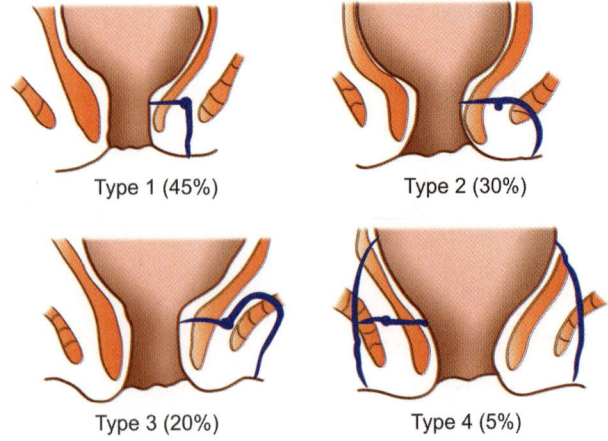

Type 1 (45%)   Type 2 (30%)

Type 3 (20%)   Type 4 (5%)

Trans-sphincteric

- Traverses external sphincter
- Communicating with the ischiorectal fossa.

Suprasphincteric

- Extends cephalad over the external sphincter and perforates the levator ani—rare

Extrasphincteric

- Extends from rectum to perianal skin
- External to the sphincter apparatus—rare
- Iatrogenic—needs colostomy

A—Intersphincteric fistula types
1 Simple
2 High blind tract
3 High blind tract with rectal opening
4 High tract without perineal opening, may or may not be rectal opening
5 High with pelvic extension
6 High fistula with primary pelvic pathology—no opening at dentate line

- B1—trans-sphincteric—uncomplicated
- B2—trans-sphincteric—high blind tract—may extend into pelvic cavity
- C—suprasphincteric
- D—extrasphincteric from skin to ischiorectal fossa to levator muscle to rectum above the sphincter
- Suprasphincteric—above the continence apparatus
- Extrasphincteric—from iatrogenic injury—completely outside sphincter apparatus

Simple Fistula

- Submucosal tract
- Low intersphincteric (traversing <30% of anal sphincter muscle)

Complex Fistula

- With multiple external openings
- High trans-sphincteric, suprasphincteric, extra sphincteric
- Horseshoe fistula
- Anterior fistula in female
- Crohn's
- Radiotherapy associated fistula

Physical Examination

- Careful digital rectal examination—fistulas palpated—fibrous tracts 3 to 7 mm thick
- Malleable anorectal probes and crypt hooks delineate the fistula via the internal or external opening
- Multiple complex fistula tracts—"watering-pot perineum"
- Internal opening—indurated nodule
  - Most often at the dentate line
- Intersphincteric fistula open close to anal verge
- Trans-sphincteric and others—away from anal verge
- Sometimes external opening may be inside anal canal
  - Internal opening—most often near dentate line which are cryptoglandular because most of the anal glands are locate in posterior midline, so 60–70% opening seen in posterior midline

The Goodsall Rule

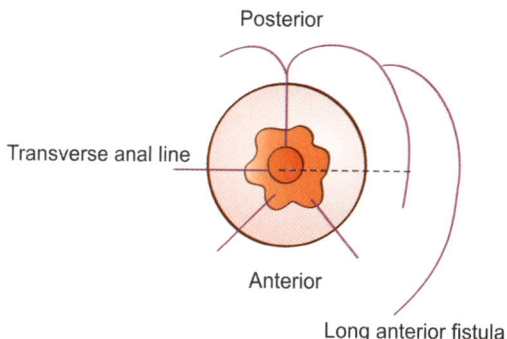

- Locating the internal opening.
- States that an external opening anterior to an imaginary transverse anal line in the coronal plane most likely communicates with an internal opening lying at the end of a radial line drawn to the nearest crypt at the dentate line.
- If external opening is posterior to line, internal opening will be in posterior midline with curved tract.

Exceptions

- Anterior openings more than 3 cm from the anal verge
- Presence of multiple external openings.
  - The internal opening most likely be in the posterior midline

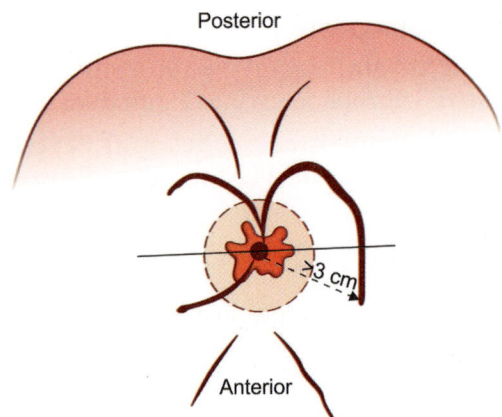

Diagnosis

- Sigmoidoscopy and colonoscopy to rule out neoplasms, inflammatory bowel disease, or associated secondary tracts in the rectum must be sought. Such findings may dictate the need for full colonoscopic evaluation.

Fistulography

- Recurrent fistulas or when a prior procedure has failed to identify the internal opening.
- Fails to give exact location of fistulous opening in relation to sphincter
  - Anorectal ultrasonography—to assess muscular anatomy and fistula 360 degree probe or linear probes used
  - Hydrogen peroxide injected into fistulas as an image enhancer in complex fistulas
  - 3D endoanal ultrasonography—with or without H_2O_2 enhancement
  - Vaginal endosonography—increase diagnostic yield by 25%

MRI

- More accurate in recurrent and complex tracts and to see internal openings
- Combinations of EUS, MRI and EUA—more helpful
- Gold standard and choice

CT

- Assess pelvic pathology in patients with supralevator abscesses
- Complex anal fistulas.
- No role in simple fistulas

Anorectal manometry—assess continence control following surgery

- Fistuloscopy—flexible ureteroscopes are used

Treatment

- Should undergo surgery—rarely heal spontaneously
- Lithotomy, prone or jackknife positions
- Left lateral position in pregnancy

Fistulotomy

- In simple fistulas—low trans-sphincteric and intershincteric, involving <30% of voluntary musculature
- Marsupialization
- In normal adults division of a portion of internal and some fibers of external sphincter would not result in incontinence
  - Sphincter saving techniques in anterior fistulas in women—any amount of sphincter division may result in incontinence, due to thin sphincters, so fistulotomy is not done

Seton (Seta Means Bristle)
Indications

- In complex fistulas with risk of incontinence or poor healing
  - Crohn disease
  - Immunocompromised
  - Incontinent patients
  - Chronic diarrheal states
- Anterior fistulas in women
- Involve more than 30% of the sphincter
- High trans-sphincteric fistulas
  - 60 to 100% success rate

Technique

- Penrose drains, silastic vessel loops, rubber bands, polypropelene, braided steel wires all these are used.
- Marking—encircling the tract to assess amount of muscle present if adequate muscle is there above the fistula, fistulotomy can be done
  - Cutting seton at 2-week interval—seton is progressively tightened, dividing the muscle by a process of ischemic necrosis and fibrosis and skin over the tract is divided.

Kshara-Sutra

- Seton with medication burns through the tissue
- Chemical cautery
- Equivalent to one-stage fistulotomy in patients with intersphincteric and distal transphincteric fistulae

Draining seton—long-term draining setons—tied loosely used in management of complex fistulas associated with Crohn disease
- Staging seton—"high" fistula is converted to "low" fistula. After dividing only superficial portion of the tract seton is applied, distal tract is encircled with seton for later division
- In second stage fistulotomy is done

Fibrin Glue

- In complex cases
- Promote the closure of fistulas without division of sphincter muscle
- Pooled plasma fibrinogen and thrombin applied after curetting or porcine derived fistula plug can also be used.

Fistula Plug

- Bioprosthetic—lyophilized porcine intestinal submucosa or synthetic absorbable biomaterial
- Acts as a scaffolding for tissue ingrowth
- Preserves anal function and is associated with a low morbidity
- Success rate of 35 to 85%

Anorectal Advancement Flaps

- In high fistulas or other persistent fistulas
- Sliding advancement flap
- Made of mucosa, submucosa, and part of internal sphincter to cover the internal opening.
- Base should be wider than apex
- 10 to 50% success rate
- Done in one stage and causes limited sphincter damage
- Crohn's, smoking, multiple prior surgeries, use of fibrin glue in these situations carry higher risk of flap failure.

Anocutaneous Advancement Flap

- In high fistulas and dense scarring due to prior surgeries
- Pedicled flap from anal margin—advancement into anal canal
- Too much advancement of anoderm into anal canal can cause pruritus

LIFT (Ligation of the Intersphincteric Fistula Track)

- 60% to 90% success rate
- Incision at intersphincteric groove and identify the fistula tract with the help of probe—and ligate

- Internal opening is closed; external opening is curetted and left open

Failures

Type-1—residual track from intersphincteric groove without internal opening

Treated by curettage and antibiotics

Type 2—downstage tract from intersphincteric groove to internal opening

Treated by fistulotomy

Type 3—complete failure extends from previous internal opening to external opening

Treated by other modalities or another LIFT
- Use of bioprosthetic mesh in intersphincteric groove called **Bio-LIFT**
- Placing fistula plug through external sphincter is called **LIFT plug**

Fistula Laser Closure (FiLaC)

- Laser emitted by a radial fiber
- Destroys epithelium and closes the tract
- Simple diathermy can damage sphincter and fails to close the sphincter
- May be combined with anorectal advancement flap

VAAFT—Video Assisted Anal Fistula Treatment by Meinero

- Visually identify the tract and any residual abscess cavity using fistuloscope and tract ablation
- Tract cauterised using bipolar energy
- Debris removed by endobrush
- Stapler or mucosal advancement flap or cyanoacrylate closure of internal opening

Stem Cells from Adipose Tissue

- Use of stem cells derived from autologous sub-cutaneous fat—20 million cells are used
- Collected after liposuction
- Immunomodulatory and anti-inflammatory
- Results are not very good

11.4 RECTAL PROLAPSE

- Mucosal or full thickness
- Usually mucosal in children
- Full thickness prolapse: Procidentia

History

- 1912: Alexis Moschcowitz: Rectal prolapse is caused by sliding herniation of pouch of Douglas through pelvic floor fascia
- 1968: Broden and Snellman: It is a full thickness rectal intussusception starting 3 inches above the dentate line. It is the most accepted theory.

Etiopathology

- More common in females (6:1)
- Age groups: Men—20s and 30s
  - Women: After 6th decade
- Association with bowel habits
- 65% are constipated
- 15% has diarrhea
- 70% has incontinence

Associated Anatomic Defects

- Weak levator ani
- Weak anal sphincter muscles
- Redundant rectosigmoid
- Deep cul-de-sac
- Loss of fixation of rectum to sacrum

Associated Conditions

- Connective tissue disorders
- Pelvic outlet obstruction
- Pelvic floor laxity
- Spina bifida, multiple sclerosis
- Cystic fibrosis
- Anorexia and bulimia nervosa
- Excess straining, valsalva maneuver
- History of mental illness (4 times higher risk).

Clinical Features

- Mass or lump in the perineum, which initially comes out after bowel movements
- Incontinence
- Sensation of chronic moisture
- Mucous discharge
- Bleeding, ulceration (chronic)
- Incarcerated prolapsed segment

Differential Diagnosis

- Prolapsed hemorrhoids—folds are radial (concentric for rectal prolapse)
  - Extremely painful
  - Fever, urinary retention may be present

Evaluation

- Detailed history
- Examination—rule out other pelvic floor defect as rectocele, cystocele

- If no prolapse on examination, ask patient to squat and observe
  - Still hidden, do defecography
- Colonoscopy: To rule out synchronous or causative neoplasm

Additional Evaluation

- If incontinence is present: Ultrasonography
- Anal manometry
- Pudendal nerve terminal motor latency to record baseline anorectal function
  - X-ray of sacrum—to identify occult spina bifida
  - Colonic transit time—for constipated. Rectopexy will worsen constipation, while resection improves
  - IVP—to identify course of ureter when perineal approach is planned and associated urinary or uterine prolapse is present .

Management

Acute Management

- Early reduction—reduce gently and tape the buttocks
- If not easily reducible and rectum is viable—sedate patient, place in the Trendelenburg position, apply salt or sugar topically to reduce edema. Hyaluronidase injection may also help
- For incarcerated rectal prolapse—emergency perineal proctosigmoidectomy

Surgery

- Definitive management is by surgery
- More than 100 methods have been described
- Approaches: Perineal and abdominal
- Abdominal may be open or laparoscopic. Laparoscopic is preferred now.
- Approach is decided by age, comorbidities of patient and surgeons experience

Perineal Approach

- Preferred for elderly and debilitated
- Less postop morbidity, less pain
- Reduced hospital stay
- Increased recurrence rate.

Abdominal Approach

- Open or laparoscopic
- Preferred for young patients
- Lesser recurrence
- Increased rate of infertility or impotence.

Abdominal Procedures

Rectopexy

- Mobilise rectum on both sides and posteriorly down to levator ani plate

- Ripstein repair—placement of mesh around mobilized rectum, with attachment of mesh to the presacral fascia
- **Wells modification**—places Ivalon sponge posteriorly leaving a 2 cm gap anteriorly
- Other recommended materials to secure rectum: Fascia lata, marlex, teflon., polyglycolic acid
- Recently it is suggested that mobilization of the rectum is sufficient to produce enough fibrotic scar to fix the bowel to sacral curvature.

Complications

- Worsens or new onset constipation
- Large bowel obstruction
- Erosion of mesh through the bowel
- Ureteric injury or fibrosis
- Small bowel obstruction
- Rectovaginal fistula
- Fecal impaction

Resection

- Help to decrease constipation
- Mobilize rectum up to coccyx, resect redundant rectosigmoid and reanastomose.
- Anastomosis should be at the level of sacral promontory
- Do not mobilize splenic flexure as it may lead to recurrence.

Resection-Rectopexy

- Described by Frykman and Goldberg
- Removes excess bowel and restore normal rectal angulation
- Improves symptoms of continence and constipation
- Recurrence rates are low

Perineal Approaches

- Preferred for elderly with comorbidities and young males with fear of infertility after abdominal procedures

- Altemeier's procedure—perineal proctosigmoidectomy
- Delorme procedure—anorectal mucosectomy with muscular plication
- Thiersch procedure—anal encirclement

Altemeier's Procedure

- Resection of prolapsed bowel via perineum
- **Prasad modification**—approach to correct associated anatomic defect.

  Pull the rectum to completely prolapse it—inject dilute epinephrine 1 to 2 cm proximal to dentate line—at this level, circumferentially incise the rectal wall in full thickness—ligate vessels to rectum and sigmoid—fix the nonprolapsing bowel to presacrococcygeal fascia with suture—posterior levatoroplasty to fix widely open pelvic floor—resect excess bowel and do coloanal anastomosis

Delorme Procedure

- No bowel resection and anastomosis

Thiersch Procedure

- For patients with severe comorbidities.
- Can be done quickly
- Two peri anal skin incision, 180 degrees apart lateral to midline—connect them with a tunnel through ischiorectal fossa—place a 1.5 cm wide prolene mesh around the deep external sphincter—tighten and suture mesh to itself until anal diameter admits only 1 finger in the anus
  - Complications—mesh erosion, recurrence, impaction

Management of Recurrence

- First procedure dictates re-operative surgical approach.
- Initial perineal resection—repeat perineal resection or abdominal rectopexy
- Abdominal resection—reoperate via abdomen
- Abdominal rectopexy reoperate through perineal proctosigmoidectomy.

Spleen

12.1 ANATOMY

- Weight 75–250 gm (avg 150 gm), 7–13 cm long
- Develops from mesenchymal cells of dorsal mesogastrium—during 5th week
- Protected by 9, 10, 11 ribs—in long axis on 10th rib
- Peritoneal reflections—splenophrenic, gastrosplenic, splenorenal, splenocolic
- Splenophrenic and splenocolic ligaments—avascular—except in portal hypertension
- Gastrosplenic ligament has—short gastric vessels on superior and left gastroepiploic on inferior aspects
- Splenorenal ligament—carries splenic artery and vein and tail of pancreas
- Thought to be associated with emotions—in ancient times
- Additional function—plays a role in embryogenesis of pancreas—serves as a reservoir of islet cell precursors
- Splenomegaly is when—weight >500 gm or length >15 cm
- Massive splenomegaly—weight >1500 gm
- Spleen is palpable when its size is at least twice the normal
- In children spleen capsule is thicker than adults, contain myoepithelial cells—helps in hemostasis
  - In children due to efficient contraction of arterioles and lack of atherosclerosis—better hemostasis
  - Ribs are more elastic—recoil—less force on spleen and less rupture
- Tail of pancreas abuts splenic hilum—in 30%
  - Within 1 cm of hilum in 70%
- So need to stay within 1 cm from hilum during splenectomy to avoid injury to pancreas

Spleen: Blood Supply

- Receives 5% of cardiac output via splenic artery
- Overall blood flow about 300 ml/minute
- Also via left gastroepiploic artery

Splenic Artery

Two variations Michels

- Magistral type—divides into terminal and polar branches near hilum—occurs in 30%
- Distributed type—branches early and away from hilum—in 70%
  - Divisions
  - Superior polar artery—anastomose with SGA
  - Superior, middle and inferior terminal arteries
  - Inferior polar artery

Magistral Type

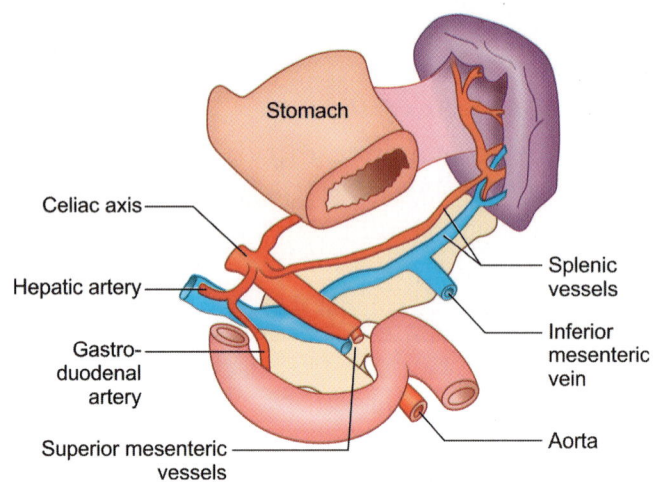

Distributed Type

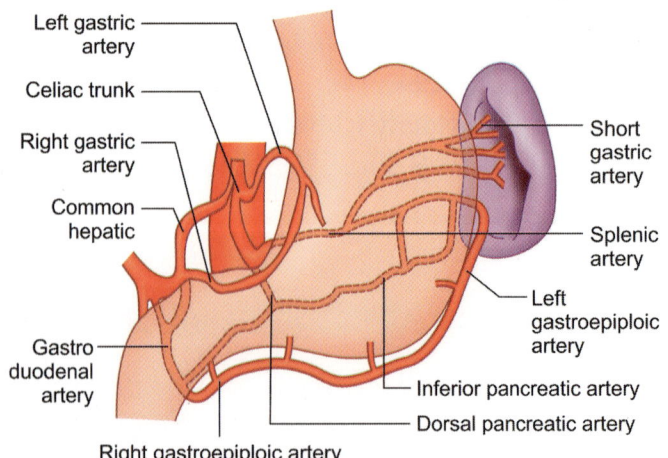

- Splenic segmental arteries—have little collaterals so occlusion leads to infarction of that region

  SA division—segmental arteries—trabecular arteries—perpendicular branches—central arteries

- Segmental blood supply—helps in partial splenectomy

- Two segments—superior and inferior segments in 84%

- Three segments—superior, inferior and middle segments in 16%

- Segments are separated by avascular planes—pass obliquely to the longitudinal axis—do not traverse full thickness from visceral to parietal surfaces

- Three zones by Dixon—hilar, intermediate and peripheral

- Bleeding from peripheral zones—controlled by topical agents—from intermediate and hilar zone by ligation

- Encased in fibroelastic capsule—trabeculae pass from capsule—compartmentalize spleen

- Spleen is also segmented by branches of splenic vessels

- Arterioles become small vessels where adventitia is replaced by lymphatic sheath and form capillaries—lymphatic sheath make up white pulp

- In the marginal zone, arterioles—lose lymphatic tissue and form sinusoids and merge to form venules and then veins

Filtration

- Closed system—blood flows directly to veins

- Open system—(90%) arterioles drain to sieve like parenchyma of reticuloendothelial cells and form splenic sinuses and form venous system. Here cellular cleansing takes place (removal of senescent cells, parasites), sequestration of RBCs and platelets

- Closed system—fast—blood flow from arterioles to venules directly—involves predominantly plasma

- Open system—slow—exposes circulating cells and RBC to splenic macrophages in red pulp

Histology

- Red pulp and white pulp are separated by thin marginal zone

- Red pulp—is 75% of spleen—predominantly made of splenic cords, capillaries and venous sinuses—function as a filter of blood

- White pulp—consisted by lymphoid follicles (mainly B lymphocytes), and periarterial lymphoid sheath (PALS) (mainly T lymphocytes)

  – Responsible for immunologic function

Functions of Spleen

- RBC quality control and removal of defective RBC

  – In red pulp

  – By pitting and culling

- **Pitting**—removal of nondeformable intracellular contents from deformable cells—rigid elements removed and deformable cytoplasmic contents returned to circulation, e.g.

  – Howell-Jolly, Heinz bodies, Pappenheimer bodies

- Normally there is <2% pitted cells

- **Culling**—removal of old RBC by 120 days of cycle

  – RBCs lose its integrity of membranes and deformability—phagocytosis by splenic macrophages

  – Spleen is not the only site for RBC destruction—no difference in RBC survival after splenectomy

  – Platelets and WBCs are not mainly removed by spleen when they age, they die in other tissues

- **Pooling**

  – In healthy state—not a reservoir for blood

  – Major reservoir for platelets—one-third of platelet mass is in spleen

- In splenomegaly up to 80% platelets pooled in spleen and leads to destruction—both cause thrombocytopenia

- Platelet count increases after splenectomy

Hematopoiesis

- In fetal life this function is transferred to bone marrow by second trimester

- In fetal life spleen produces white and red cells—taken over by bone marrow by 5th month of gestation beyond this, there is no hematopoietic function

- In myclofibrosis, and hemolysis—extramedullary hematopoiesis in spleen occurs—more immature cells

- Spleen contains about 8% of RBCs

- Antibody synthesis happens in white pulp—especially IgM

- Contains 67% of T cells and 10–15% B lymphocytes

Filtration

- Macrophages in marginal zone—catch cellular and non cellular material from blood and also encapsulated bacteria—destroy them (opsonisation)
- Spleen acts as a filter
- Produces properdin and tuftsin—the opsonins
- Normal RBCs are biconcave—deform easily—allow passage through microvasculature and exchange of oxygen
- Abnormal RBCs with inclusions like nucleoli, Howell-Jolly bodies (nuclear remnant), Heinz bodies (denatured hemoglobin), Pappenheimer bodies (iron granules), acanthocytes (spur cells), codocytes (target cells)—undergo cleansing in spleen
- Aged RBC >120 days—loss of plasticity and hence trapped and destroyed
- Abnormal RBCs in sickle cell, thalassemia—destroyed produce anemia and splenomegaly leads to autoinfarction of spleen
- In ITP—platelet destruction

Congenital Abnormalities of Spleen

- **Splenic agenesis**—in 5% children with congenital heart disease
- **Polysplenia**—rare—due to failure of fusion

Accessory Spleen (Splenunculi)

- Seen in 20% of population—one or more
- Most common anomaly of spleen
- In hematologic pathologies—may be seen in 30%
- Usually located near splenic hilum—in 50%, related to splenic vessels and behind tail of pancreas in 30%
- Other sites—pancreas, omentum, pelvis, reproductive glands
- Tc 99 labelled RBC scan—to localise

12.2 SPLENIC ARTERY ANEURYSM

- Constitute 60% of all visceral artery aneurysm—most common visceral artery aneurysm
- Third most common intra-abdominal aneurysm after AAA and iliac artery aneurysm
- Usually saccular type, 2–3 cm
- Situated in distal third of artery in 75%
- Rarely intrasplenic
- May be thrombosed—without affecting vascularity

Causes

- Atherosclerosis
- Arterial degenerative syndromes
- Collagen vascular disease—Marfan's, Ehlers-Danlos
- Associated with sepsis, pancreatic necrosis
- More common in pregnant ladies due to hormonal influence (estrogen, progesterone, relaxin) which causes internal elastic laminal disruption and medial fibrodysplasia
- In liver disease and portal hypertension
- Women—more arise from middle to distal portion of SA
- Situated in main trunk
- Usually asymptomatic can produce bruit
- Treated with embolisation, or surgery with splenectomy and ligation
- Rupture into lesser sac can cause collapse and shock but can result in tamponade due to containment of blood in lesser sac leads to transient stability. Later extravasation of blood into peritoneum leads to loss of tamponade, shock and death, called double rupture phenomenon
- Rupture into peritoneal cavity—more common in pregnant women in third trimester leads to 95% mortality of fetus

Diagnosis

- X-ray—signet ring-shaped calcification left upper quadrant
- USG—preferred in pregnant
- CECT—the choice
- MRI
- Angiogram—therapeutic also

Treatment

- Depend on size, growth and clinical setting
- Symptomatic aneurysms are treated—irrespective of size
- In asymptomatic >2 cm—need treatment
- Women of child bearing age and pregnant—are treated even if <2 cm
- Growing in size while on surveillance—treated

Endovascular Techniques

- Stent grafts—maintain patency
- Best for proximal lesions where pancreas make surgery difficult

- Embolization—can cause splenic ischemia, abscess

Surgery

- Distal lesions—ligation with splenectomy with or without distal pancreatectomy
- Proximal lesions—ligation with or without grafting
- Middle lesion—aneurysectomy alone with or without reconstruction—preserve spleen

Evaluation of Spleen

USG

- In normal spleen—cannot differentiate red pulp and white pulp—seen as homogenous texture

CT

- Normal spleen—40–60 HU
- CECT heterogenous—as flow through red and white pulp vary
- CT volumetry of spleen

X-ray

- Calcifications
- Splenomegaly

MRI

- Homogenous on noncontrast
- With contrast—heterogenous during arterial phase

Angiography

- With selective arterial embolization—in trauma, preoperatively to reduce bleeding and size, in PHT
- In large spleen, as in ITP—more pain and complications like pancreatitis can occur

Nuclear imaging

- Tc99m sulfur colloid—to locate and assess the size—in accessory spleen
- No advantage in preoperative localization
- In platelet sequestration—indium labelled autologous platelet scanning (ILAPS) demonstrates the sequestration in spleen, liver or both—decides benefit of splenectomy
- Autologous platelets are used after labelling
- Tc99m—phytate scintigraphy
- Liver to spleen uptake is altered in NASH—not in NAFLD—so can differentiate

12.3 CYSTS AND TUMORS OF SPLEEN

Splenic masses		
Solid masses		*Cystic masses*
Lymphoid		**Primary or 'true'**
• Hodgkin		• Parasite
• Non-Hodgkin		• Nonparasite
		• Congenital
		• Neoplastic
Nonlymphoid		**Pseudocysts**
• Benign		• Post-traumatic
• Malignant (primary or metastatic)		• Other

- Nonlymphoid tumors are mainly vascular tumors
- Characterized by USG, CT, MRI
- Usually asymptomatic

Cystic Lesions

- Most common in 2–3 decades
- Usually asymptomatic
- Large mass—symptoms due to compression
  - Pain—referred to left shoulder
  - Not related with food
- Risk of rupture—25% if size >5 cm
- Worldwide—most common primary cysts are parasitic—echinococcus most common
- Treatment of choice for hydatid cyst—splenectomy

Congenital Cysts

- 10% of all splenic cysts and 25% of nonparasitic cysts
- Seen in children and young
- Arise from invaginations of mesothelium lined splenic capsule

Neoplastic Cyst

Not common

- Most common—endodermoid cysts. They are not true cysts and include hemangiomas and lymphangiomas
- <5 cm—observed. >5 cm surgery
- 75% of nonparasitic cysts—secondary cysts (pseudocysts)
- Usually due to trauma—also infarction, infection
- Seen in young, females—hormonal influence
- Hematoma once absorbed can cause pseudocyst
- <5 cm observed, >5 cm—surgery
- In primary cysts—CEA and CA 19–9 may be elevated

Solid Tumors
Lymphoid Tumors
- Lymphoid tumors—HD and NHL
- May be primary or secondary
- Lymphoid lesions are first seen in white pulp
  - Diffuse in nodular lymphoma
  - Localised in large cell lymphoma
  - Cystic lesions

Nonlymphoid Tumors
- Primary or secondary
- Most common nonlymphoid primary—vascular tumors—benign and malignant hemangiomas, lymphangiomas, hemangioendotheliomas
- Most common benign tumor—hemangioma
- Secondary—most common from—melanoma, breast, lung
- Though spleen is very vascular—metastatic lesions are rare

Hemangiomas of Spleen
- Most common benign tumor
- Most are asymptomatic and incidentally detected
- Can be single/multiple/involving entire spleen
- If large can cause compression symptoms mainly renal
- May rupture
- Can cause consumptive coagulopathy due to platelet trapping
- Littoral cell angioma—arise from cells of red pulp causing splenomegaly
- CECT shows contrast pooling (lakes)

Lymphangiomas
- Congenital malformations of lymphatic system
- May fill with eosinophilic, proteinaceous material leads to increased weight of spleen and mass effect—usually symptomatic
- No "lakes" seen unlike hemangiomas
- Hemangioma and lymphangioma if large—splenectomy
- Small are observed

Primary Malignant Tumors
- Primary hemangiosarcoma—most common primary malignancy

Features
- Cachexia
- Mets to lymph nodes, lung, liver, BM

- May rupture
- Treatment—splenectomy

Metastatic Disease
- Incidence 0.3% to 7.3%
- Rarity—reasons
  Anatomic—acute angle of splenic artery makes it difficult for tumor emboli
  - Lack of afferent lymphatics
  Functional
  - Rhythmic contractions of spleen
  - High antitumoral activity of splenic lymphoid tissue
- Rare to have isolated splenic metastasis, so look for other sites for metastasis
- May rupture
- Treatment—splenectomy—to relieve symptoms
- *N. menigitidis*, *H. influenzae*, *S. pneumoniae*—vaccines are given in complete splenectomy
- In primary tumors and staging—complete splenectomy is preferred
- FNAC/biopsy are not recommended for fear of bleeding, tumor seeding

Partial Splenectomy
- Suitable for only splenic cysts
- At least 25% of spleen is required to protect against OPSI with *S. pneumoniae*—most common organism
- Immunisation—polyvalent pneumococcal vaccine (PPV23), *H. influenzae* type b meningococcal. Given 10 days to 2 weeks prior or within 2 weeks of surgery
  - Booster dose in 5 to 10 years

Pathogenesis of Postsplenectomy Infection
Due to
- Loss of splenic macrophages
- Diminished tuftsin
- Loss of reticuloendothelial screening function
- Dysregulated coagulation
- Normally—these work to eliminate opsonised bacteria from blood
- These defence mechanisms help in removal of encapsulated bacteria, their polysaccharide coating is a defence against opsonisation (*S. pneumoniae*, *H. influenzae*, etc.)

- **In postsplenectomy—more infection with**
  - Protozoa invading RBC—ehrlichia, plasmodium, babesia seen
  - Group A streptococci, enterococcus, bacteroides, salmonella
- In the absence of spleen—elimination of these is by liver which is less effective

OPSI

- Most common—*S pneumoniae*
- Others—*H. influenzae*, menigococci
- Greater risk in first 2 years
- Can present late 2 to 5 years after splenectomy
  - Risk >200 times than other population
- Fever, sepsis—DIC—coma—death
- More common in children
- More common when done for malignancy and hematologic conditions than for trauma
- More risk in children <5 years and adults >50 years
- Need lifelong vigilance
- Vancomycin and ceftriaxone as treatment are preferred
- Some suggest life long antibiotic prophylaxis
- Overall incidence 3.2 to 3.5%
- Mortality 40–50%
- Post vaccination—antibody titer does not correspond to clinical immunity.
- *S. pneumonia* antibody may decline in 5–10 years so may require revaccination.
- *H. influenzae*—annual vaccination is indicated in asplenic patients.

Vaccine protocol in splenectomy

Elective surgery—at least two weeks preoperatively
Pneumococcal PPV23, *H. influenzae* and meningococcal C. Children under 2 years pneumococcal 7 valent vaccine.

Emergency surgery

Immediate postop—pneumococcal vaccine

At least 2 weeks postop—*H. influenzae* and meningococcal C vaccine

Postsplenectomy Cancer

- Taiwanese population study
- Higher risk for cancers of stomach, esophagus, head and neck, liver and lymphomas
- Due to impaired immune response

Splenic Abscess

- Predisposed in immunocompromised, drug abuse, trauma
- 70% from hematogenous spread
- Also from local spread, trauma
- Gram positive and negative involved
- Present with fever, pain
- Splenomegaly—not typical
- In adults—one-third of abscesses are multilocular—majority unilocular
- In children one-third is unilocular—majority are multilocular
- CT scan is the investigation of choice
- Treatment—unilocular—can be drained percutaneously with 75–90% success
- Multilocular—splenectomy and lavage

Wandering Spleen

- Due to:
  - Congenital lack of peritoneal attachments—lack of fusion of dorsal mesogastrium (congenital atresia) to posterior abdominal wall
  - In multiparous due to hormonal reasons—laxity—acquired defect in splenic attachments.
- Present with pain, mobile mass, splenomegaly
- CT scan—diagnostic—whirled appearance and abnormal position of spleen
- Treatment—splenopexy—in children without infarction and splenectomy is preferred in adults—depending on presentation and vascularity

Partial Splenectomy

- In trauma, Gaucher's disease, spherocytosis, benign lesions
- Vessels ligated—spleen divided inside ischemic demarcation—to reduce bleeding

Hernias

13.1 ANATOMY OF ABDOMINAL WALL

Embryology

- Derived from lateral plate of mesoderm
- Mesoderm divides into
  - Somatic
  - Splanchnic structures

Boundaries

Anterior

- Xiphoid process (T9) to pubic symphysis

Superolateral

- Right and left costal margins
- Tenth costal margin, lowest at mid axillary line called subcostal plane (L3)

Lower Limit

- Iliac crest (L4)
- Anterior abdominal wall is divided by linea alba
- Umbilicus is at L3–4 level
- Transpyloric plane
  - One hand breadth below xiphisternal notch
- Trans tubercular plane
  - Tubercle at 5 cm behind anterior superior iliac spine

- Transpyloric plane—L1 vertebra
- Subcostal plane—L3 vertebra
- Plane passing from highest point of iliac crest—L4 vertebra
- Intertubercular (trans tubercular) plane—L5 vertebra

Structure of anterior abdominal wall

- Roof
  - Diaphragm
- Floor
  - Bony pelvis

- Anteriorly
  - Two recti
  - Linea alba, which is an area of weakness
  - Muscles
- Abdominal wall: 9 layers
  - Skin
  - Subcutaneous tissue
  - Superficial fascia
  - Ext oblique muscle
  - Internal oblique muscle
  - Transversus abdominis muscle
  - Transversalis fascia
  - Preperitoneal adipose and areolar tissue
  - Peritoneum
- No deep fascia in anterior abdominal wall.

Scarpa's fascial attachments

- From lower part of abdominal wall, passes over inguinal ligament and attached to deep fascia of thigh along Holden's line (8 cm approx.) passing laterally from pubic tubercle
- Medially, it passes downwards above the pubic body and becomes continuous with superficial perineal fascia of Colle. Colle's fascia attachments are:
  - Conjoint ischiopubic rami laterally
  - Posteriorly fused with posterior border of perineal membrane
- Also extends into penis and scrotum (labia majora in females)

Umbilicus

- Normal scar on anterior abdomen
- At L3-L4 level
- Anatomical importance
  - Watershed area of lymphatic drainage
    □ Supplied by T10 nerve root
  - Portocaval anastomosis

Camper's Fascia

- It is continuous with adjoining parts
- Absent in penis
- In scrotum it is replaced by dartos
- Camper's fascia is also called panniculus adiposus

Rupture of bulbar urethra—extravasated urine—fills superficial perineal pouch—extends to scrotum, penis and anterior abdominal wall inferior to umbilicus and deep to scarpas fascia. Urine will not extend into thigh as the membranous layer of superficial fascia is attached to fascia lata, along the Holden's line and pubic arch

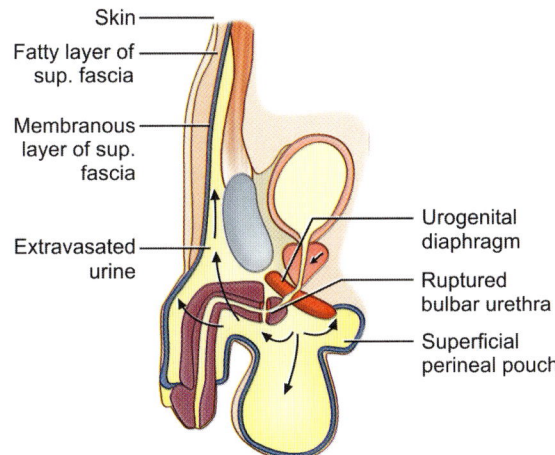

Scarpa's Fascia

- Membranous layer
- Attach with colles' fascia
- Prevent extravasation of urine
- Contiguous with fascia lata of thigh
- Approximation helps in surgical alignment
- Continues downwards and forms the fundiform ligament of penis or suspensory ligament of clitoris and continues to penis and scrotum and fuses with superficial fascia of perineum

External Oblique

- Origin—lower seven ribs
- Insertion—aponeurosis and anterior two-thirds of outer lip of iliac crest
- Nerve supply—lower 6 inter costal nerves
- Forms—inguinal ligament
  - Superficial inguinal ring

Internal Oblique

- Origin—lateral 2/3 inguinal ligament and thoracolumbar fascia

- Insertion—lower four ribs and aponeurosis
- Nerve supply—lower 6 intercostal nerves
- Cremaster muscle is formed from fibers of this muscle
- Form conjoint tendon along with transversus abdominis

Transversus Abdominus

- Origin—lateral 1/3 inguinal ligament, anterior 2/3 of iliac crest, thoracolumbar fascia
- Insertion—xiphoid process, linea alba, conjoint tendon
- Nerve supply—lower six intercostal nerves
- Neurovascular plane is between internal oblique and transversus muscle, where the neurovascular bundle of abdominal wall is situated

Rectus Abdominis

- Origin—lateral head from lateral part of pubic crest
  - Medial head from anterior pubic ligament
- Insertion
  - Xiphoid process, 5, 6, 7 costal cartilage

Nerve Supply

- Is derived from the anterior rami of the lower six thoracic and first lumbar nerves
- Thoracic nerves are the lower five intercostal and the subcostal nerves
- First lumbar nerve is represented by the iliohypogastric and ilioinguinal nerves

Blood Supply

- Skin near the midline is supplied by branches of the superior epigastric artery and the inferior epigastric artery.
- Skin of the flanks is supplied by branches from the intercostal, lumbar, and deep circumflex arteries

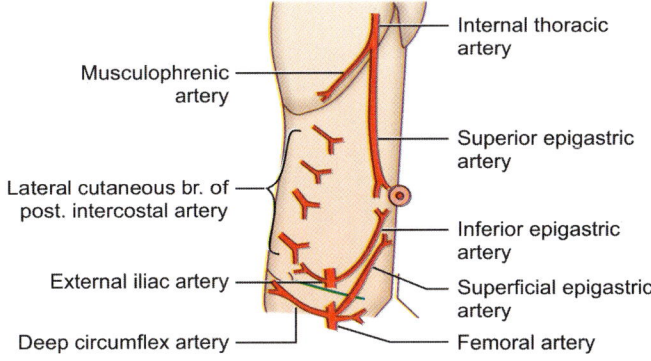

Vascular zones of abdominal wall: Huger zones I to III

SEA—superficial epigastric artery

DIEA—deep inferior epigastric artery

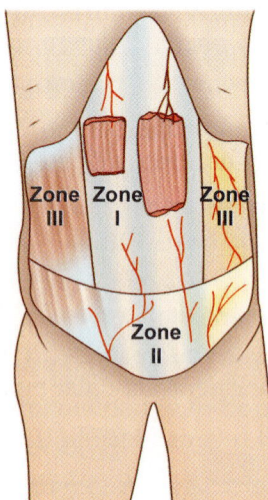

Zone I   SEA and DIEAs rectus abdominis and overlying subcutaneous tissue and skin

Zone II SIEA and superficial external pudendal artery sup. fascia and skin

Zone III Lumbar and intercostal artery

Zone I - Superficial
Zone II - Caudal
Zone III - Lateral

Pyramidalis muscle	
Origin	Pubic crest and symphysis
Insertion	Linea alba
Innervation	Subcostal nerve (T12)
Blood supply	Inferior epigastric vessels
Function	Tenses linea alba

Lymphatics

- Lymph drainage of the skin of the anterior abdominal wall above the umbilicus is upward to the anterior axillary.
- Below the level of umbilicus drains downward and laterally to the superficial inguinal nodes.

Venous System

- Venous blood is collected into a network of veins that radiate from the umbilicus
- The network is drained above into the axillary vein via the lateral thoracic vein
- Below into the femoral vein via the superficial epigastric and the great saphenous veins
- Few small veins, the paraumbilical veins form a clinically important portal-system venous anastomosis

Rectus Sheath

- Is a long fibrous sheath.
- Encloses the rectus abdominis and pyramidalis muscle.

- Contains the anterior rami of lower six thoracic nerves and the superior and inferior epigastric vessels and lymph vessels
- Formed mainly by aponeurosis of three lateral abdominal muscles
- Linea alba is formed in the midline and is widest at xiphoid
- Weakest at umbilicus
- Umbilicus is the weakest part of abdominal wall

Patterns of midline decussations of aponeurosis varies at different sites. Decussations may be between aponeurosis of one muscle, two muscles or three muscles and can be only anteriorly, posteriorly or both.

Fascia Transversalis

- Also called endo abdominal fascia
- It has two laminae—anterior and posterior

Linea Semilunaris (Semilunar Line or Spigelian Line)

- Curved fibrous line at the lateral border of rectus sheath
- From tip of 9th costal cartilage to pubic tubercle
- Formed by the aponeurosis of internal oblique before it splits to enclose the rectus muscle and is reinforced anteriorly by external oblique and posteriorly by transversus abdominis above the arcuate line (linea semicircularis or Douglas line)

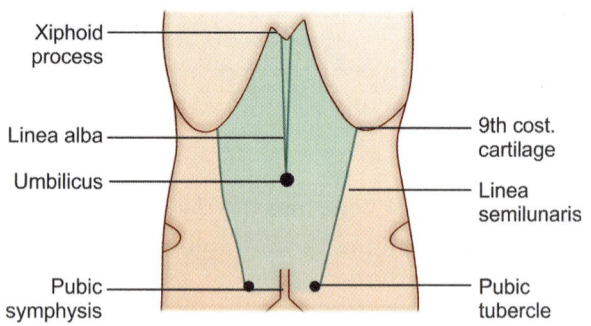

Spigelian Fascia

- Its a true aponeurosis formed by the fusion of aponeuroses of internal oblique and transversus abdominis and extends from cartilage of 8th rib to pubis. It is lateral to rectus muscle and medial to semilunar line

- Below umbilicus this fascia runs parallel and can be separated easily while dissection.

- This is weakest at the level of semicircular line of Douglas

- Also the inferior epigastric vessels traverse the rectus abdominis at this area—contributing to the weakness

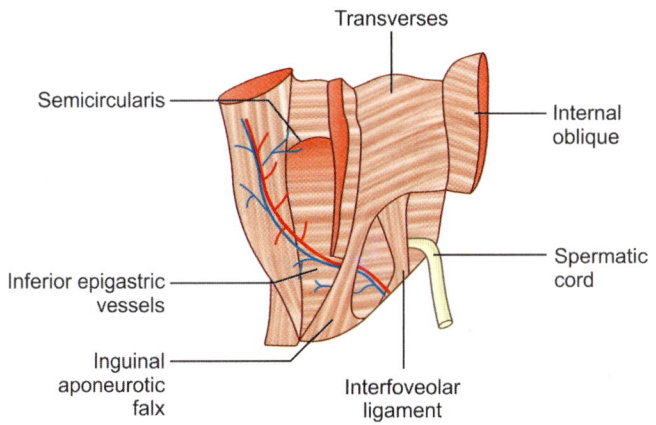

Linea Semicircularis (Arcuate Line, Douglas Line)

- Lower limit of posterior layer of rectus sheath

- Inferior epigastric artery pierce rectus abdominis here

- Above arcuate line posterior rectus sheath is formed by posterior lamina of internal oblique and transversus abdominis

- Below this line, internal oblique and transversus. Abdominis form only anterior sheath and there is no posterior rectus sheath thereby rectus abdominis muscle rests directly on transversalis fascia

- It is situated midway between umbilicus and pubic crest

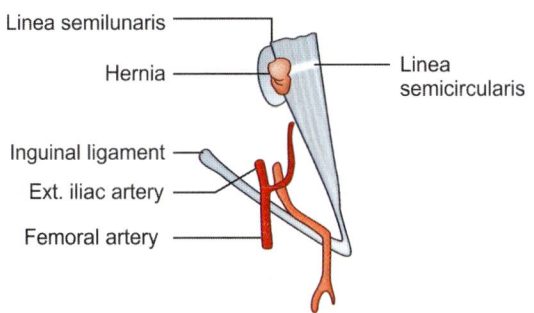

Anatomy of Posterolateral Abdominal Wall

- Boundaries

  - Superior—12th rib

  - Inferior iliac crest

  - Medially—erector spinae

- Eight muscles are arranged in three layers

Superficial Layer

- Constituted by external oblique and latissimus dorsi

- The triangular space between these two muscles and iliac crest is called Petit's triangle or inferior lumbar triangle

Middle Layer

- Constituted by erector spinae, internal oblique and serratus posterior inferior

- Superior lumbar triangle (Grynfeltt) is located in this layer

  - Bounded superiorly by 12th rib, serratus posterior inferior and superior lumbocostal ligament

  - Inferiorly internal oblique

  - Medially erector spinae

Deep Layer

- Three muscles—quadratus lumborum, psoas major and transversus abdominis

Inguinal Canal

- 4 cm long
- Boundaries

Anterior Wall
Whole Extent

- External oblique aponeurosis

- Skin

- Superficial fascia

Lateral One-third

- Fibres of internal oblique muscle

Posterior Wall

Whole Extent

- Fascia transversalis
- Extraperitoneal tissue
- Parietal peritoneum

Medial Two-thirds

- Conjoint tendon
- Medial end by reflected part of inguinal ligament

Lateral One-third

- Interfoveolar ligament extending between lower border of transversus abdominus and superior ramus of pubis

Roof

- Arched fibres of internal oblique and transversus abdominus

Floor

- Inguinal ligament

Inguinal Canal: Anatomy

- **Skin and subcutaneous tissue**—and below this, superficial circumflex iliac, superficial epigastric and external pudendal arteries and veins—which arise from and drain to proximal femoral vessels.
- **External oblique aponeurosis**—inferiorly and medially directed fibres. Inferior edge forms inguinal ligament (Poupart ligament) which continues downward to superior ramus of pubis as lacunar ligament (Gimbernat)—fan-shaped medial expansion and forms the medial border of femoral canal and expands laterally along pectineal line, the Cooper's ligament
- **Superficial ring**—superior and lateral to pubic tubercle—spermatic cord exits through this
- **Internal oblique and transversus abdominis muscle**—inferior fibers run in inferior direction in inguinal region
- Conjoint tendon is formed by fusion of medial aspect of internal oblique aponeurosis and transversus abdominis aponeurosis
- Internal oblique forms cremasteric muscle
- Conjoint tendon seen in only 5–10%
- **Transversus abdominis muscle and aponeurosis**—strength and continuity are important for prevention and treatment of inguinal hernia

- **Shutter mechanism**—transversus abdominis contracts—conjoint tendon approximates.
- **Transversalis fascia**—endoabdominal fascia—component of inguinal floor, denser in inguinal region, though still it is thin.

Iliopubic Tract

- Thickened transversalis fascia and transversus abdominis aponeurosis laterally
- Posterior to inguinal ligament
- Extends from pubic tubercle and inserts on anterior superior iliac spine and iliac crest
- Composes the inferior margin of anterior repairs.
- Contributes to anterior and medial walls of femoral sheath and a portion of inferior crus of deep inguinal ring
- At its insertion of pubic tubercle, blends with Cooper's pectineal ligament
- In laparoscopic repair—staples or tacks should not be applied lateral to and below the internal ring
- **Pectineal (Cooper) ligament**—consists of pubis periosteum and aponeurotic tissue along superior ramus of pubis—and it is the posterior border of femoral canal
- 75% patients have aberrant obturator artery crossing the lateral border of Cooper ligament—arising from inferior epigastric vessels to join normal obturator vessels—**corona mortis**.

Transversalis Fascia

- Inner surface of abdominal muscles which is separated from peritoneum by extraperitoneal connective tissue
- 1.2 cm above midinguinal point there is a defect, the deep inguinal ring
- Important in inguinal anatomy
- Also known as deep or endoabdominal fascia
- Covers the internal surface of transversus abdominis, iliacus, psoas, obturator internus and periosteum
- It is bilaminar—posterior fatty preperitoneal component or preperitoneal fascia and anterior lamina
- Crura of ring has a valvular action which prevents indirect hernia.
- Derivatives from transversalis fascia are iliopectineal arch, iliopubic tract, crura of deep inguinal ring (shaped like "monk's hood"), internal spermatic fascia

Structures Passing through Canal

- Spermatic cord in males
- Round ligament in females
- Ilioinguinal nerve

Contents of Spermatic Cord

Contains three layers of spermatic fascia, three arteries, three veins, two nerves, pampiniform plexus, lymphatics and vas deferens, and obliterated processus vaginalis.

3 Coverings

- External spermatic fascia derived from external oblique
- Cremastric fascia from internal oblique
- Internal spermatic fascia from transversalis fascia

3 Arteries

- Testicular, cremastric artery, and artery of ductus deferens

3 Veins

- Testicular vein, cremasteric vein and vein of vas deferens
- Lymph vessels from testis

Nerves

- Genital branch of genitofemoral nerve, sympathetic nerve, ilioinguinal nerve (ilioinguinal nerve is external to spermatic cord)

Fascial structures/spaces—other names
Fatty layer of superficial fascia; panniculus adiposus; Camper fascia
Investing fascia of external abdominal oblique; fascia innominate
Membranous layer of superficial fascia; Scarpa fascia
Retro inguinal space; space of Bogros
Retropubic space; space of Retzius
Ligamentous structures
Iliopectineal ligament; iliopectineal arch
Lacunar ligament; Gimbernat ligament
Pectineal ligament; Cooper ligament
Iliopubic tract; Thomson ligament (band)
Inguinal ligament; Poupart's ligament
Aponeurosis—derived structures
Arcuate ligament; semicircular line; linea semicircularis; line of Douglas
Reflected inguinal ligament; Colle's ligament
Semilunar line; linea semilunaris

13.2 VENTRAL HERNIA

- Only areas of natural weaknesses are lumbar triangles and posterior wall of inguinal canal

Zollinger ventral wall hernia classification
Congenital
Gastroschisis
Omphalocele
Umbilical (infant)
Acquired
Midline
Diastasis recti
Epigastric
Umbilical
Paraumbilical
Median
Supravesical—anterior, posterior, lateral
Paramedian
Spigelian
Interparietal
Incisional
Midline
Paramedian
Transverse
Others
Traumatic
Penetrating
Blunt
Focal
Destructive
Extensive

European Hernia Society classification for primary ventral hernia			
	Small<2 cm	Medium 2–4 cm	Large >4 cm
Umbilical epigastric			
Spigelian lumbar			

- Protrusion through anterior abdominal wall fascia
- Diastasis of recti are not true hernias, present as bulge in midline
  - Here linea alba is stretched and causes bulge at the medial margins of rectus muscles
  - There is no fascial ring or hernia sac
- Incisional hernia account for 15–20% of abdominal wall hernias
- Umbilical and epigastric hernia—10%

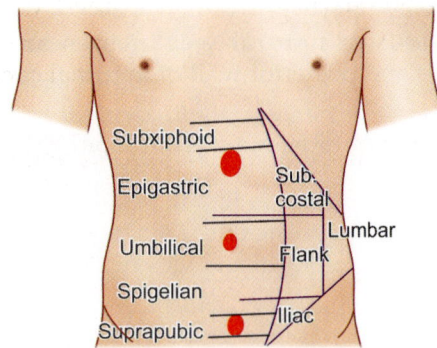

Umbilical Hernia

- Umbilicus is formed by umbilical ring of the linea alba

   Intra-abdominal connections

   – Superiorly—round ligament (ligamentum teres) and paraumbilical veins

   – Inferiorly—median umbilical ligament (obliterated urachus)

In Infants

- Are congenital
- More common in premature babies
- More common in blacks
- Umbilical ring close spontaneously by two years, >80% close by age 5
- Only abdominal wall defect which is genetically programmed to close
- If persist beyond 5 years, are repaired (2 years—bailey)
- Complications of hernia are rare

Associations in Children
- Beckwith-Wieldmann syndrome
- Down's syndrome
- Mucopolysaccharides storage diseases

In Adults

- In >90% are acquired due to raised abdominal pressure
- More common in women and in with raised abdominal pressure like ascites, obesity, pregnancy
- More common in with single decussation of fibers at linea alba (normally decussation from all three lateral abdominal muscles)

- Strangulation is rare—more commonly seen in patients with ascites

Adults—indications for repair
- Symptomatic
- Large size
- Incarceration
- Thinning of overlying skin
- Uncontrollable ascites—can have spontaneous rupture and peritonitis
- Small asymptomatic hernias need not be repaired

Umbilical Hernia—Repair

- Small defects—closed primarily after separation of sac from overlying umbilicus and fascia
- Defect size >3 cm repaired using mesh
- Preperitoneal, sublay
- Laparoscopic

Epigastric Hernia

- 3–5% of population have epigastric hernia
- Two to three times more common in men
- Located between xiphoid and umbilicus, within 5–6 cm of umbilicus, where perforating neurovascular bundles travel though the fascial layers that form the linea alba
- More common in single aponeurotic decussation
- Can cause incarceration of preperitoneal fat which cause pain out of proportion to their size
- Can be multiple in 20%
- Placed in midline in 80%
- Epigastric hernia begin with a transverse slit in the midline raphe, so the defect is elliptical
- Usually contain extra peritoneal fat
- Shape of a mushroom
- Initially only extra peritoneal fat, later peritoneal sac can form
- Most common cause of recurrence—failure to identify multiple defects

Surgical Repair

- Excision of incarcerated preperitoneal fat and simple closure of the defect
- Large defects—mesh repair
- These hernias are better repaired anteriorly as the defect is small and the fat which has herniated from peritoneal cavity is difficult to reduce
- Difficult to visualize the sac laparoscopically

Spigelian Hernia

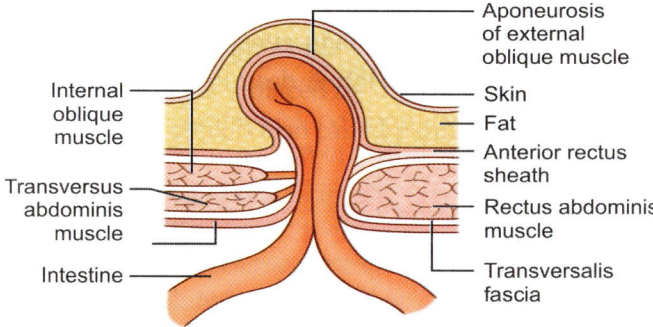

- Adriaan van den Spiegel, Belgian anatomist—first to describe the semilunar line, a concave region lateral to rectus muscle formed by aponeurosis of internal oblique

- Klinkosh in 1764 described spigelian hernia

- Occurs through spigelian fascia—that is composed of aponeurotic layer between rectus muscle medially and semilunar line laterally

- They occur at or below the arcuate line, absence of posterior rectus sheath cause the weakness in this area

- 90% occur through 'spigelian belt'—a 6 cm area of aponeurosis extending from the line between anterior superior iliac spines

- But they can occur anywhere along spigelian line

  - This area is bound laterally by semilunar line, inferior epigastric vessels medially and arcuate line superiorly

- They are interparietal, hernial sac is posterior to external oblique aponeurosis

- They are small defects (1–2 cm) in size

- The defect is almost always above arcuate line

- More common in 4–5 decades of life

- Account for 0.1 to 2% of abdominal wall hernias

Clinically

- Localized pain without a bulge—most common—as the hernia is beneath the external oblique aponeurosis

- Associated with obesity, multiparity, COPD, BPH

- USG or CT—can diagnose

- >50% are diagnosed intraoperatively

- Due to small neck, 20–30% need emergency intervention

- So even incidental spigelian hernias should be repaired

- Repair is done as there is a risk of incarceration due to narrow neck

  - Site marked preoperatively

  - Transverse incision—sac opened and contents reduced

  - Repaired by simple suture of transversus abdominis and internal oblique muscles and later external oblique aponeurosis

- Larger defect—may need mesh repair

- Spigelian hernia is also described in infants—this may be congenital due to incomplete differentiation of the mesenchymal layers of abdominal wall

Obturator Hernia

- Represent 0.05 to 1.4% of all hernias

- Obturator means a device which closes a defect

- Formation of obturator canal is by the joining of pubic bone and ischium

- This canal is covered by a membrane (obturator membrane). This is pierced by obturator nerve and vessels at the medial and superior border

- Weakening of the membrane—cause enlargement of the canal and hernia sac, can lead to incarceration of bowel and strangulation. Defect is usually located anterior and medial to the neurovascular bundle

- The sac can take the path of either the anterior or posterior division of obturator nerve

- Sac may contain fat, bowel, bladder, uterus

- Pain in the anteromedial aspect of thigh due to compression of obturator nerve and its genicular branch—*Howship-Romberg sign*. This pain is relieved by flexion of thigh. Exacerbated by extension, adduction and medial rotation of thigh

- **Hannington-Kiff sign** is the absence of adductor reflex of the thigh with an intact patellar tendon reflex. This is a more specific sign

- This hernia is more common in thin, females >60 years called "**the little old lady's hernia**"

- Swelling of hernia is deep within thigh between pectineus and adductor longus muscles

- Seldom causes swelling in scarpas triangle, but swelling becomes more obvious if the limb is flexed, abducted and rotated outwards
- May be bilateral, also can be associated with other hernias—most commonly femoral hernia
- More common on right side, because left side sigmoid colon prevents occurrence
- PV or PR examination—hernia may be felt as a tender swelling at obturator foramen
- Can undergo strangulation: Richter type hernia
- Present with bowel obstruction in >50%, most commonly small bowel
- CT—diagnostic. Rarely diagnosed preoperatively

Surgery
- Laparotomy or laparoscopy preferred
- Other approaches retropubic, preperitoneal, inguinal
- In strangulation abdominal approach is preferred
- Full Trendelenburg position is used
- Sac reduced, obturator foramen opened posterior to nerve and vessels
- Incision of fascia is made parallel to neurovascular structures
- Obturator foramen repaired with mesh-not by suture to protect neurovascular structures
- In bowel gangrene—need laparotomy
- If laparoscopy is done, TAPP can be done, mesh is placed with glue, not with tacks or sutures

Lumbar Hernia
- Can be congenital or acquired developed after a surgery
- Superior lumbar triangle hernia (Grynfeltt-Lesshaft triangle) is more common
    - **Boundaries**—12th rib, paraspinal muscles, and internal oblique muscle
- Most common site of hernia:
    - Just below the 12th rib where the transversalis fascia is not covered by external oblique
    - Area of penetration of 12th intercostal nerve

- Inferior lumbar triangle (Petit's triangle) hernia—less common
    - Bound by iliac crest, latissimus dorsi muscle and external oblique muscle
- Weakness of lumbosacral fascia lead to protrusion of extraperitoneal fat and hernia
- Secondary lumbar hernia—secondary to trauma, mostly surgical or infectious (e.g. spinal tuberculosis with paraspinal abscess)

Clinical Features
- 20% are congenital and the remaining are acquired
- Extreme thinness, obesity, COPD are causative factors
- Spontaneous hernia may occur through superior triangle
- Secondary hernia usually involves inferior triangle—due to trauma, fractures
- Lumbar hernias usually do not cause incarceration
- Small hernias are asymptomatic
- Larger ones cause back ache, mass effect
- CT diagnostic
- Repair—with mesh
- Fixing mesh may be difficult due to bones as boundaries, but usually enough fascia will be there
- Lumbar pseudohernia—due to lumbar incisional hernia, neuropathic injury causing muscle atrophy and diffuse bulge need mesh repair

Gluteal and Sciatic Hernia
- Most infrequent pelvic hernia
- Most commonly hernia occurs through greater sciatic foramen, the gluteal hernia. This can occur above or below the pyriformis muscle
- Hernia through lesser sciatic foramen—sciatic hernia is rare
- Mostly asymptomatic and later present with bowel obstruction
- Other than obstruction—most common presentation—slowly growing swelling in the gluteal or infragluteal region
- Sciatic nerve pain may be there—a rare cause of sciatic neuralgia
- Can present with intestinal obstruction

- Hernia sac may contain ureter. This can cause obstructive features of ureter. Retrograde pyelogram or CECT shows 'curlicue ureter'

Types of Sciatic Hernia

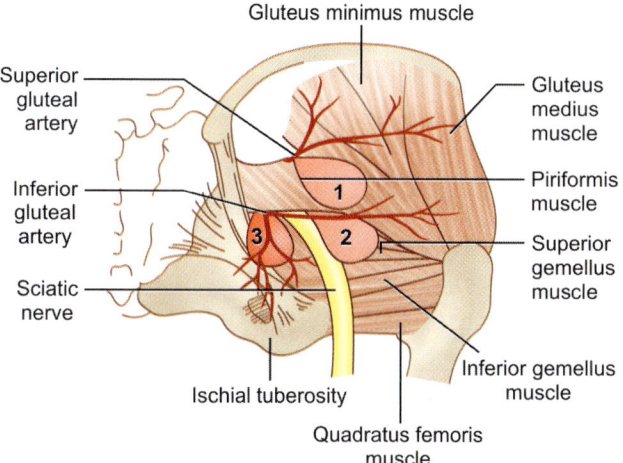

1—suprapiriform, 2—infrapiriform, 3—subspinous

Surgery

- In obstruction, transperitoneal approach is preferred
- Hernia reduction and mesh placement
- Transgluteal approach in:
  - When diagnosis is certain
  - Hernia is reducible
  - Surgery in prone position, incision from greater trochanter across hernia, gluteus maximus opened, sac tackled and repaired with sutures or mesh
- DD—lipoma, TB abscess, gluteal aneurism

Perineal Hernia

- May be congenital or acquired—rare
- Can occur after APR or perineal prostatectomy
- Hernia protrudes through perineal diaphragm
- Primary hernias seen in old women as a mass perineum.

4 Types

- Postoperative after APR
- Median sliding perineal hernia this is complete prolapse of rectum
- Anterolateral perineal hernia, occurs in women presents with swelling on labium majus
- Posterolateral passes through levator ani to enter ischiorectal fossa, occurs in both sexes

- Surgery is done transabdominal route or combination of abdominal and perineal route
- Defect sutured or mesh is placed
- Patient is operated in semi-Trendelenburg position

Suprapubic Hernias

- Due to the disruption of the musculo tendinous elements of lower abdominal wall insertion to pubic symphysis
- Usually after blunt trauma or pelvic surgery
- Traumatic hernia through the rupture of rectus muscle at or near its insertion to pubic bone
- Incisional type results from apical osteotomy of pubic bone or iatrogenic detachment of rectus muscle from pubic insertion during pelvic surgery
- Most common cause—radical prostatectomy

Surgery

- Primary repair—primary herniorrhaphy should be done without delay because with time muscle may retract.
- Mesh repair is preferred. But challenging due to proximity to vascular, neural structures and bladder

Traumatic Hernia

- Through nonanatomical defects—post-trauma

Athlete's Pubalgia/Sports Hernia

- Do not have hernia but only a weakness of posterior inguinal floor
- Involves the balance of lower abdominal muscles and adductors of thigh
- Seen almost exclusively in men, pain radiates to scrotum and upper thigh
- Tenderness in inguinal canal and over pubic tubercle, at site of insertion of adductor muscle
- Pain may be due to adductor strain or pubic symphysis diastasis
- Pain due to muscle tearing is called *Gilmore Groin*
- To rule out other causes
- MRI is the choice

Treatment

- Conservative with analgesics, steroids, rest
- Surgery—last resort, mesh hernia repair
- Need multispecialty evaluation

Interparietal Hernia

- Sac lies between the layers of abdomen wall
- Preperitoneal—between peritoneum and transversalis fascia
- Interstitial—between layers of abdominal muscles
  - Inguinal interstitial hernia—majority are this type
  - Inguinal crural hernia—sac passes behind inguinal ligament in the region of femoral ring
- Cause—congenital abnormalities like failure of testicular descend and congenital pouches
- Diagnosis—CT/USG may help
  - Pain—the main symptom, rarely cause obstruction, may be detected on surgery only

Other types
- Littre's hernia—inguinal and femoral hernia containing Meckel's diverticulum
- Amyand hernia—inguinal hernia containing appendix
- De Garengeot hernia—femoral hernia containing appendix

Perivascular hernias
- Laugier's hernia—perivascular hernia occurring through a defect in lacunal ligament
- Cloquet hernia—hernia through pectineal fascia
- Velpeau hernia—hernia anterior to femoral vessels but behind inguinal ligament
- Serafini hernia—hernia behind femoral vessels
- Hernia lateral to femoral artery
  - Anterior—Hesselbach hernia
  - Posterior—Partridge hernia

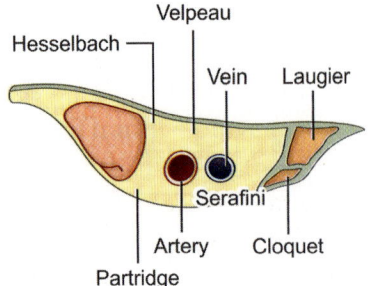

13.3 INCISIONAL HERNIA

Definition

- Hernia developing as a result of failure of fascial tissues to heal and close following laparotomy
- Hernia needs a fascial defect and a sac of eventeration and diastasis

Etiology

- **Mechanical factors**—intra-abdominal pressure overwhelming a weakness in the abdominal wall.
- Pathologic changes in collagen that adversely affect wound healing.
- Reduced ratio of type I to type III collagen
  - Type I collagen is dominant in a mature scar
  - Type III collagen dominates in the early stages of wound healing

Controllable Factors

- Obesity
- Incision
- Sutures
- Suture technique:
  - Tension
  - Wound infection

Uncontrollable Factors

- Age
- Sepsis
- General debility
- Pulmonary complications
- Steroids
- Vitamin/nutritional deficiency

Type of Incisions

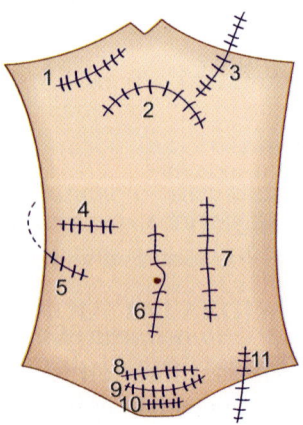

1. Kocher
2. Gable
3. Thoracoabdominal
4. Transverse muscle splitting
5. Rutherford Morison
6. Midline
7. Paramedian
8. Maylard
9. Pfannenstiel
10. Cherney
11. McEvedy

- Maylard—true muscle cutting incision 3–8 cm above pubic symphysis.
- Cherney—rectus muscle divided at tendinous insertion to pubic symphysis—access to space of Ritzius. During closure—muscle sutured to rectus sheath—not to bone to avoid osteomyelitis.

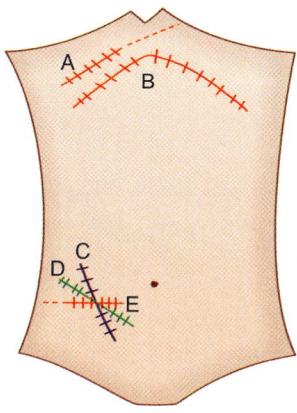

- **A**—saber slash extension to costal margin
- **B**—Bilateral Kochar/bucket handle/chevron/ gable/roof top
- **C**—McBurney incision
- **D**—Lanz incision/modified McBurney/Langer's line
- **E**—Rockey-Davis—transverse
  - Medial extension—Fowler-Weir extension
  - Lateral oblique and upward extension—Rutherford Morison

Incisional Hernia
- More in vertical incision—up to 20% develop

Type of Incision
- Vertical incision can cause more incisional hernias due to distraction of wound edges

Jenkin's Rule
- For closure of abdominal fascia with interrupted sutures, use suture material 4 times the length of the wound. Sutures are placed 1 cm apart and 1 cm from wound edge

Rate of resorption of different suture materials	
Material	Time for resorption (in days)
Rapidly resorbed	
Catgut	15
Chromic catgut	90
Polyglactin 910 (Vicryl)	60–90
Slowly resorbed	
PDS	180
Polyglyconate (Maxon)	180
Nonresorbable	
Polyamide (Ethilon)	
Polypropylene (Prolene)	
Polyethylene (Ethibond)	
Nylon (Nurulon)	

PRIMA trial
Trial comparing primary suture closing with mesh to reduce incisional hernia

STITCH trial
Trial evaluating the effects of small stitches on incidence of incisional hernia in midline closure
- Sutures 5 mm apart and 5 mm from fascial end
- "Small bite" technique

- Currently recommended for abdominal closure:
  - Delayed absorbable—PDS
  - Nonabsorbable—polypropylene

Incisional hernia staging system		SSO %	Recurrence %
Stage I Low recurrence and SSO	<10 cm, clean	12%	10%
Stage II Moderate recurrence and SSO	<10 cm if contaminated 10–20 cm if clean	18–20%	14–16%
Stage III High recurrence and SSO	≥ 10 cm if contaminated > 20 cm in any case	40%	20%

SSO—surgical site occurrence

European Hernia Society (EHS)

Classification of ventral incisional hernias: European Hernia Society			
Midline	Subxiphoid	M1	
	Epigastric	M2	
	Umbilical	M3	
	Infraumbilical	M4	
	Suprapubic	M5	
Lateral	Subcostal	L1	
	Flank	L2	
	Iliac	L3	
	Lumbar	L4	
Recurrent	Yes	No	
Width cm	W1 <4 cm	W2 ≥4–10 cm	W3 ≥10 cm

Midline/Medial Hernias

- **Cranial:** The xyphoid
- **Caudal:** The pubic bone
- **Lateral:** The lateral margin of the rectal sheath

Lateral Hernias

- **Cranial:** The costal margin
- **Caudal:** The inguinal region
- **Medially:** The lateral margin of the rectal sheath
- **Laterally:** The lumbar region.

EHS Classification (Chevrel)

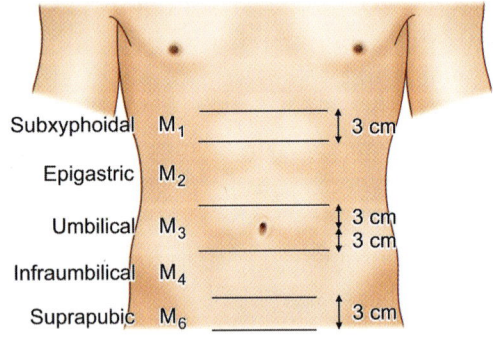

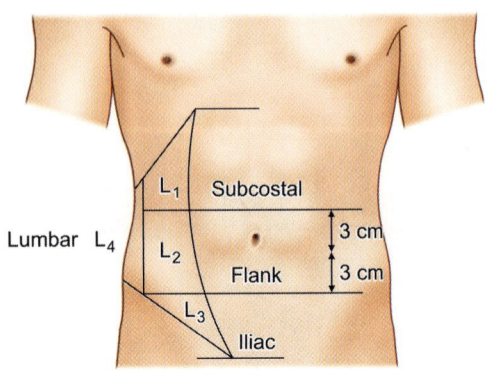

- **M1:** Subxiphoidal (from the xiphoid till 3 cm caudally)
- **M2:** Epigastric (from 3 cm below the xiphoid till 3 cm above the umbilicus)
- **M3:** Umbilical (from 3 cm above till 3 cm below the umbilicus)
- **M4:** Infraumbilical (from 3 cm below the umbilicus till 3 cm above the pubis)
- **M5:** Suprapubic (from pubic bone till 3 cm cranially)
- **L1:** Subcostal (between the costal margin and a horizontal line 3 cm above the umbilicus)
- **L2:** Flank (lateral to the rectal sheath in the area 3 cm above and below the umbilicus)
- **L3:** Iliac (between a horizontal line 3 cm below the umbilicus and the inguinal region)
- **L4:** Lumbar (laterodorsal of the anterior axillary line)
- W1—width <4 cm
- W2—4–10 cm
- W3 >10 cm
- Multiple defects are measured by the point of greatest distance in either axis

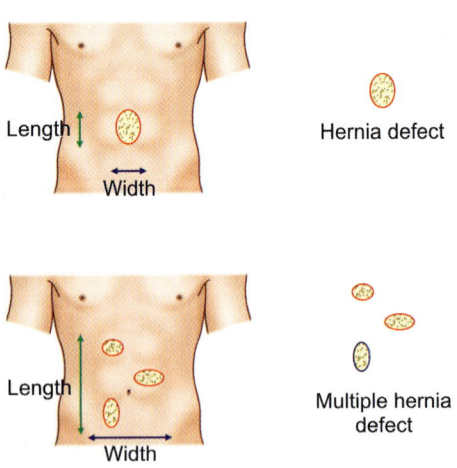

Port Site Hernia

- Port sites >5 mm trocars—better closed
- Difficult to diagnose
- May occur infra-fascially
- More Richter type

Management of Incisional Hernia

– *Indications:*
  □ Loss of abdominal domain
  □ Pain and discomfort
  □ Intestinal obstruction
  □ Irreducibility
  □ Strangulation
  □ Intertrigo
  □ Blunt trauma

Principles of Repair

- Tension free repair
- Incision—chosen to provide good exposure of the defect
- Do not expose bowel to reactive mesh
- Clear adequate margins of the defect
- Skin hygiene
- Antibiotic prophylaxis
- Choice of anesthesia
- Avoid counter-incisions

Preoperative Management

- Weight reduction
- Optimal skin hygiene
- Treatment of DM, HTN, RTI, IHD
- Delayed repair—repair is planned ideally after 1 year
- Nutritional replacement
- Low dose heparin
- Treatment of ulcers and infections
- Skin pinch test—skin can be separated from underlying abdominal viscera on palpation

Operative Technique

Assessment

- Assessment of patient is done in lying/standing
- Size
- Reducibility
- Condition of skin
- Isolation of healthy fascia

Closure of Hernial Sac

- Plication
- Keel procedure
- Excision

Closure of Hernial Defect

- Direct closure is done if defect <2–3 cm
  – If >3 cm, mesh is used with 4–5 cm overlap
- Shoelace repair
- Mayo's operation—'vest over pants' or double breasting
- Prosthetic mesh repair
- Laparoscopic

Ventral Hernia Working Group

- Grade 1—healthy, no comorbidities, infection
- Grade 2—comorbid without infection
- Grade 3—comorbid, potential for infection, stoma
- Grade 4—active infection, contamination
- In grade 3 and 4—synthetic mesh is not advised

Onlay

- **Advantages**
  – No contact with viscera
- **Disadvantages**
  – Large subcutaneous dissection
  – More seroma
  – Superficial mesh-get infected
  – Repair under tension

Intraperitoneal Mesh

- Placed at least 4 cm beyond fascial margin
- Mesh in contact with bowel

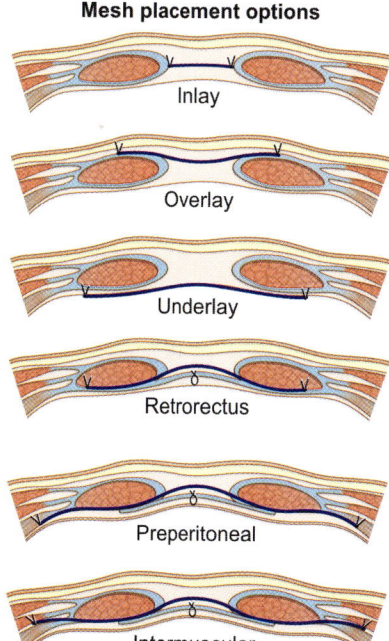

Mesh placement options

Inlay

Overlay

Underlay

Retrorectus

Preperitoneal

Intermuscular

Laparoscopic

- IPOM—intraperitoneal mesh
- TAPP
- eTEP technique
- Robotics

Myofascial Releases: Component Separation

- To re-establish linea alba—functional abdominal wall—protects mesh from superficial wound infection—more durable repair
- Abdominal wall and rectus muscle are bounded by several myofascial bundles—by releasing them, we can advance the rectus muscle to the midline
- Creates a local advancement flap of rectus muscle
- Should protect the neurovascular bundle to rectus muscle

Myofascial Releases

- Posterior rectus sheath incision and retromuscular mesh placement
- Posterior component separation
- Anterior component separation
- Endoscopic component separation
- Ramirez technique—anterior separation
- Fabian technique—also includes internal oblique aponeurosis. All components of posterior rectus sheath is brought anteriorly and sutured to anterior rectus sheath

Anterior Component Separation (ACS)

- Done on both sides—can yield up to 20 cm for advancement
- External oblique aponeurosis is divided 2 cm lateral to linea semilunaris and a few cm above costal margin
- Has to raise large skin flaps—from above costal margin to inguinal ligament and laterally to midclavicular/anterior axillary line—can cause devascularization of skin flap

Periumbilical Perforator-Sparing ACS-Dumanian

Based on the principle that deep epigastric vessels divide into musculocutaneous perforating branches near umbilicus which provide vascularity to central abdominal wall

Transversus Abdominis Release (TAR)

- Extensive release of posterior rectus sheath and more medial advancement of posterior rectus sheath. This allows medialization of rectus muscle and reconstruction of linea alba and placement of mesh

Pascal's Law

- Intraperitoneal mesh placement is based on this law
- Defects >12–15 cm better treated by open surgery
- Failed onlay repair—better treated with laparoscopic technique
- Previous sublay/TAR better treated with open surgery

Complications of Incisional Hernia Repair

- Enterotomy
- Wound infection
- Mesh infection
- Persistent seroma
- Prolonged pain
- Ileus
- Bleeding/hematoma
- Recurrence
- Respiratory distress
- Abdominal compartment syndrome or IVC compression

Seroma

- Develops almost always
- Resolves spontaneously
- Not considered a major complication unless it stays >8 weeks postop

13.4 INGUINAL HERNIA

Introduction

- Word meaning in Latin = rupture
- 75% of hernias are—inguinal hernia of which, 2/3rd are indirect, remainder are direct hernias
- 3% of all groin hernias are femoral hernia
- Men 25 times more likely to develop groin hernia
- Indirect hernia most common in both males and females

- Femoral hernia and umbilical hernia occur more common in females
- 10% of women and 50% men with femoral hernia will develop inguinal hernia
- Most common hernia—indirect inguinal hernia
- In females most common hernia—indirect inguinal hernia
- Indirect inguinal and femoral hernias occur more on right side
- Right side—slower testicular descent and delay in processus vaginalis atrophy, thus causing indirect inguinal hernia
  - Tamponading effect of sigmoid colon on left side prevent femoral hernia of left side
- Prevalence of hernia increases with age
- Strangulation incidence increase with age.
  - Occur in 1–3% of groin hernias, more common in extremes of age
  - Most common strangulated hernia—indirect inguinal hernia
  - Femoral hernia have highest rate of strangulation—15–20% of all hernias

Pathology

- Russel's saccular theory is that presence of the patent processus vaginalis cause—indirect hernia
- Increased intra-abdominal pressure and relative weakness of posterior inguinal wall
- Fruchaud's concept—failure of the transversalis fascia to retain the peritoneum.
- Bendavid—unified theory—multiple etiologies with common denominator of altered collagen matrix
- Disturbances in collagen metabolism:
  - Decrease in hydroxyproline
  - Decreased collagen type I to III ratio
  - Reduced fibroblast proliferation
  - Metastatic emphysema—increased elastase and decreased elastase inhibitory activities (smokers)
  - Alteration in metalloproteinases (mmps) [mmp-2 and mmp-13 overexpression]

Anatomy

Extra Peritoneal Space of Bogros

- Between the posterior lamina of transversalis fascia and peritoneum (preperitoneal space). Contains preperitoneal fat and areolar tissue. Mesh should be placed in this space superficial to vas deferens
  - Medial most aspect of preperitoneal space which lies superior to bladder is space of Ritzius

Myopectineal Orifice of Fruchaud

Boundaries

- Superior—arch of the internal oblique muscle and transversus abdominis muscle
- Lateral—iliopsoas muscle
- Medial—lateral border of rectus muscle
- Inferior—Cooper ligament
- Inguinal ligament divides this space

Myopectineal Orifice

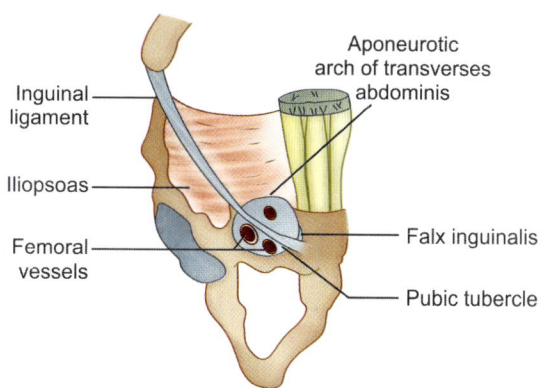

- Vascular space is between the two laminae of transversalis fascia—and it contains the inferior epigastric vessels

Laparoscopic Anatomy

Three Umbilical Peritoneal Folds

- Single median umbilical fold
- Medial umbilical fold
- Lateral umbilical fold

Three Fossae

- Supravesical fossa—supravesical hernia
- Medial fossa—direct hernia
  - Lateral fossa—congenital or indirect hernia
- Medial umbilical fold—obliterated urachus
- Medial umbilical ligament—obliterated umbilical artery

- Lateral umbilical ligament—contains inferior epigastric artery

- Supravesical hernia—between median and medial umbilical ligament

- Direct inguinal hernia—between medial and lateral umbilical ligament

- Indirect inguinal hernia lateral to lateral umbilical ligament

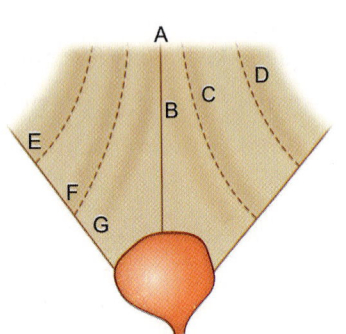

A. Umbilicus
B. Median umbilical
C. Medial umbilical
D. Lateral umbilical ligament
E. Lateral fossa
F. Medial fossa
G. Supravesical fossa

Triangle of Doom

- Borders—vas deferens medially, vessels of spermatic cord laterally, apex at deep ring, inferior aspect is arbitrary and is the margin between dissected and non-dissected peritoneum

- Contents—external iliac vessels, deep circumflex iliac vein, femoral nerve and genital branch of genitofemoral nerve

- Inadvertant application of sutures, cautery or tacks in this space during lap hernia repair—can cause bleeding and nerve injury

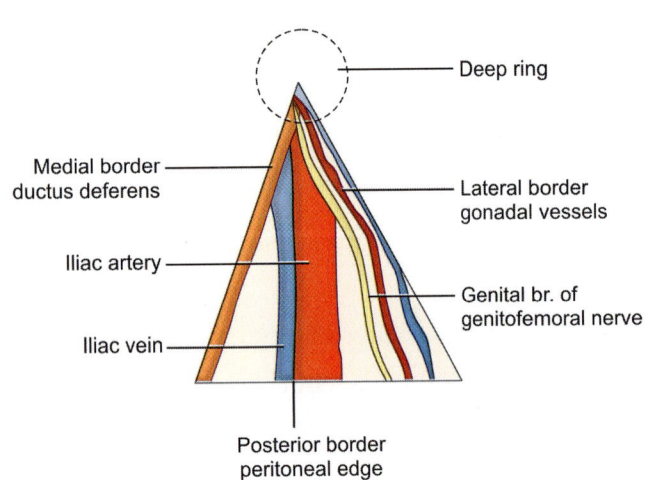

Deep ring
Medial border ductus deferens
Lateral border gonadal vessels
Iliac artery
Genital br. of genitofemoral nerve
Iliac vein
Posterior border peritoneal edge

Triangle of Pain

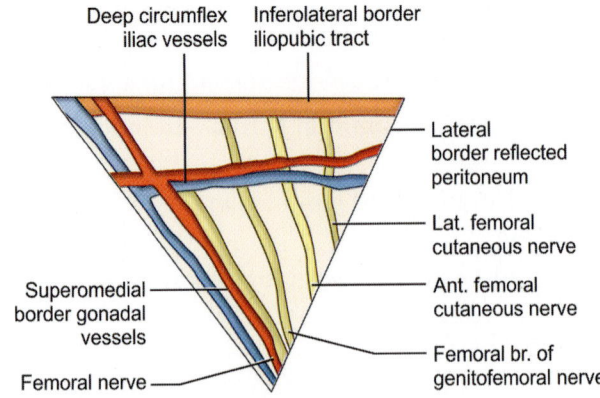

Deep circumflex iliac vessels
Inferolateral border iliopubic tract
Lateral border reflected peritoneum
Lat. femoral cutaneous nerve
Ant. femoral cutaneous nerve
Superomedial border gonadal vessels
Femoral br. of genitofemoral nerve
Femoral nerve

- Borders—iliopubic tract and gonadal vessels. Lateral and inferior borders are nebulous and include the entire area lateral to internal spermatic vessels

- Contains—lateral femoral cutaneous nerve, femoral branch of genitofemoral nerve, femoral nerve

- Application of suture or tacks in this area can cause prolonged postoperative pain

Circle of Death (Crown of Death)
Corona Mortis

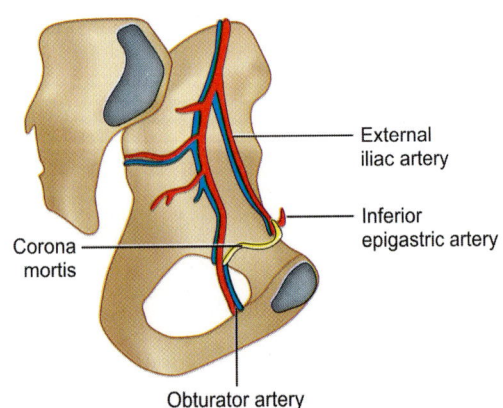

External iliac artery
Inferior epigastric artery
Corona mortis
Obturator artery

- Seen in 70–75%.

- Anastomosis between accessory obturator artery from obturator artery which is a branch of internal iliac artery and inferior epigastric branch of external iliac artery

- Found 3–5 cm from pubic symphysis

- Can cause torrential bleeding, if injured

Hesselbach's triangle: Bounded medially by rectus sheath, laterally by inferior epigastric vessels and inferiorly by inguinal ligament. This area is only supported by peritoneum and transversalis fascia. On abdominal contraction, the arching fibers of transversus abdominis protect this area. Through this area direct hernia develops

Nerves in Relation

- Ilioinguinal and iliohypogastric nerves arise together (L1)
- Ilioinguinal nerve—emerges from lateral border of psoas major muscle, just medial to anterior superior iliac spine, it pierces transversus and internal oblique and enters inguinal canal, then exits through superficial inguinal ring serving as the somatic sensation to upper and medial aspect of thigh, base of penis and scrotum, mons pubis and labium majus
- Iliohypogastric nerve (T12, L1) passes between internal oblique and transversus abdominis and supplies both. It then divides into lateral and anterior cutaneous branches
- Genitofemoral nerve (L1, L2). Genital branch traverses superficial inguinal ring supplies ipsilateral scrotum, cremaster mons pubis and labium major. Femoral branch supplies skin of anterior thigh
- Lateral cutaneous nerve of thigh (L2, L3) passes inferior to inguinal ligament supplies lateral thigh

Pathophysiology

- Adult hernias are acquired defects in abdominal wall
- Pediatric hernias are due to developmental defects
- Processus vaginalis usually closes by 36–40 weeks of gestation. Persistence can cause hernia especially in preterm babies

Risk factors

- Smoking
- Positive family history
- A patent processus vaginalis
- Collagen diseases—Ehlers-Danlos syndrome, ADPKD, Marfan's syndrome, CHD, etc.
- Abdominal aortic aneurysm
- History of appendectomy or prostatectomy
- Ascites
- Peritoneal dialysis
- COPD
- Pregnancy
- Smoking cessation is the only proven prevention method.

Classification systems of inguinal hernia

- Cooper—direct and indirect
- Harkins—grades—I–IV
- Casten
- Halverson and McVay
- Zollinger—*modified traditional classification system*
- Ponka
- **Gilbert**
- **Nyhus and Stoppa**
- **European Hernia Society**
- Schumpelick/Aachen

Nyhus classification

Type I

Indirect inguinal hernia: Normal inguinal ring (pediatric hernia)

Type II

Indirect inguinal hernia: Internal inguinal ring dilated, posterior inguinal wall intact; inferior deep epigastric vessels undisplaced

Type III

Defect in the posterior wall

A: Direct inguinal hernia
B: Indirect inguinal hernia: Internal ring dilated, medially infiltrating transversalis fascia of Hasselbach triangle (scrotal, pantaloon or sliding)
C: Femoral hernia

Type IV

Recurrent hernia

A: Direct
B: Indirect
C: Femoral
D: Combined

Gilbert classification

Type I	Snug internal ring, peritoneal sac passes out as indirect hernia
Type II	Moderately dilated internal ring, admits one finger
Type III	Large internal ring defect, >2 finger breadth admitted
Type IV	Direct hernia with large full blow out of the posterior wall, internal ring intact
Type V	Direct hernia protruding through punched out hole in transversalis fascia, internal ring intact
Type VI	Pantaloon/double
Type VII	Femoral hernia

European Hernia Society classification

EHS classification	Primary	Recurrent
Size	0 1: <1 finger 2: 1–2 fingers 3: 3 or more fingers	X: Diffuse defect in the transversalis fascia, imbrication not possible
L: Lateral M: Medial—direct hernia where repair by imbrication of transversalis fascia is possible F: Femoral		

Aachen/Schumpelik-Arit (1995) classification

Classification	Type	Size
L	Lateral (indirect) hernia	I orifice <1.5 cm
M	Medial (direct) hernia	II orifice 3 cm
Mc	Combined hernia	III orifice >3 cm
F	Femoral hernia	

Diagnosis

- Clinical
- Ultrasonography—for occult hernias
- Herniogram
- MRI—for athletic pubalgia

Clinical Features

- Pain—is due to compression of nerves by the sac which may be localised, generalised or referred to thigh or scrotum
- In case of chronic constipation, urinary retention and cough, evaluate to rule out malignancy
- Femoral pseudohernia—a prominent inguinal pad of fat in a thin patient, may be wrongly diagnosed as femoral hernia
- MRI is the most accurate investigation

Sliding Hernia

- Acquired type due to weakness of muscles
- Occurs at deep inguinal ring lateral to inferior epigastric vessels. Retroperitoneal fat is pushed down first and later hernial sac is created
- Wall is formed by the content usually posterior and lateral walls

- Sac is created secondarily contrast from classic indirect hernia
- On left side sigmoid and on right side cecum is pulled down
- Wall of the bowel may not be covered with peritoneum. So, can be injured

Treatment

- **Fitzgibbon**—watchful waiting can be advised in asymptomatic or in mildly symptomatic, older patients, small hernias. Not for women
- Risk of incarceration reduces over time as the defect gradually increases which help spontaneous reduction
- Large volume of hernia is not a marker for morbidity
- Truss—spring and elastic. Spring better
- **Complication of truss**—testicular atrophy, ilioinguinal or femoral neuritis, hernia incarcerations
- Femoral hernias and symptomatic inguinal hernias should be repaired electively

Operative Repairs

Open repair—anterior repair and preperitoneal repair
- Anterior repairs have both **tissue repair** and **mesh repair**
- Preperitoneal repair needs mesh reinforcement.
- Laparoscopic repair—approach
  - Total extraperitoneal (TEP)
  - Transabdominal preperitoneal (TAPP)
- During open surgery ilioinguinal and iliohypogastric nerves should be left in their natural bed to avoid injury
- Indirect sac is seen on the anteromedial aspect of spermatic cord
- Genital branch of genitofemoral nerve is seen on inferolateral surface of cord adjacent to external spermatic vein

Tissue Repairs
Indications

- Operative field contamination
- Emergency surgery
- Doubtful viability of contents
  - **Iliopubic tract repair**—approximation of transversus abdominis aponeurotic arch to iliopubic tract with interrupted sutures

– **Shouldice repair**—multilayered imbricated repair of posterior wall with continuous suture of monofilament nonabsorbable suture

– **Bassini repair**—conjoint tendon to inguinal ligament

– **McVay repair**—transversus abdominis to Cooper ligament—for direct, large indirect, recurrent, femoral hernias

Bassini Repair

- Transversalis fascia is incised from pubic tubercle to internal ring
- Triple layer repair—internal oblique, transversus abdominis and the transversalis fascia are sutured to the edge of inguinal ligament and the periosteum of pubic tubercle with interrupted sutures
- In the lateral aspect of repair, the internal ring is reinforced

Shouldice Repair

- Genital branch of genitofemoral nerve is routinely divided
- Transversalis fascia is double breasted. Starting at pubic tubercle, initial suture approximates iliopubic tract to rectus sheath and then the transversalis fascia edge of lower flap to undersurface of upper flap. At internal ring sutured backwards and tied at pubic tubercle
- Next layer begins at internal ring. Aponeuroses of internal oblique and transversus abdominis sutured to external oblique aponeurosis in two layers. Suture tied at internal ring

McVay Repair

- Addresses both inguinal and femoral hernias
- Transversalis fascia incised and dissected
- Cooper's ligament is dissected
- A relaxing incision of 2–4 cm made on surface of anterior rectus sheath, this is called Tanner slide incision
- Superior transversalis flap is sutured to Cooper's ligament to occlude femoral ring. Lateral to femoral ring transversalis fascia is sutured to inguinal ligament

Desarda Repair

- Mesh free repair using a strip of external oblique aponeurosis
- External oblique aponeurosis incised, medial leaf is sutured to inguinal ligament from pubic tubercle to

internal ring using nonabsorbable monofilament sutures. Each suture is first taken from inguinal ligament, then transversalis fascia and then external oblique aponeurosis

- A splitting incision is made on external oblique aponeurosis, separating a strip. The free border of this strip is sutured to conjoint tendon

Darning Techniques

- Abramson
- Moloney
- Creates a mesh-like structure using sutures which is tension free

Nyhus/Condon Repair

- Using iliopubic tract
- Transversus aponeurotic arch is sutured to iliopubic tract and Cooper ligament
- In femoral hernia—Cooper ligament is sutured to iliopubic tract
- Can be reinforced with mesh

Krugel/Ugahary Operation

- Two incisions of 2–3 cm each, 2–3 cm above internal ring
- Devised as an alternative to laparoscopic surgery
- Special prosthesis is used for repair

Tension Free Anterior Repair

- Lichenstein repair
- Plug and patch technique
- Sandwich technique—bilayered device
- Preperitoneal self-expanding patch repair
- Stoppa-Rives repair

Lichenstein Repair

- In 1986
- Tension free, flat
- Polypropylene mesh—8*15 cm placed over posterior wall and suture fixating with conjoint tendon and inguinal ligament
- Very low recurrence rate
- Complication—chronic pain

MESH

Mesh: Principle

- Due to the porous nature-promotes neovascularization and fibroblast proliferation and gets incorporated into the tissues, thus strengthening the abdominal wall

- Macroporous mesh—>75 micrometer pore size

Mesh characters
- Woven, knitted or sheet
- Synthetic or biological—mostly synthetic
- Light, medium or heavyweight—lightweight better option
- Intraperitoneal use or not, non-adhesive on one side
- Absorbable or not—mainly nonabsorbable

- MESH—is a prosthetic—either net/sheet
- Bridge a defect, plug a defect, augment a repair
- There should be 2–5 cm overlap over the defect as mesh can shrink even more than 50% due to the contraction of the fibrous tissue
- Types:
  - Net This can be woven or knitted-Allows fibrous ingrowth and become integrated to host tissues
    - Flatsheets—encapsulated by fibrous tissue, e.g. PTFE. They will not allow any tissue ingrowth
    - Synthetic—polypropylene, polyester, polytetra-fluoroethylene (PTFE)

Weight of a Mesh

- Heavyweight mesh cause more fibrosis
  - Lightweight mesh <40 g/m^2 (35 g/m^2 in shack)
  - Medium weight 40–80 g/m^2 (35–60)
  - Heavyweight >80 g/m^2 (>60)

Synthetic Mesh—nonabsorbable

- Polypropylene:
  - Strong, monofilament
  - Hydrophobic
  - Both these features impede bacterial ingrowth

- **Polyester**—they are hydrophilic and helps rapid vascular and cellular infiltration and can cause more infection
- **PTFE**—they are flat sheets and provide nonadhesive barrier between tissue layers. They are not incorporated into tissues.
- **Biological mesh**—they are decellularised and non-immunogenic
  - Prepared from human/animal dermis/bovine pericardium or porcine intestinal submucosa
  - Act as a scaffold—aids ingrowth of tissues
    - Host enzymes break down them and replaced by host tissue
- Some degrades with infection
- The one with labyrinthine microstructure—resist infection
- Provide matrix for neovascularization and native collagen deposition
- Useful in infected fields
- Better used as fascial reinforcement—than bridge or interposition
- They can be crosslinked or noncrosslinked
- Sterilized by gamma rays or ethylene oxide
- New material—poly-4-hydroxybutyrate (P4HB) created using genetically engineered *E.coli* to produce a protein substrate which is refined and woven into a mesh. absorption period of 12–18 months

Absorbable mesh made of polyglycolic acid fibre.
- Used in temporary abdominal wall closure, buttress sutured repair
- They induce minimal collegen deposition
- No role in hernia repair as they induce minimal collagen response

Tissue Separating Mesh

For intraperitoneal use

Dual type—one side macroporous and the other side is microporous made of same material—ePTFE (expanded)

PTFE is not incorporated into tissue unlike polypropelene

Composite mesh: Double layer.

One side is made of polypropylene, other side by PTFE

Or macroporous mesh with absorbable barrier composed of collagen hydrogel, omega 3 fatty acids or oxidized cellulose applied on the surface facing peritoneum

- **Plug and patch**—Rutkow-Robbins repair-shaped plug inserted into defect-fixed along with flat anterior mesh component. In case of indirect hernia, plug is placed into internal ring. In direct hernia, plug is placed into the hernial defect and fixed to Cooper's ligament, inguinal ligament and internal oblique aponeurosis

- **Sandwich technique**—bilayered hernia system—an underlay patch + connector + onlay patch

- **Stoppa-Rives repair**—subumbilical midline incision—large mesh into preperitoneal space covering up to pre-vesical space beyond obturator foramen-distributes natural intra-abdominal pressure across a broad area. Can be employed in large recurrent or bilateral hernias

- Mesh should overlap for 1.5 to 2 cm over the pubic tubercle and overlap 2–5 cm on all sides of defect

Preperitoneal Repair

- Open and Lap

- Open—recurrent, sliding, femoral, some strangulated

- Avoids mobilization of spermatic cord and injury to the sensory nerves

Laparoscopy—TEP and TAPP and IPOM
Total Extraperitoneal Repair

- Create a preperitoneal space with balloon dissector—identifies inferior epigastric vessels—Cooper ligament cleared—iliopubic tract identified—lateral dissection up to ASIS—spermatic cord skeletonized-hernia reduced—12*14 cm mesh inserted—covers direct, indirect and femoral spaces—fixed to Cooper ligament

Transabdominal preperitoneal repair

- Preperitoneal space reached transabdominally—peritoneal flap from median umbilical ligament to ASIS avoiding triangle of pain and triangle of doom

- Mesh fixation techniques

  - Suturing, stapling, tacking—may cause pain

  - Fibrin glue

  - Self-fixing meshes

Complications
Laparoscopy

- Risk factors—large defect and scrotal hernia

- TEP have more risk of complications in recurrent hernias

- Vascular injuries—mainly during trocar placement

- Bowel injury—more common small bowel

- Bladder injury

- Urinary retention

- Recurrence—13% (VA trial)

- Ischemic orchitis

- Groin pain—lap have lesser incidence of early post-operative pain. Chronic pain equivalent to open

Open Repair

- SSI—5%

- Recurrence 1–2%—direct hernias—near pubic tubercle

- Inguinodynia—chronic pain—15–33%

- Cord and testicular injuries

- SSI—may result in chronic draining sinus

Nerve Injuries

- **Nerve injuries** and **chronic pain syndromes**—most common complication—postoperative and long term.

- **In open surgeries:**

  - Ilioinguinal nerve

  - Genital branch of genitofemoral nerve

  - Iliohypogastric nerve

- **Laparoscopic surgery:**

  - Lateral femoral cutaneous nerve

  - Genitofemoral nerve

- Nerve entrapment syndrome—may need re-exploration + neurectomy + mesh removal

- Laparoscopy— avoid tacks below and lateral portion of iliopubic tract.

Recurrence

- Causes—excessive tension

  - Missed hernias

  - Not including aponeurotic arch

  - Improper mesh size

– Failure to close internal ring properly

– Others—chronically elevated intra-abdominal pressure (chronic cough), deep incisional infections, poor collagen formation

- More common with direct hernia and recurrent hernias

- 5–10% patients with recurrence have femoral hernia

- Treated by placing a second prosthesis through a different approach

- Use of mesh reduces recurrence by 60% with no difference in lap or open approach

Pain

Nociceptive Pain

- Most common, due to muscular or ligamentous trauma and inflammation

- Pain is aggravated by muscle contraction

- Treated by rest, analgesics

Neuropathic Pain

- Due to nerve damage or entrapment

- Localised, sharp

- Treated by analgesics, local injection of steroids or anesthetics

Visceral Pain

- Due to sympathetic injury—pain during ejaculation

- Pain conveyed through afferent autonomic fibers

- Poorly localised

Postherniorrhaphy Inguinodynia

- 10% will have chronic postoperative pain

- Independent of hernia repair method

- Analgesics, local neurolysis of ilioinguinal, iliohypogastric and genital nerve with mesh removal and rerepair of hernia is the choice in refractory cases

- If pain is still persisting—laparoscopic neurectomy of these three nerves can be done in the lumbar plexus

Entrapment Pain

- Greatest risk for ilioinguinal and iliohypogastric nerves in anterior repairs and genitofemoral nerve in laparoscopic repairs.

- Meralgia paresthesia—injury to lateral cutaneous nerve of thigh results in persistent paresthesia of lateral thigh

- Treated by rest, analgesics, steroid injections, gabapentine

Oteitis Pubis

- Inflammation of pubic symphysis

- Causes medial groin pain aggrevated by thigh adduction

- Should avoid periosteal sutures while hernia repair to avoid this

- Bone scan is confirmatory test

- Treated with analgesics initially—may need orthopedic intervention in refractory cases

Cord and Testes Injury

- Ischemic orchitis is most commonly due to injury to pampiniform plexus, not to testicular artery

- Occurs in <1% and most are self-limiting

- Testicular necrosis—may need emergency orchidectomy

- Testicular artery injury leads to testicular atrophy, taking a protracted course, not necrosis. This is because of the collaterals from inferior epigastric, vesical, prostatic and scrotal arteries

- Proximal ligation of hernial sac and avoiding manipulation of cord reduces the risk

Laparoscopic Complications

- Vessel injury—most common vessels injured inferior epigastric and external iliac vessels

- Urinary retention-most common cause is general anesthesia

Results

- Among tissue repairs, most commonly done is Shouldice technique

- Recurrence about 1%

- Lichenstein technique—most commonly done procedure

  – Recurrence 0.2%

- Higher incidence of intra-abdominal injury in TAPP

- Rerecurrence 4–5%

Emergency Inguinal Hernia Surgery

- 5% present as emergency
- Open surgery is preferred over laparoscopic

13. 5 FEMORAL HERNIA

A femoral hernia is the protrusion of a viscus from the abdominal or pelvic cavity, through the femoral ring into the femoral canal.

The (peritoneal) hernia sac may contain pre-peritoneal fat, bladder, omentum, small bowel, or other structures.

The sac cannot pass into the thigh as the superficial fascia of the abdomen (Scarpa's fascia) is attached to the fascia lata of the thigh at lower border of the fossa ovalis. Hence, the sac passes through fossa ovalis and becomes subcutaneous and becomes retort shaped.

Epidemiology

- 2–8% of all adult groin hernias
- 2–5 times more common in women
- More in 40–70 years of age
- About 25% emergency femoral hernia repairs require bowel resection
- Mortality is tenfold higher than elective inguinal hernias

Femoral Canal

- Elliptical shaped inverted cone
- 2 cm in legnth from femoral ring superomedially to femoral orifice inferolaterally

Boundaries

- Anterior—iliopubic tract
- Posterior—Cooper's ligament
- Laterally femoral vein
- Medially—junction of iliopubic tract and Cooper ligament (lacunar ligament)
- Apex—pubic tubercle
- Usually contains lymphatics and connective tissue, Cloquet's LN—femoral hernia occurs in this space
- Femoral canal is enveloped by fascia lata—superficial layer forms the anterior wall and deep layer-posterior wall
- Femoral canal usually ends blindly—if hernia occurs—femoral orifice is created

Femoral Sheath

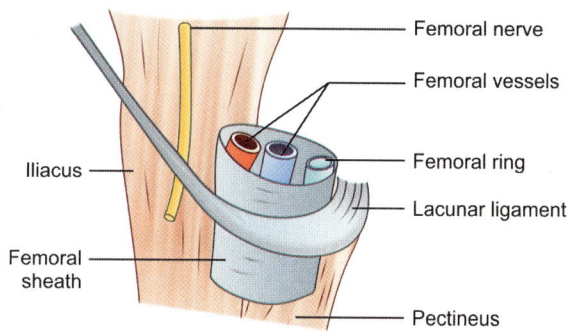

Pathology

- Enters through femoral canal and becomes superficial through saphenous opening.
- Because of its irregular pathway and narrow neck, it is more prone for obstruction and strangulation.
- During surgery, precaution should be taken about the femoral vein and pubic branch of obturator artery (or accessory obturator artery) which often may get injured leading to torrential haemorrhage.

Etiology

- **Pregnancy:** Increased intra-abdominal pressure
- **Wide femoral canal:** Due to narrow insertion of iliopubic tract into pectineal line of pubis
- History of recent loss of weight
- Constipation
- Bronchitis
- Iatrogenic—Bassini repair under tension—damages femoral ring

Incidence

- Uncommon
- More common in female
- Right more common, bilateral—15–20%
- More common in parous women
- >65 years
- 3% of all hernias
- 7% of groin hernia

Presenting Symptoms

- Nonacute—50%
- Acute—50%
- Strangulation—15–20%
- 50% of men with femoral hernia—have associated direct inguinal hernia

- Only 2% of women have associated direct inguinal hernia
- Recurrence rate—2%
- Rerecurrence rate—10%

Nonacute

- Pain or discomfort in groin
- Groin lump—below and lateral to pubic tubercle
- Impulse on coughing
- Mild pain exacerbated by bending or lifting
- Gurgling sound during reduction
- Mild tenderness

Acute Emergency

Obstruction

- Vomiting
- Abdominal distension
- Constipation
- Blood in stools
- Lump irreducible
- Lump tender
- Colicky, abdominal pain

Strangulation

- Lump very tender
- Skin red/inflamed
- Signs of shock

Difficulties With Diagnosis

- 1/3 of patients do not complain of symptoms directly attributable to a hernia
- A groin lump is not always present.
- Obesity
- Elderly—have to think about other diagnoses

Differential Diagnosis

- Inguinal lymph node
  - Lymphoma, lymphogranuloma venerium
- Femoral artery aneurysm
- Saphena varix
- Psoas abscess
- Psoas bursa

- Ectopic testis
- Lipoma
- Pseudohernia

Treatment: Surgery

- Femoral approach
- Inguinal approach
- Preperitoneal approach
- Dissection of the sac
- Inspection/reduction of the contents
- Ligation of the sac
- Closure of femoral ring
- Approximation of the inguinal and pectineal ligaments
- Mesh patch

Open Surgery

Classically 3 Approaches:

- Lockwood's infra-inguinal approach
- Lotheissen's trans-inguinal approach
- McEvedy's high approach
- In incarceration or strangulation—avoid femoral and laparoscopic TEP approaches

Lockwood-low operation: (Femoral approach) Here sac is approached below the inguinal ligament through groin crease incision (or over the swelling) so that fundus of sac is dissected by direct vision and repair is done from below and inguinal ligament is sutured to Cooper's ligament.

McEvedy

High operation: An incision is made over the femoral canal extending vertically above the inguinal ligament.

- Sac is dissected from below, neck from above and repair is done from above.
- It is done in strangulated femoral hernia.

Lotheissen's Operation

It is through inguinal canal approach. Transversalis fascia is opened and neck of the sac is identified in femoral ring. Sac is dissected from above, neck is ligated and repair is done.

Complication: Bleeding, hematoma, abscess formation

AK Henry's Approach

- Repair of bilateral femoral hernia through lower abdominal incision.

Laparoscopic Mesh Repair

- Totally extraperitoneal approach (TEP)
- Transabdominal preperitoneal approach (TAPP)

Open Surgery or Laparoscopic Surgery

- Bladder may be involved in medial part of hernia sac
- Repair suturing the inguinal ligament to the pectineal ligament with non-absorbable sutures
- Avoid any pressure on the femoral vein

Incarcerated Hernia

- Avoid femoral approach or laparoscopic TEP approach
- Lap TAPP preferred over femoral approach
- If strangulation is present—avoid mesh placement due to bowel resection

Presenting as an Emergency

- Increased morbidity and mortality
- Increased rates of bowel resection
- Increased complications
- Wound infection
- Cardiovascular and respiratory complications

Miscellaneous

14.1 BLIND LOOP SYNDROME

- In a stagnant bowel bacterial overgrowth takes place

Manifestations

- Diarrhea, steatorrhea, megaloblastic anemia, deficiencies of fat-soluble vitamins, neurologic disorders
- Caused by stricture, fistula and diverticula-jejunoileal and Meckel's
- Excessive proliferation of aerobic and anaerobic bacteria, compete for vitamin B_{12} and induce deficiency of B_{12}—megaloblastic anemia

Diagnosis

- Evaluation of bacterial growth
  - Culture—collected through intestinal tube
  - Indirect method—C14-xylose or C14-cholylglycine breath tests—bacterial use of C14 substance produce C14-CO_2 which is assessed
  - Schilling test—Co57-labelled vitamin B_{12} absorption-reveal urinary excretion of B_{12} similar to pernicious anemia—urinary loss 0–6%—(normal is 7–25%)
- Addition of intrinsic factor—will not alter vitamin B_{12} excretion but a course of antibiotic will bring it to normal level

Treatment

- Parenteral B_{12} and antibiotics—tetracycline
- Rifaximin and Metronidazole—also effective:
  - Single course may bring long lasting results
- Surgical correction of cause

14.2 MECKEL'S DIVERTICULUM

- Described by German anatomist—Johann Meckel
- Most common congenital malformation of small intestine

Rule of 2s

- 2 inches long
- 2 ft (60 cm) from IC valve
- Affect 2% of population

- Twice as often in males
- Contain one or two types of heterotopic mucosa
- Present in first 2 decades of life—most common in first 2 years of life

Embryology and Anatomy

- 3rd week of gestation—patent Vitelline duct (omphalomesenteric duct)—allows communication of yolk sac with the gut
- Between 5th–9th week, it obliterates—placenta replaces yolk sac as source of nutrition
- Proximal persistence causes Meckel's diverticulum it is a
  - True diverticulum—only true diverticulum of small intestine
- Occurs in antimesenteric border, <100 cm from I-C valve
  - In older age, occurs farther away
- Blood supply—vitelline artery
- Cells lining the vitelline duct is pluripotent—so, can have heterotopic mucosa
- 60% Meckel's—have heterotopic mucosa
- Most common heterotopic tissue—pancreatic (Sabiston-gastric—50%, pancreatic 5%)
- Most common heterotopic tissue in symptomatic—gastric tissue (shack)

Other Anomalies

- Ileal-Umbilical fistula—duct remains patent
- Vitelline duct cyst—failure of umbilical side of duct to obliterate
- Fibrous cord—connecting ileum to umbilicus
- Most common vitelline duct anomaly—Meckel's diverticulum—90%

Clinical Presentation

- Rarely symptomatic
- Symptoms in 2–4 %
- Most commonly seen as diverticulum of about 5 cm long and with diameter of 2 cm
- 80% found at operation—asymptomatic
- Symptomatic presentation decreases with age

Complications

- Obstruction, intussusception, diverticulitis, perforation, ulceration, malignancy (rare)
- GI bleeding—bright red or painless slow intermittent melena
- Remnant of left vitelline artery can persist and form meso diverticular band which tethers the diverticulum to the ileal mesentery

Obstruction

- In adults—most common complication—obstruction—in 35–40%

Due to

- Anatomically longer, narrow based
- Lead point for intussusception
- Point of fixation for volvulus
- Adhesive band, small bowel entrapment
- Stenosis (diverticulitis)

Bleeding

- Acid secretion from ectopic gastric mucosa
- Ulceration and bleeding from ileal mucosa
- Episodic, painless GI haemorrhage

Diverticulitis

- In 20%
- Similar to appendicitis
- Can present in femoral or inguinal hernia—Littre hernia

Tumors in Meckel's Diverticula

- In .5 to 3.5% of symptomatic cases can have tumors
- Most common carcinoid (80%), adenocarcinoma (11%), lymphoma (1%)

In Children

- Bleeding is the most common complication—due to gastric heterotopic mucosa which produce acid and pepsin and ileal ulceration—bleeding
  - 50% of complications in age <18
  - Rare after 30 years as the gastric mucosa atrophies
- Risk of complications inversely proportional to age—4–5% at age 2,1% at 41 and 0% at 74
- Long, narrow-based diverticula can cause obstruction or inflammation

Diagnosis

- <10% preop diagnosed
- CT/USG have limited role
- In bleeding—Tc-99 pertechnate scintigraphy—(Meckel's scan)—heterotopic gastric mucosa take up the tracer—visualised at the same time stomach is visualised. Not seen if gastric mucosa is atrophic

More sensitive in children as in adults contain less gastric mucosa

- Cimetidine increases sensitivity—reduce peptic secretion, not radionuclide uptake
- False negative in—inadequate gastric mucosa, inflammatory edema, outlet obstruction of diverticulum, low hemoglobin
- Angiography with tagged RBCs
- If Meckel's scan negative and with doubt of Meckel's can do SPECT/CT

Operative Diagnosis: Gold Standard

Management

- Symptomatic—surgical resection
- Incidentally detected—specific indications to remove
  - <50 yrs.
  - >2 cm length
  - Presence of fibrous band
  - Evidence of heterotopic mucosa
- **Contraindicated** in Crohn's disease
- If presents with bleeding, may have gastric mucosa. So ileal resection is preferred
- If no bleeding, V-shaped diverticulectomy can be done

Principles of Resection

- **In bleeding**
  - Diverticulum + band + ileal segment

Simple Diverticulectomy

- In the absence of bleeding, V-shaped diverticulectomy + transverse closure to avoid narrowing lumen
- 2-layer closure

14.3 INTUSSUSCEPTION

Proximal segment (intussusceptum) invaginates into distal (intussuscipiens)

- Lead point seen in 80–90% in adults
- Enteric type—only bowel

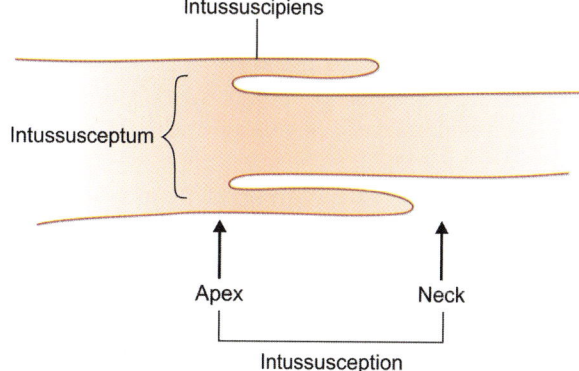

- Colonic—ileocolonic, colocolonic
- Colonic—55% associated with malignancy
- Enteric—20% associated with tumors

Other causes—idiopathic, polyps, HIV, sprue
- Entering inner tube—intussusceptum
- Returning middle tube
- Sheath or outer tube—intussuscipiens
- In children—most common—ileocolic
- Adults—colocolic more common

Presentation

- Accounts for 1% of bowel obstruction
- Complete obstruction in <20%
- In children—triad—pain, mass, bloody stool (red current jelly)
  - Adults—most common—pain
- Vomiting, distention
- Empty RIF—sign of dance
- Distension is not marked initially
- Per rectal examination—blood stained mucus, palpable apex

In Children

- Lymphoid hyperplasia seen near i-c junction
- In older children—lead point is seen in 12%—most common Meckel's diverticulum
- Occurs in 3 months to 3 years of age, two-thirds <1 year
- Sausage-shaped mass palpable with concavity towards umbilicus

Diagnosis

X-ray—intestinal obstruction

Barium

- In enteric type—'stacked coin' or "coiled spring" appearance
- In colonic—cup-shaped filling defect (claw sign)—representing distal extent of intussusceptum
- No hydrostatic reduction in adults because of fear of malignancy and also if gangrene/perforation are suspected

CT

- Most accurate and is the choice
- **Target sign**—intussusceptum and associated mesentery seen within lumen of intussuscipens—in axial view
- Sausage-shaped mass with layering effect
- "Bowel within bowel"—mesenteric vessels are seen compressed within walls of small bowel—pathognomonic
- Donut sign

USG

Less diagnostic but more useful in children
- **"Target sign" and "donut sign"**—in transverse view
- "Pseudokidney" sign—seen in longitudinal view

Endoscopy

- In suspected malignancy
- In case of chronic ischemia, biopsy or polypectomy are not recommended

In Children: Treatment

- Reduction using air or barium—success is achieved by reflux of air or barium into small bowel and resolution of symptoms
- Contraindicated if gangrene/perforation suspected
- Success rate—70%
- Recurrence—in 10% after nonoperative reduction—usually in 24 hours—can try one more hydrostatic reduction
- If not successful—surgery—reduction by gentle compression-not pulling
- Not viable or lead point seen—resection

Treatment: Adults

- Surgery—choice
- No role for non-operative management in adults
- Resection—formal oncologic resection preferred
- So reduction of intussusception—not indicated
- In postop adhesion and intussusception—reduction may be advised

14.4 COLONIC VOLVULUS
Occurrence

- Sigmoid—Ileocolonic—cecal bascule—transverse colon, in that order
- Primary—due to congenital malrotation or bands—volvulus neonatorum, cecal volvulus, sigmoidvolvulus
- Secondary—more common around an acquired adhesion or stoma
- Latin word 'volvere' means to twist upon
- Presents with pain, distension, diminished stool output, nausea and vomiting
- May develop ischemia within affected segment of colon

Physical Finding

Tympany, abnormal bowel movements, abdominal wall tenderness
- Torsion of 180 degrees can cause obstruction
  - Further torsion to 360 degree induce venous congestion—gangrene and perforation
- Perforation can occur
  - At the point of torsion
  - Within the closed loop
  - In the cecum

Sigmoid Volvulus

- First description in 1550 BC
- Hippocrates employed air insufflation and long suppository to reduce the twisted bowel
- Represent 60% of all volvulus
- Torsion occurs in anticlockwise direction
- Represent 20–30% of all intestinal obstruction.
- Endemic in India, Africa, Pakistan, Middle East and Eastern Europe
- High fibre diet thought to lengthen the colon , hence elongation of mesentery
- Genetic predisposition
- More in males—80%
- Other causes—Hirschsprung, adhesions
- Most common cause of intestinal obstruction in **pregnancy**

Pathophysiology

- Long mesentery with narrow base—'dolichomesocolic colon'
- Rotate 180 degree in anticlockwise manner around its vascular pedicle
- Cause closed loop obstruction of the sigmoid colon
- Second closed loop obstruction of proximal colon occur, if ileocaecal valve is competent
- Sigmoid volvulus—most common type mesenterico axial—counterclockwise
  - Organoaxial—rare less serious can undergo spontaneous detorsion—also known as physiological incomplete torsion—may be incidental

Etiology

- Average age—60–70 years
- In endemic areas usually in younger
- Usually occurs equally in both sexes, in endemic areas male affected more
- More in neuropsychiatric patients—drugs affect intestinal motility
- Chagas disease
- Parkinson's disease
- Chronic neurological disorder
- Diabetes
- Chronic constipation
- Laxative abuse
- High altitude
- Previous surgery involving mobilisation of colon

Clinical Features

- Sudden onset pain, distension, obstipation

- Ischemia of bowel due to
  - Distension of bowel
  - Twisting of mesentery
- May have previous history

Diagnosis
Plain Radiograph

- Absence of bowel gas in LIF
- Bent inner tube sign
- Apex of loop near right hemidiaphragm in 60%
- Coffee bean sign, omega sign
- Absence of rectal gas
- Sensitivity 75%
- Specificity 100%
- White stripe sign:
  - Due to walls of interposed loops—white stripe

Lower GI Contrast Radiology

- Bird's beak sign—show point of obstruction and torsion
- Mucosal spiral pattern
- May also be therapeutic and temporarily reduce the volvulus

CT Scan—100% Accuracy

- Sigmoid transition point—most sensitive
- Mesenteric whirl sign
- Dilated ahaustral colon
- 'X marks—the spot' sign—indicates complete obstruction. Two points of obstruction seen, one at proximal sigmoid and the other at distal sigmoid. Orientation of loops is like "X"
- "Split wall" sign—represents partial obstruction of sigmoid loops. Can see transition point with mesenteric fat separating the two sigmoid walls in 'twist tie configuration'—diagnostic, but seen in only 50%
- Dilated sigmoid extends beyond the level of transverse colon—**northern exposure sign**
- Clinical suspicion should be given more importance in deciding on ischemia—than radiological signs

Treatment
Non-operative

- Endoscopic reduction attempted in patients without signs of necrosis or perforation
- Rigid scopy is performed with minimal air insufflation

- Better because it helps to visualise mucosa
- A well lubricated large diameter rectal tube (no. 30 to 36 French) is inserted through sigmoid across the twisted segment and secured to skin for several days
  - Success rate nearly 60%
- Flexible endoscope using minimal air insufflation can also be used, guidewire can be used to pass rectal tube
- After reduction—confirm position by radiograph
- Rectal tube taped to thigh and kept for 1–2 days
- Recurrence rate—70%
- Elective sigmoidectomy is indicated even if volvulus is reduced

Alternatives to Resection After Detorsion

- Percutaneous endoscopic colostomy
- Endoscopic T-fastener fixation
- Used only in high risk patients
- Resection is the choice with or without anastomosis

Operative

- After detorsion, mechanical bowel preparation is done
- Resection and primary anastomosis can be attempted in a semi-elective manner
- Laparoscopic resection can be attempted, but colon will be distended
- In necrosis—resection of gangrenous bowel followed by:
  - Paul Mikulicz procedure
  - Hartmann's procedure
  - Primary anastomosis with covering stoma

Ileosigmoid Knot

- Loop of ileum wraps around the base of a redundant sigmoid loop, and is called compound volvulus
- Cause double obstruction, both colon and small bowel
- More common in Middle East, Africa, India
- Distended redundant sigmoid—small bowel descend into pelvis and knots
- Seen with Meckel's and pregnancy
- Sigmoid and ileal necrosis seen in 80%

Etiology—Not Known

- Hypermobile small bowel with an elongated mesentery

- A short, redundant omega-shaped sigmoid
- High fibre diet followed by fasting is a predisposing factors
  - **X-ray**—dilated sigmoid with air fluid levels in small bowel
- Descending colon—deviated medially—due to tethering of sigmoid mesocolon towards ileal mesentery

CT—dilated sigmoid, ileum, whirling of sigmoid and ileal mesentery

Treatment

- Endoscopic reduction always are unsuccessful
- Resection of involved ileum, and sigmoid is treated according to its condition, vascularity and gangrene
- If gangrenous mortality after surgery—20 to 100%
- Nongangrenous bowel after surgery—mortality 6 to 8%

Cecal Volvulus

- Isolated cecal volvulus is rare—actually most of them are cecocolic volvulus
- Represent nearly 25% cases of colonic volvulus
- Represent 1% of all intestinal obstruction

Etiology

- Persons with lack of retroperitoneal fixation of right colon are predisposed to axial rotation of ileocolic junction.
- Axial rotation of terminal ileum, cecum and ascending colon with twisting of mesentery
- Factors causing caecal volvulus—pregnancy, previous surgery, obstructing lesion in left colon, malrotation, chronic constipation
- Most common type—organoaxial—90%
- Hypermobility—predisposes to torsion—in congenital
- Females are more affected than males
- 4th decade

Clinical Presentation

- Sudden onset pain abdomen, distention
- Ischemia
- Asymmetric distention—tympanitic in left upper quadrant or central abdomen
- Most proximal part of obstruction is terminal ileum—so present with small bowel obstruction
- Prior history of chronic pain abdomen—relieved by passage of gas—seen in cecal volvulus—"mobile cecum syndrome"

Abdominal X-ray

- Dilated cecum displaced to left side of abdomen—under left hemidiaphragm
- Cecum—dilated kidney-shaped or comma-shaped—concavity facing inferiorly and to the right side
- Sometimes cecum assume circular shape—with a narrow, triangular density pointing upwards and to the right
- Proximal small bowel dilatation
- Absent gas in RIF

Barium—beaking of ascending colon
- Enema reduction of volvulus—contraindicated
  - **CT**—whirl sign—torsion of engorged mesenteric vessels pointing towards collapsed cecum
- Beaking of cecum
- SB obstruction

Cecal Bascule

- Variant of caecal volvulus (10% of volvulus) where a mobile cecum folds interiorly and superiorly over a fixed ascending colon without rotation on a vascular pedicle.
- Flap valve obstruction
- Gangrene is rare—as there is no vessel obstruction
- Produce intermittent obstruction—relieved spontaneously
- Whirl sign is not seen
- Barium enema is useful in diagnosing caecal bascule
- X-ray—dilated cecum overlies mid-abdomen or the pelvis
- CT shows central cecum—no whirl sign

Treatment
Nonoperative
- With endoscopy is less successful
- Colonoscopy successful in 30% patients—less than sigmoid volvulus
- Attempts at reduction using barium insufflation pressure enema is contraindicated.

Operative—in almost all cases is the choice
- Detorsion alone—high recurrence
- Detorsion with cecostomy—high recurrence
- Right hemicolectomy is the choice—in volvulus and basule
- In cecal bascule—cecopexy may be considered

Outcomes
- Recurrence after resection is 0%
- 30 to 40% recurrence for cecopexy or detorsion alone

- Cecopexy is suturing right colon to lateral peritoneal surface
- Recurrence in cecostomy range from 0 to 30%

Transverse Colon Volvulus
Etiology
- Rare
- Associated with c/c constipation, distal obstruction, previous surgery, pregnancy, hypermobile colonic flexure
- Mental retardation, cerebral palsy Hirschsprung disease
- Absent gastrocolic, lienocolic, phrenocolic ligaments

Clinical Features
- Vomiting is early symptom because transverse colon will compress DJ flexure.

Diagnosis
- X-ray—"inverted coffee bean sign"—dilated transverse colon—apex pointing to pelvis
- **CT**—may also show similar features—nonspecific
- Misdiagnosed as sigmoid volvulus and in attempted endoscopic reduction will fail to show the torsion

Treatment
- Nonoperative
  - Colonoscopic decompression not used now

Surgical Therapy is the Choice
- Resection
- Extended right hemicolectomy
- Partial left colectomy
- Segmental transverse colectomy
- Subtotal colectomy with ileocolic anastomosis

14.5 COLONIC PSEUDO-OBSTRUCTION
- Also called Ogilvie syndrome (Sir William Heneage Ogilvie)
- Distension of colon with signs and symptoms of obstruction without actual cause of obstruction.
- Primary and secondary
- Acute or chronic

Primary
- A motility disorder—familial visceral myopathy (hollow visceral myopathy syndrome)
- A diffuse motility disorder—affecting autonomic nerve fibres—disturbance of intestinal hormones.

Secondary Pseudo-obstruction

- Commoner

Etiology

- Medication—neuroleptic, opiates
- Severe metabolic illness
- Myxedema
- Diabetes mellitus
- Uremia
- Hyperparathyroidism
- Lupus, scleroderma
- Parkinson disease
- Traumatic retroperitoneal hematoma

Mechanism not Clearly Known

- One theory—sympathetic overactivity overriding the parasympathetic system
- Acute variety—patients with any of the chronic organ failure diseases.
  - Only colon involved
- Chronic—other parts of GI tract also get involved. Multiple bouts of subacute and partial obstruction recur periodically

Clinical Features and Diagnosis

- Acute pseudo-obstruction. In medically ill patients present with acute abdominal distension—tympanitic—nontender—with bowel sounds.
- Plain abdominal radiogram—distended colon—right and transverse colon more affected
- Investigation of choice (if suspecting Ogilvie syn.)—water soluble contrast enema
- Colonoscopy—risk of perforation—treatment and diagnostic

Treatment

- Nasogastric decompression, IV fluids, electrolyte correction
- Stop all medication suspected to cause this condition like opiates, antihistamines
- Ambulate the patient—as soon as patient is stable and fit
- Monitored daily with serial abdominal examination and abdominal X-ray
- Water-soluble enema—rule out mechanical obstruction

If Cecum is More than 12 cm

- Neostigmine
  - 2.5 mg over 3 minutes—resolution happens in less than 10 min
  - Parasympathomimetic
  - Competes with acetylcholine for acetylcholinesterase binding sites
  - Recurrence—20%
- Epidural anaesthesia
  - Both not effective
- Colonoscopic decompression
- If not relieved—surgery is indicated
  - If no ischemia—treated with loop colostomy
  - In case of gangrene—resection, mucus fistula

Cecum Size Less than 12 cm

- Observe for 12–24 hrs
- No resolution—treat as cecum with more than 12 cm

14.6 SHORT BOWEL SYNDROME

- Normal length of small intestine highly variable it could be between 300 and 850 cm
- SBS occurs when <200 cm remain
- Minimal length required to prevent lifelong TPN
  - –100 cm if colon is absent
  - –60 cm if colon is present

Etiology of short bowel syndrome
Congenital
a. Intestinal atresia
Acquired
a. Surgical resection of bowel
b. Recurrent Crohn's disease
c. Massive enterectomy secondary to a catastrophic vascular event, such as a mesenteric arterial embolism or venous thrombosis, volvulus, trauma, or tumor resection
d. Gastroschisis
e. Necrotizing enterocolitis
f. Intestinal atresia
g. Extensive aganglionosis
h. Chronic intestinal psuedo-obstruction syndrome
i. Refractory sprue
j. Radiation enteritis
k. Congenital villous atrophy

- Ultra short bowel syndrome in children—when remnant bowel is <10% (with ICV) or <20% (without ICV) of predicted SB length

Functional SBS

- Radiation enteritis
- Low grade malignancies—pseudomyxoma peritonei
- Refractory sprue
- Congenital villous atrophy
- Most common etiology—mesenteric ischemia
- In adults 75% occur from resection for mesenteric ischemia, CD, malignancy
- Multiple resections in CD contributes to 25%
- Neonates—most common cause—resection due to necrotizing enterocolitis and atresia
- Prime determinant of mortality—nutritional failure

Risk factors of development of short bowel syndrome after massive small bowel resection

- Small bowel length <200 cm
- Absence of ileocecal valve
- Unhealthy remaining bowel as in Crohn's disease
- Ileal resection
- Absence of colon

Determinants of Nutritional Failure and Mortality

- Active presence of underlying pathology
- Presence/functional continuity of colon
- Ileocecal valve—a marker of greater ileal or colon resection
- Resection of jejunum is better tolerated than ileum. Ileum is involved in absorption of B_{12}, bile salt
- Ileum has tighter intercellular junctions for better fluid absorption and can assume functions of missing jejunum—not vice versa
- Ileocecal valve—delays transit—prolong contact of mucosa and nutrients
- Assessment of postabsorptive levels of plasma citrulline, a nonprotein amino acid produced by intestinal mucosa acts as an indicator to differentiate transient from permanent intestinal failure

Prevention

- Crohn's disease—minimal resection
- Mesenteric ischemia—minimal resection—second look laparotomy

Normal Intestinal Physiology and Pathophysiology

- Absorptive gradient decrease proximal to distal
  - Duodenum > Jejunum > Ileum
- Luminal diameter duodenum is more than Ileum

- Consequences due to loss of absorptive surface
  - Loss of site specific absorption, as in loss of IC valve
  - Decrease in area of hormone production
- In major resection, larger volumes of undigested nutrients reach intestine which is hyperosmolar—can cause diarrhea

Absorption and Secretion Sites

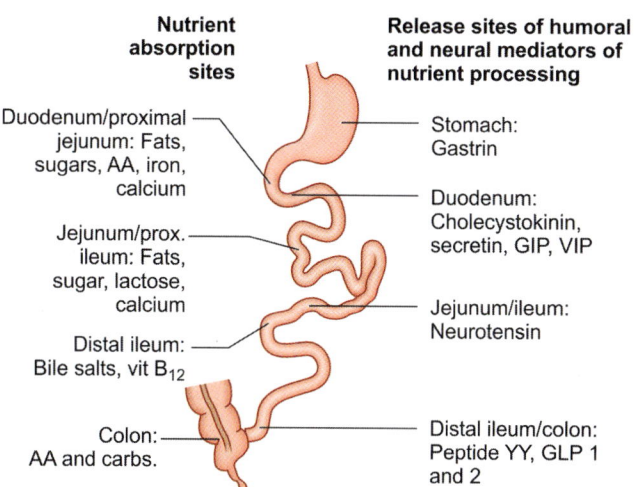

Three anatomical subtypes of short bowel syndrome

1. Jejunoileal anastomosis—majority jejunum resected.
2. Jejunocolic anastomosis—part of jejunum, whole ileum and part of colon resected.
3. End jejunostomy—part of jejunum, whole ileum and colon removed with end jejunostomy

Type 1

- Adapt best
- Need for permanent PN, transplant—if <40 cm jejunum left
- Loss of CCK cause—increased gastric acid—rapid transit of fluids
- Acid inactivate pancreatic enzymes. So need PPI
- Less chance of dehydration—colon absorbs water
- When duodenum and 40 cm jejunum preserved—water soluble vitamin absorption less affected

Type 2

- When <65 cm of jejunum remains with no ileum—may need permanent PN
- Vit B_{12} supplementation needed
- Fat malabsorption occurs

- Presence of unabsorbed bile salts in colon—increase colonic motility and secretion—steatorrhea
- Dry skin, night blindness—due to vit A deficiency
- Osteomalacia, rickets—due to vit D deficiency
- Macular degeneration—due to vitamin E deficiency
- Spontaneous hemorrhage—due to vit K deficiency

Type 3
- Most challenging
- When less than 100 cm is remaining—also lead to loss of gastric and intestinal secretions
- Need permanent PN/IV support
- Ileum has more tight junctions and narrower luminal surface area—permeability to water less—less water enters ileal lumen in response to hyperosmotic load
- Colon increase absorption by 400%—(from 1.8 L to 5 L per day)

Intestinal Adaptation
- Starts within 24 hours up to 2 years
- Keller—3 phases
  - **Acute phase**—up to 4 weeks—stabilize malabsorption, diarrhea
  - **Adaptive phase**—1 to 2 years—goal is to achieve adaptation—gradual increase in nutritional exposure
  - **Maintenance phase**—long term
- Absorptive capacity increased by—increased mucosal surface and increased absorption
- Increase in blood flow lead to increase in number of crypts and villi
- In colon—a process of hyperfermentation of undigested carbohydrates by colonic bacteria which produce SCFA, then absorbed
- Enteral nutrition induces more adaptation
- Long chain TG induce more intestinal hyperplasia
- Glutamine with growth hormone cause more hyperplasia

Medical Management
- Nutritional absorption
- Fluid electrolyte balance
- Vitamin and trace elements supplementation
- Weight maintenance

Acute Phase
- Fluid electrolyte balance
- PPI
- Somatostatin—to reduce secretions
- Cholestyramine—to reduce cholerectic diarrhea
- Metronidazole—to reduce small bowel bacterial overgrowth
- Enteral feeding started on 4–5 days
- Goal of 30–40 kcal/kg/day. But due to malabsorption need to give more in acute phase
- Enteral feeding structured
  - Isotonic salt—glucose solutions, elemental diet with glutamine, Medium chain TG (if preserved colon, but not in type 2 and 3)
- 30–40% lipids and 40–50% carbohydrates

Adaptive Phase
- **After 4 weeks**
  - Diet expansion—Long chain TG, FFA, maltose, pectin-proteins comprise 20% of diet
- If colon is preserved, carbohydrate rich diet avoiding fat is given. Carbohydrate is degraded to SCFA which is an added source of energy
- Oral calcium
- Metabolic acidosis prevented by bicarbonate
- Novel drug—Teduglutide—human analogue of glucagon like peptide (GLP-2) intestine trophic hormone—promote villous height and crypt cell mass

Other Hormones
- Human growth hormone—short-term improvement in weight
- Somatotropin—recombinant human growth hormone—anabolic—currently indicated with nutritional support
- IGF-I

Intestinal Rehabilitation Center (IRC)
- Multidisciplinary

Complications of SBS
Small Bowel Bacterial Overgrowth (SBBO)
- Normally there is less bacteria due to bactericidal action of gastric acid, enzymes, antegrade peristalsis and IC valve

- In SBS—SBBO—due to villous atrophy, loss of gut associated lymphoid tissue, reflux of colon bacteria in the absence of ICV and rapid intestinal transit time
- SBBO—symptomatic presence of >10 5 colony forming units (CFU)/ml in intestine
- Features—pain, bloating, diarrhea—nutritional deficiency
- Endoscopic CFU study
- Hydrogen breath test—produced by bacteria on carbohydrates

Treatment: SBBO
- Antibiotics, metronidazole
- Correction of factors like fistula
- Reduce carbohydrates
- Antimotility drugs should not be used
- Probiotics useful

Catheter Related Infections
- From central venous catheters 3–6% life span risk
- Most common coagulase negative Staph, *S. aureus*, gram negative bacilli

Liver Disease
- Cholestasis—steatosis—fibrosis—cirrhosis—endstage liver disease

Factors Affecting Liver Disease
- PN >1 year
- Central line infection
- Intestinal length <60 cm
- Cholecystectomy
- Lack of enteral feed—decreased entral hormones—stasis, loss of GB contractility—SBBO—cholestasis—stone formation in liver and GB—increased lithocholic acid

Prevention
- Routine enteral feeding
- Antibiotics to prevent SBBO
- PN mixtures with balanced carbohydrates and fat with taurine and cysteine
- Easiest way to assess intestinal failure when patient is on EN—urine output and urinary sodium
- Metabolic problems after EN—oxalate nephropathy and lactic acidosis

Surgical Management
- Conserve as much intestine as possible
- Preserve IC valve
- Note the preserved length, stoma
- Not to do any adjunctive procedures at initial surgery—75% of SBS patients—adaptation is sufficient—no need for surgery
- Patients who fail to achieve PN independence will require surgery

Autogenous Intestinal Reconstruction Surgery (AIRS)
- To improve intestinal function
- Optimize bowel motility
- Increase mucosal absorptive area

To Improve Intestinal Function
- Stricturoplasty, adhesiolysis, segmental resection
- Stoma takedown and re-establishing intestinal continuity
  - Improves bowel function—absorbs and prolongs transit time
  - Restoring colonic continuity—like adding another foot of small bowel
- Procedures to prolong transit or improve motility

Reversal of Intestinal Segment
- 5–15 cm of segment in reverse fashion peristalsis—slows myoelectrical activity
- Colonic interposition
  - Iso or antiperistaltic
  - Proximally placed isoperistaltic segment and distal antiperistaltic

Intestinal Tapering and Plication
Tapering

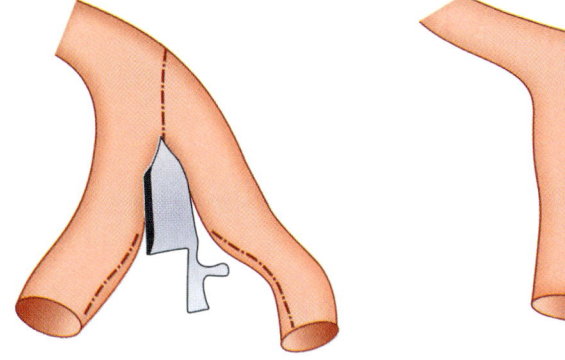

- When dilated loops—causing malabsorption and infection with adequate intestinal length
- In plication—no bowel wall resected—absorptive mucosal border is not lost

Procedures to Increase Absorption

Longitudinal intestinal lengthening and tailoring (LILT) and serial transverse enteroplasty (STEP)

Longitudinal Intestinal Lengthening and Tailoring

- First done by Bianchi in 1980 in pigs
- Depend on bifurcated blood supply within mesentery—bowel can be split longitudinally
- Criteria for selection
  - Intestinal diameter >3 cm
  - Length of residual bowel >40 cm
  - Length of dilated bowel >20 cm
- Difficulty—when blood supply on one side of mesentery only and in thickened short mesentery

LILT-Iowa Procedure—1993 by Kimura

- When mesentery is shortened
- Only short gut remaining is dilated duodenum

Two Step

Step 1

- Deseromyotomizing the antimesenteric surface of dilated segment to a host organ
  - To deperitonealized abdominal wall (Iowa model 1)
  - To decapsulated liver (Iowa model 2)
  - To adjacent bowel with incised serosa (model 3)
- Allow vessel collaterals to co-apt

Step 2

- Longitudinal split of the bowel with the developed own blood supply and end to end anastomosis is done
- Need multiple laparotomies
- Takes time for the results
- LILT cannot be repeated on same intestinal segment
- If cannot be weaned off PN after LILT—small bowel transplantation has to be done

Serial Transverse Enteroplasty (STEP)

- Kim—2003
- Relies on the principle that small bowel blood supply from mesentery runs perpendicular to the long axis of SI
- Placing alternating and opposite transverse staple fires parallel to mesentery and create zigzag-shaped elongated bowel
- Distance between staple lines 1.5 times the diameter of remaining lumen
- Can be done on any bowel and after LILT
- STEP increase length by 1–2 fold

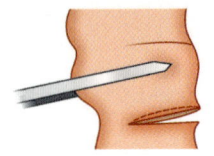 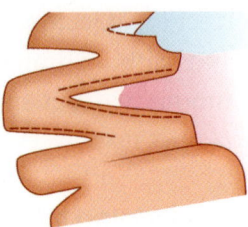

Spiral Intestinal Lengthening and Tailoring (SILT)

- Cserni—2013
- Cutting the bowel and its associated mesentery along 45–60 degree spiral line, then longitudinally lengthening
- No manipulation of mesentery and no change in orientation of muscle fibers—a cause for redilatation in STEP

Creation of intestinal valve, retrograde pacing and loop recirculation

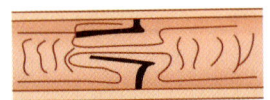 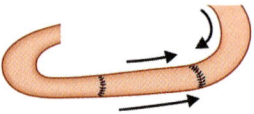

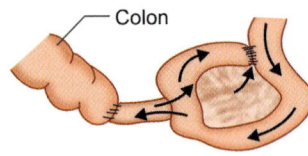
Colon

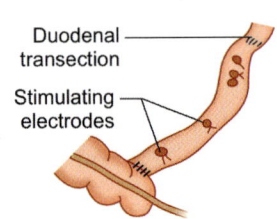
Duodenal transection
Stimulating electrodes

Small Bowel Transplantation
Indications in SBS

- Intestinal failure associated liver disease (IFALD)
- PN failure, recurrent CRI (catheter related infection)

- Fungemia, shock
- Thrombosis of 2/6 central lines
- Growth failure
- Impending liver failure

14.7 SUPERIOR MESENTERIC ARTERY SYNDROME

- Other names—cast syndrome, Wilkie syndrome, aortomesenteric duodenal compression
- First described by Carl von Rokitansky in 1842
- Obstruction of D3 between aorta and SMA
- More in females, 10–18 years of age
- In rapid weight loss—hyperdisorders, on chemotherapy
- Following hip spica application
- Following proctocolectomy

Clinical Features

- Need high index of suspicion
- Pain, nausea, vomiting—bilious
- Relief on knee to chest position and lying on the stomach. These open the aorto mesenteric angle

Diagnosis

- Upper GI scopy—can show obstruction
- Barium or hypotonic duodenography—abrupt or near total cut-off of flow from duodenum to jejunum
- CT angiography with or without oral contrast is the choice. This show
  - SMA compressing D3
  - Aortomesenteric angle <22 degrees (normal 38–65 degrees)
  - Aortomesenteric distance <8 mm (normal 10–28 mm)

Treatment

Conservative Treatment: The Choice

- Acute phase—NPO, nasogastric aspiration, nasojejunal feed

  Surgery
  - For complications—mass, vascular aneurism
  - Haye's maneuver—pressure is applied below the umbilicus incephalad and backward direction. This elevates root of small bowel mesentery which relieves obstruction temporarily

Surgery

- Goal—to improve narrow aorto mesenteric angle
- Strong's procedure—mobilization of D4 and ligament of Treitz (duodenal derotation)
- Duodenojejunostomy is the choice
  - And also GJ

14.8 PNEUMATOSIS INTESTINALIS

- Multiple gas filled cysts in GIT
- Located in subserosa, submucosa and rarely muscularis layer
- Size vary from a few mm to cm
- Can occur anywhere in GIT
- Most common site—jejunum
  - Also ileocecal region and colon
- Mesentery, falciform ligament and peritoneum also involved
  - Equal in both sexes, 4–5 decades
- In children associated with necrotizing enterocolitis

Theories

- Mechanical
- Mucosal damage
- Bacterial
- Pulmonary hypothesis

Associations

- COPD
- Immunocompromise—AIDS, leukemia, lymphoma, transplantation, on chemotherapy and steroids
- Intestinal—infection, obstruction
- Iatrogenic—endoscopy, jejunostomy
- Diabetes
- Not associated with any lesion—primary pneumatosis—in 15%
- Secondary pneumatosis in 85%
- Cysts resemble lymphangiomas or hydatid cysts
- Histology—honeycomb appearence
- Thin walled—can break and cause pneumoperitoneum

  Symptoms:
  - Of primary condition
  - Pain, diarrhea, distension, vomiting
  - Bleeding

Complications

- Occur in 3%
- Volvulus, perforation, obstruction
- Pneuomoperitoneum—more with SI cysts
- Peritonitis—unusual
- Produce sterile pneumoperitoneum

Diagnosis
X-ray

- Radioluscent areas within bowel wall—linear, curvilinear, grape-like or like tiny bubbles

  Barium and CT—to confirm

  USG—can visualise cysts

  CT—the choice

- Worrisome findings
  - Wall thickening
  - Free peritoneal fluid
  - Soft tissue stranding
  - Extensive pneumatosis
  - Location and presence of free peritoneal air—do not indicate severity

Treatment

- No treatment is needed
- Indicated in-complications
  - Bleeding, volvulus, tension pneumoperitoneum
- Directed towards the cause
- To rule out intestinal ischemia related pneumatosis

Gastric Pneumatosis

- Rarer
- Submucosal or subserosal
- Develop in benign and life-threatening conditions
- If associated with portal venous gas—life threatening

Two Types
Emphysematous Gastritis

- By direct infection with gas forming organism or blood borne
  - *C. perfringens, E. coli,* Pseudomonas—most common

- In immunosuppression, diabetes, steroids, NSAIDs
- Patients—have peritonitis and are sick and may have sepsis

Gastric Emphysema

- Noninfectious
  - Air enters by traumatic, pulmonary or obstructive reasons
- Also after OGD scopy, vomiting
- Pulmonary cause from rupture of emphysema and gas track through mediastinum and intogastric wall
- Present with nausea vomiting—usually resolve by itself

14.9 LOWER GI BLEED

- **Definition:** Bleeding site distal to DJ junction (ligament of Treitz)
- Less frequency for hospitalization than upper GI bleed
- **Mortality:** 3% (increases with age)
- **Incidence:** Increases with age
- 95% cases source of bleeding is colon

Etiology

- Unknown 10–25%
  - Most common etiology of lower GI bleeding—carcinoma
  - Most common etiology of acute symptomatic lower GI bleeding—diverticulosis

Colonic bleeding 95%
- Diverticular disease 30–40%
- Anorectal disease 5–15%
- Ischemia 5–10%
- Neoplasia 5–10%
- Infectious colitis 3–8%
- Postpolypectomy 3–7%
- IBD 4%
- Angiodysplasia 3%
- Radiation proctitis/colitis 1–3%

Small bowel bleeding 5%

- **Angiodysplasia**
- **Erosion or ulcers (Potassium, NSAIDs)**
- **Crohn's disease**
- **Radiation**
- Meckel's diverticulum
- Neoplasia
- Aortoenteric fistula

LGI bleeding—ASGE—4 types

- Occult GI bleeding
  - No gross bleeding—test positive stool/anemia
- Melena
  - Dark, tarry, sticky—first evaluate UGI
- Scant intermittent hematochezia
  - Most common pattern—intermittent passage of small amounts of bright red blood PR
  - Anorectal source—anoscopy
  - Colonoscopy—in age >50 and in features of neoplasia
- Severe hematochezia
  - Active bleeding

In acute bleeding LGI scopy is done within 24 hours after stabilising the patient

Vascular Ectasias

- Angiodysplasia, AV malformation—most common vascular lesions of colon—bleeding after age 60
- Arise from age related degeneration of colonic vessels, dilated tortuous submucosal veins.
- Located in cecum and ascending colon
- <5 mm and multiple
- Endoscopy—small flat red lesion with ectatic vessels radiating from central lesion
- SMA, IMA angiography may show blush of contract
- Present with recurrent self-limiting episodes of bleeding—gross blood/occult
- >90% spontaneous resolution

- 15%—massive bleeding—may need intervention endoscopically, interventional radiology or by surgical resection
- Risk increase with number of lesions
- **Heyde syndrome**—angiodysplasia of colon and aortic stenosis association

Vascular Lesions of the Colon

- Hemangioma, vascular ectasia, arteriovenous malformation, colonic varices, telangiectasia
- Syndrome related lesions (Klippel-Trénaunay—Weber syndrome, Maffucci syndrome)

Others

- Vascular disease of liver disease
- Degenerative phlebectasia of older adults
- Vasculitis
- Ulcerative, Crohn's, and ischemic colitis
- Neovascularity of radiation colitis
- Angiosarcoma (as in Kaposi sarcoma)

LGI Bleeding is Discussed in Diverticular Disease

14.10 OSTOMIES AND STOMA CARE

- Important for Wide variety of colorectal conditions
- Social implication
- Either temporary means of fecal diversion or permanent orifices for passage of stool or urine
- Permanent colostomies usually created from descending colon or proximal sigmoid colon
- With development of ilial pouch anal anastomosis, permanent ileostomies are far less common

Indications of permanent—colostomies:

- Rectal cancer
- Radiation proctopathy
- Incontinence
- Refractory anorectal infections
- Ischemia
- Diverticular diseases
- Sacral decubitus ulcer

  - If a permanent colostomy is being contemplated with transverse colon, better resect the remaining colon and make an end ileostomy—difficult to manage transverse colostomy and is associated with more complications

Indications of Permanent Ileostomies

- IBD
- FAP
- Multiple synchronous colorectal cancer

Types of diverting stomas

- End/loop sigmoid colostomy
- Transverse loop colostomy
- Loop ileostomies

PREOPERATIVE CONSIDERATIONS

- Preoperative education
- Enterostomal therapist consultation
- Appropriate abdominal wall site
- Marked prior to surgery
- Ostomy triangle
  - Anterior superior iliac spine, pubic tubercle and umbilicus—ostomies are better placed within this
- 5 cm away from all bony prominences, umbilicus and scar or skin folds

Proper Marking of Stoma

- Sit up to ensure
- Avoid in patients beltline
- If the patient is in wheelchair, mark when he is in wheelchair
- Pass through rectus muscle
- Free from creases
- Visible to patient
- Explain the purpose
- Examine in various positions
- Identify lateral edge of rectus muscle by lying down and raising head
- 2 inches from midline
- Make sure patient has seen the site
- In case of large protuberant abdomen
  - Placement in upper abdomen may be considered.
  - Preoperative mechanical and antibiotic preparation is given

Operative Techniques

- **END ileostomies**
  - Skin disc removed
  - Expose anterior rectal sheath
  - Cruciate fashion incision
  - Avoid medial extension
  - Rectus muscle is split in line to expose posterior rectal sheath
  - Ileum is prepared
  - Mesentery cleared from the terminal 5 to 6 cm
  - Leave 1 cm strip of mesentry—it carries a vessel parallelling the ileal wall
  - Ileum oriented with cut mesenteric edge cephalad
  - Protrude 5 to 6 cm
  - Ileostomies must be everted and matured
  - **Tripartite sutures**

    Through dermis of skin, seromuscular layer at the level of fascia and full thickness cut edge of ileum (Brooke's technique)
  - Three or four sutures applied to evert the ileum-additional sutures 4–8 between cut edge of ileum and dermis
  - Should appear pink and should protrude 2 to 3 cm above skin edge

End Colostomies

Indications
- APR
- Hartmann
- Rectourethral/rectovaginal fistula
- Necrotising soft tissue infections
- Severe rectal trauma

- If IMA ligated, take descending colon for ostomy
- Closure of lateral gutter or fixing to posterior abdominal fascia—do not prevent hernia/prolapse
- Suture the free edge of colon mesentery to lateral abdominal wall
- Tripartite sutures kept—sutured with minimal eversion because contents are solid and not irritating

- **Prophylactic mesh placement**—to prevent hernia

    – Two methods—modified sugarbaker (intraperitoneal) and keyhole technique

    – Another method—create extraperitoneal tunnel

    – Retroperitoneal colostomy

    Tunelling of colon under posterolateral peritoneum—to exit through the marked colostomy site—reduces hernia and prolapse—more technically demanding

- **Loop end stoma**

    – Variation of end stoma

    – In obese and with short mesentery—difficult for the stoma to reach the skin

- Brought out as a loop, with distal end stapled and closed

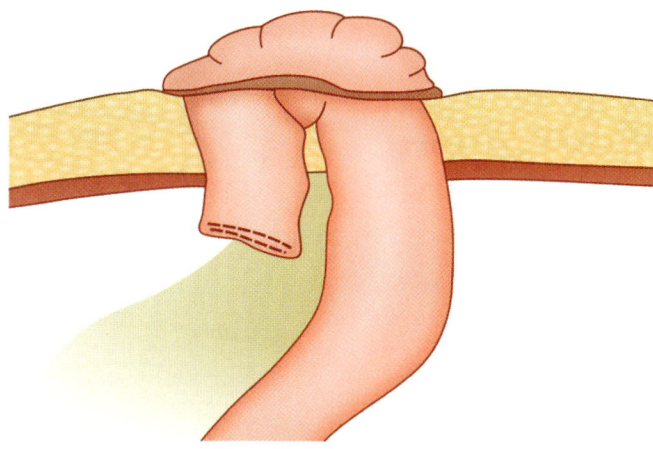

Diverting Stomas

- Loop ileostomies
- Loop colostomies
- Loop end ileostomies

Loop Ileostomies

- Terminal ileum is selected
- 20 to 30 cm proximal to ileocecal valve
- Abd wall defect is created
- Distal end is marked with a suture-for proper orientation
- Distal aspect of ileum just above wall is transected circumferentially 80% (from mesentery to mesentery)

- Distal end is matured by sutures between cut end and dermis
- Tripartite suturing done for proximal end
- Functioning loop should protrude and occupy 80% of the defect

Loop Colostomies

- Left lower quadrant
- Eversion is not necessary
- Sigmoid colon is ideal

Transverse loop colostomy—Liquid effluent, more chance of prolapse but provides temporary complete diversion

Sigmoid/descending colon loop colostomy. Effluent is thick, less fluid loss and less chance of colostomy prolapse

- Supporting rod in loop colostomy removed usually on 5th postop day.
- Spur is the posterior wall of the loop colostomy stoma. After about 6 weeks, spur may retract and feces from proximal end can spillover to distal end.

End Loop Stomas
Three Types
- End loop ileostomy
- End loop colostomy
- End loop ileocolostomy

End loop Ileostomy

- Ileum transected using cutting stapler
- Proximal end brought out as standard end ileostomy.
- Distal-nonfunctioning end

    – Brought out and sutured to functioning bowel—completely diverts the bowel

    – Antimesenteric end of the distal end only is opened and matured. Remaining bowel wall is closed and buried

        ☐ Functioning end matured

        ☐ A single suture connects both limbs

- Act as end ileostomy

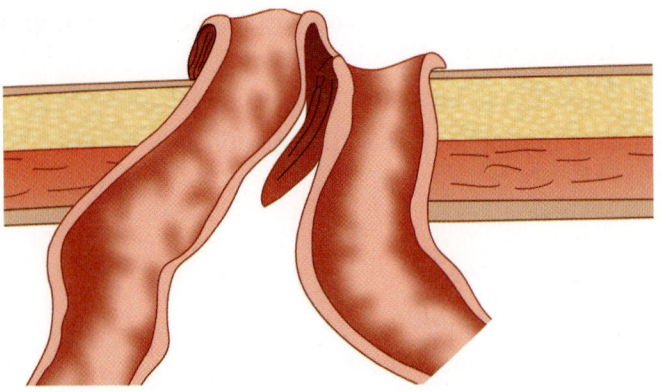

End loop Ileocolostomy

- After right hemicolectomy—when primary anastomosis is not ideal
- Usually in right upper quadrant
- Ileum brought out
- Transverse colon—antimesenteric border of staple line resected—sutured to skin edge
- Ileum opened—matured—sutured to colon
- Easy to close—both loops are close together

Benefits

- Stoma management easy
- Can be made by remote sections of intestines
- No formal laparotomy is needed to close the ostomy

Modified Abdominoplasty (Abdominal Wall Contouring)

- In stomal retraction—in rapid weight loss—lax abdominal wall
- Short gut
- Peristomal skin problems
- **In rapid weight gain**—retraction of stoma can happen
- Options are
  - Weight reduction
  - Stoma revision
  - Liposuction

Enterostomal Therapy

- Stoma therapist
- Ileostomy emptied—4–6 times/day

- Colostomy once or twice/day—even other day
- Entire appliance changed every 4–7 days
- Pouches changed when stoma is least active—often after a period of fasting
- Avoid food which creates gas
- Odor proof pouches, charcoal filters, pouch deodorants
- Oral deodorants—bismuth subgallate and chlorophyllin complex

Closure

- Proctogram done—to rule out distal obstruction/continuing problem
- Closure done after maturing—2 months
- Circumferential incision around colostomy 3 mm from mucocutaneous junction
- Close defect transversely

Blowhole Colostomy

- Described by Turnbull
- Indication— toxic megacolon
- Along with loop ileostomy—decompress the colon
- Usual location transverse colon
- Can be done under local anesthesia
- Incision in midepigastrium
- Incise fascia and peritoneum
- Expose serosa of transverse colon
- Interuppted sutures between seromuscular layer of colon and peritoneum
- Decompress gas in dilated colon with large bore needle
- 2nd layer of interrupted sutures are placed between fascia and seromuscular layer
- Incise colon and suction out of gaseous and stool that is under pressure
- Place interrupted sutures between full thickness of bowel wall edge to skin
- In very toxic patients with toxic megacolon just suturing the anterior wall of colon to rectus sheath, peritoneum and skin

Without mobilising colon, which can perforate the colon due to the thin wall and dilated condition of colon.

- Blow hole colostomy can be done at multiple sites
- a covering ileostomy is also done.
- Once the patient improves, definitive procedure can be undertaken

Anti-adhesion Barriers and Stoma

- Carboxy methyl cellulose and sodium hyaluronate are used in order to facilitate less adhesions and easy reversal
- Ileum can be wrapped at time of creation

Complications of Stomas

- 10 to 70%
- Early—peristomal skin irritation (most common), leakage, high output, ischemia
- Late—skin irritation (most common) parastomal hernia, prolapse, obstruction and stenosis

Skin Irritation

- More common in ileostomy due to liquid and caustic effluent
- 35% due to leakage
- 55% due to reaction to adhesive
- Obesity is a risk factor—can place stoma in upper abdomen where there is less fat and patient can see better
- Avoid frequent change and too long change
- Fungal infections

High Output Stoma

- More common with ileostomy
- Seen in 5–20% of ileostomy patients
- Output peaks on 4th postop day
- Can cause hyponatremia and dehydration
- High output decreases when small bowel adapts by mucosal hyperplasia
- Managed by oral rehydration
- High incidence of *Clostridium difficle* enteritis in ileostomy.

Treatment

- Oral fibre supplements and cholestyramine
- Histamine receptor antagonists and PPI
- Anti motility agents
- Stomatostatin analogues

- Foods that slowdown and thicken ileostomy output like peanut butter, cheese, banana, bread, potato, tapioca
- In ileostomy there is more chance of urinary stones
  - 60% of them uric acid stones
  - Due to loss of fluid, bicarbonate and sodium and reduction urinary pH and volume

Bowel Obstruction

- In 23% of ileostomy patients
- Most common cause is adhesion
- Other causes—volvulus and internal hernia
- Food bolus obstruction
- Red rubber tube catheter inserted and saline irrigation initiated

Ischemia

- Due to oedema and venous congestion
  - Usually self-limiting
  - Results from error—in dividing sigmoid vessels to gain length—instead of this should divide IMA or mobilize splenic flexure to gain length and preserve sigmoid arcades
- Careful scopy is done and if bowel is viable at fascial level—may be observed—if not immediate laparotomy
- Sometimes laparotomy and stoma revision is required

Parastomal Hernia

- Most common complication requiring operative intervention
- In 2–30% of end ileostomy
- In 4–50% of end colostomy
- Can be managed with belted appliances but surgical repair with mesh maybe needed
- Results of surgical correction is poor
  - Maximum nonsurgical treatment

European Hernia Society classification of parastomal hernia

Type I: <5 cm hernia without concomitant incisional hernia

Type 2: <5 cm parastomal hernia (PH) with incisional hernia

Type 3: >5 cm hernia without incisional hernia

Type 4: >5 cm PH with incisional hernia

Each is divided into primary PH and recurrent PH

Prevention of Parastomal Hernia

- Make smallest possible opening
- Lateral space closure
- Fascial fixation
- Stoma through rectus muscle
- Prophylactic sublay mesh

Treatment

- Primary fascial repair—involves hernia reduction and primary fascial reapproximation after peristomal incision. This carries very high rate of recurrence
- Stoma relocation. Laparotomy and relocates the hernia to a new site

Prosthetic Repair

- **Key hole fashion**—biologic or synthetic mesh is placed around the new stoma site
- **Mesh is placed as a flat** sheet lateralizing the stoma: Sugarbaker technique
- **Laparotomy, stoma is taken down** and re-sited to contralateral side, posterior component separation done and a large mesh is placed in a retromuscular fashion covering old stoma site, midline and new stoma in a key hole fashion
  - Direct simple repair—almost 100% recurrence
  - Mesh repair—least recurrence
  - Mesh—inlay method—best results—Sugarbaker
    □ Can be sublay or onlay also
  - STORRM—Stapled Transabdominal Ostomy Reinforcement with Retromuscular Mesh
  - SMART approach—Stapled Mesh Stoma Reinforcement Technique—a prolypropelene mesh is fixed in the retromuscular plane and fixed. Cut by firing circular stapler—then colostomy is created
  - **Sugarbaker**—inlay prolene mesh—no hole was made in the mesh—colostomy is fashioned by lateralizing the colon

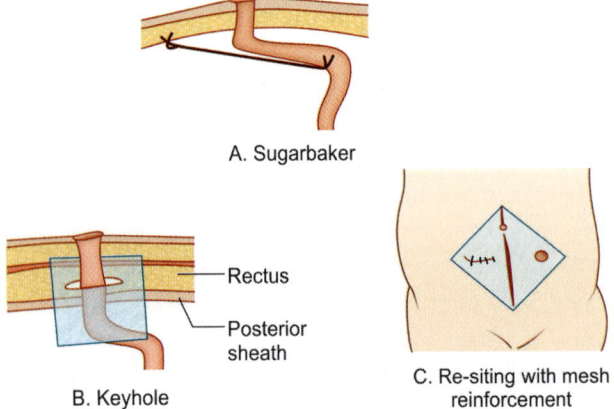

A. Sugarbaker

B. Keyhole

Rectus

Posterior sheath

C. Re-siting with mesh reinforcement

- **In modified Sugarbaker**—Mesh is fixed and colon lateralised—mesh overlaps 5 cm on all sides

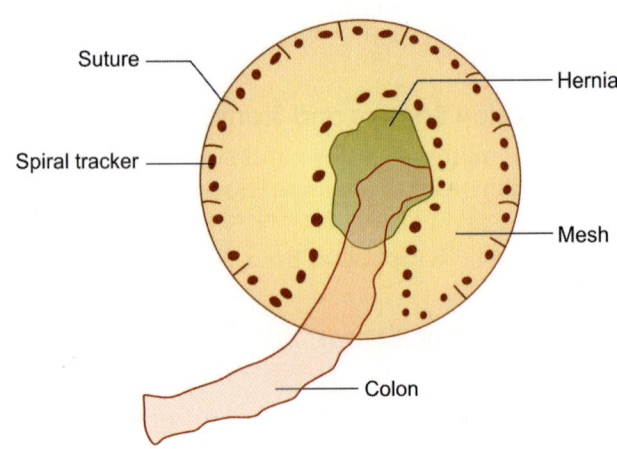

Suture

Spiral tracker

Hernia

Mesh

Colon

Stenosis

- 10% incidence
- Result from ischemia, excessive tension, retraction or IBD
- Asymptomatic—no treatment
- Skin level stenosis treated with Z or W plasty
- Digital dilatation can be tried

Prolapse

- Incidence 10–15%
- Transverse loop colostomy most common—efferent limb the offending cause
  - Reason for preferring loop ileostomy over loop transverse colostomy
  - Surgical intervention may be needed—pulled until bowel is taut and excised and new ostomy formed
  - In case of incarcerated prolapse sugar can be applied as desiccant

Peristomal Varices

- May cause life-threatening hemorrhage
- Occur at mucocutaneous border
- In liver metastasis/liver disease

Treatment

- Local pressure/suture
- TIPS

- Mucocutaneous disconnection of stoma up to fascia
- Relocation
- Liver transplantation

14.11 ENTEROCUTANEOUS FISTULA

- Abnormal communication between digestive organ and skin

Statistics

- Mortality 10%
- Iatrogenic 75–85%

Etiology

- Anastomotic leak
- Injury to bowel
- Erosion by suction catheter
- Laceration by mesh
- Crohn's
- Malignant disease
- Radiation
- Diverticulitis
- Sepsis
- Trauma

Webster and Carey

Classification of small bowel fistula

- **Congenital**
  - Vitello intestinal duct
  - Fecal matter discharge—from umbilicus
- **Trauma**
  - Fish bone, toothpick
  - Iatrogenic
- **Infection**
  - TB, coccidiomycosis, salmonella
  - Actinomyces (appendicectomy)
- **Perforation**
- **Inflammation**
- Irradiation or tumor
- For gastric fistula—most common cause—anastomotic leaks
- Most common type of small intestinal fistula—ECF

Classification

- Low output (<200 ml). Intermediate output (200–500 ml). High output (>500 ml)

Anatomy

- Gastric
- Small bowel
- Colon
- Rectum

Clinical Presentation

- Febrile postop patient
- Erythematous wound
- Purulent or bloody discharge
- Leakage of enteric content
- **Triad**
  - Sepsis
  - Fluid imbalance
  - Electrolyte imbalance

Enteroatmospheric Fistula

- Fistula associated with large abdominal defect

Björck's Classification of Open Abdomen

Grade	Description
1A	Clean OA without adherence between bowel and abdominal wall or fixity (lateralization of the abdominal wall)
1B	Contaminated OA without adherence/fixity
2A	Clean OA developing adherence/fixity
2B	Contaminated OA developing adherence/fixity
3	OA complicated by fistula formation
4	Frozen OA with adherent/fixed bowel; unable to close surgically; with or without fistula

Diagnosis

- Clinical
- If uncertain, give oral
  - Activated charcoal
  - Indigo carmine

Factors Preventing Closure

- High output fistula
- Severe disruption of intestinal continuity (>50%)
- Active inflammatory bowel disease
- Cancer
- Radiation enteritis
- Jejunal origin of fistula
- Foreign body in fistula
- Tract <2.5 cm in length
- Epithelization
- Undrained abscess cavity

Prevention

- Gentle handling
- Serosal tear repair
- Not to break interloop adhesions in repeat laparotomy

Most Common Abnormalities

- Hypovolemia
- Hypokalemia
- Metabolic acidosis—due to loss of pancreatic bicarbonate in proximal fistula

Malnutrition

- Fluid rich in ingested nutrients and endogenous protein, enzymes and albumin—lost
- Protein calorie malnutrition
- Mg, Se and Zn depletion
- Absence of nutrients in intestine cause reduced intestinal hormones and GH release
- Gastric hypersecretory state

Intrahepatic Cholestasis

- Loss of bile salt and disruption of enterohepatic circulation
- Bacterial overgrowth

Abdominal wall and Wound Sepsis

- Delays formation of granulation tissue

Dermatitis

- Effluent dermatitis
  - Corrosive effect of intestinal content
- Fecal dermatitis
  - Erythema and desquamation of skin

Psychological

- Decreased morale of the patient

Malignancy

- Chronic fistula may become carcinoma especially in Crohn's disease

Principles of Management

SNAPP

- Sepsis control
- Nutrition
- Anatomy delineation
- Plan the procedure
- Protection of the skin

SOWATS

- Sepsis control
- Optimize nutrition

- Wound care
- Anatomy delineation
- Timing of surgery
- Strategy of surgery

Phase 1: Recognition/Stabilisation

- Resuscitation
- Early detection—fever, tachycardia, abdominal signs
- CT scan
- Fluid, electrolyte correction
- Antibiotics

Fluid and Electrolyte

- More loss in proximal fistulas
- May need bicarbonate to correct metabolic acidosis
- Urine output maintained >0.5 ml/kg/hr
- Blood/albumin transfusion
- Management of local wound infections
- Drainage of intra-abdominal collections (percutaneous)
- Laparotomy may be required for:
  - Extensive cellulitis/necrotising fasciitis
  - Incomplete percutaneous drainage of collections
  - Disruption of anastomosis
- Antibiotics as per indicated

Surgery

- Proper exposure
- Exteriorisation of dehiscent bowel
- If delayed/difficult cases consider proximal stoma
- "Defunction and drain"—in anterior resection—if <50% disruption—proximal stoma and drain
  - >50% disruption, consider—end stoma
- Repair of the fistula—not ideal
- Uncontrolled sepsis may need Parenteral nutrition
- Proper appliances
- Dressing
- 'Floating stoma'
- VAC

Nutritional Management

- Plays central role in management
- Adequate circulation and tissue oxygenation must for optimal utilization
- May be
  - Enteral
  - Parenteral

TPN Indications

- Inability to obtain enteral access
- High output fistulas

- GI intolerance with enteral nutrition
- Multiple unfavourable factors (ileus, obstruction)

Enteral Nutrition
- **Benefits:**
  - Trophic effect on bowel
  - Stimulates hepatic protein synthesis
  - Improves immune/hormonal/barrier function
  - Decreased infection rate/metabolic complication
  - Inexpensive
- 4 ft of functional bowel and distal patency are required for EN
- Lipid-based formula absorbed more efficiently
- In proximal fistulas—hypotonic fluids like water—increase fistula output. So ORS is preferred.

Fistuloclysis
- In high output fistulas
- Enteral feeding tube placed directly into the matured high output fistula
- In proximal fistula, bowel distal to the fistula is intubated
- Improves nutrition

General Guidelines
- 30–35 kcal/kg/day—in low output
- In high output fistula—1.5 to 2 times more
- Patients daily protein requirement is 1.2 to 2.0 gm kg/day.
- 20–25% of nutrition through enteral route is sufficient for its benefits
- Fluid requirement is 30 ml/kg/day

Reduction of Fistula Output
- Restrict hypo-osmolar fluids
- Encourage electrolyte mix
- Antisecretory agents
  - Proton pump inhibitors
  - Somatostatin or octreotide
- Antimotility agents
  - Loperamide
  - Codeine
- **Somatostatin Analogue**
  - Inhibit gastrin and cholecystokinin
  - Reduces splanchnic blood flow
  - Reduces rate of gastric emptying
  - Inhibit gall bladder contraction
- PPI—reduce gastric acid and secretions—in proximal fistulas
- Infliximab (TNF alfa-monoclonal antibody) (in Crohn's disease)

- Oral tacrolimus (in Crohn's disease)
- Cyclosporin—in CD

Plugging of Fistula
- Used in—long tract
  - Without epithelialization
  - Low output
- Endoscopic injection of platelet rich fibrin glue
- Radiologic guided percutaneous gelfoam embolization of enteric opening
- Absorbable fistula plug

Techniques of Skin Care
- Wound pouch dressings
  - One/two piece design
  - Clip closure or urostomy type
  - May be attached to a bed side bag or suction catheter

Sump Drainage
- For fistulae draining with open abdominal wound
- Large bore drains or sumps
- High pressure suction

VAC
- Removes chronic edema, leading to increased localized blood flow, and the applied forces result in the enhanced formation of granulation tissue

Phase 2: Investigations
- CT with GI contrast
  - Localise, and characterise fistula
  - Evaluate for distal obstruction
- Fistulogram down the tract
- **Objectives of investigation plan in 7–10 days: To define:**
  - Precise anatomical location
  - Is the bowel in continuity or is disrupted
  - Abscess cavity
  - Condition of adjacent bowel
  - Is there a distal obstruction
  - Etiological disease process
- **Definition of Anatomy**
  - CT
  - Fistulography
  - Small bowel follow through
  - Contrast enema
  - Endoscopy—not in acute perforation
  - May be in internal fistulas—OGD/colonscopy
  - Diagnostic laparotomy

Phase 3: Decision

- If infection and nutrition taken care of—90–95% fistula close in 4–8 weeks
- Early intervention only to control sepsis, if not amenable to percutaneous intervention
- Ideal time for intervention—either within 10 days or after 4 months after patient stabilization
- Spontaneous closure unlikely after 4–6 weeks

Failure of Spontaneous Closure of ECF
FRIENDS

- Foreign body
- Radiation
- Inflammation/infection
- Epithelialization
- Neoplasm
- Distal obstruction
- Steroids
- Average time to close
  - Oesophageal—15–25 days
  - Duodenal—30–40 days
  - Colonic—30–40 days
  - Small bowel—40–60 days
- No signs of imminent closure after 4–6 weeks, then patient should be prepared for surgery
- Unfavourable characteristics since beginning

Factors	Favorable	Unfavorable
Origin	Oropharyngeal, esophageal, deodenal, PB, jejunal	Gastric, lateral duodenal, ligament of teris, ileal
Etiology	Postop, appendicitis, diverticulitis	Maligancy, IBD
Output	Low	High
Sepsis	Absent	Present
Fistula	Tract >2 cm, defect <1 cm sq	Tract <1 cm, defect >1 cm sq,
Misc	Same institution	Referred
State of bowel	Healthy adj tissue, intestinal continuity, absence of obstruction	Abscess, bowel discontinuity, irradiation epithelialization of tract
Nutrition	Well nourished, transferrin >200 mg/dl	Malnourished, transferrin <200 mg/dl

- Uncontrolled sepsis urgent drainage of sepsis
- General condition very poor, then only abscess drainage
- In case of malignancies early operation should be done

Phase 4: Definitive management

- Well-healed abdominal wall without inflammation should be there
- Assess distal bowel

Surgical Wisdom in ECF
Approach

- Abdominal wall closure is most warranted
- Window of doom—10 days to 6 weeks following initial surgery-adhesions—more chance of injury
- Optimal nutrition parameters
- Free of sepsis
- Well-healed abdominal wall without inflammation
- Prophylactic antibiotics
- Tapering of tube feeding
- Operative approach preferably through a new incision or extending the old incision and entering through an unoperated area
  - Midline
  - Transverse
- Prevent contamination of abdominal wall tissues
- Repair enterotomies
- Repair serosal tears—Lembert sutures (5–0 prolene)
- Stomas with mucus fistula or exteriorization
- **Bowel refunctionalisation**
  - Free all adhesion
  - Drain any abscess
  - Relieve any obstruction
- **Dissection/Adhesiolysis**
  - Start with least dense adhesion
  - Sharp Dissection
  - Wet laparotomy pads
  - Saline injection (hydrodissection)
  - Extrafascial dissection
- Best results are with definitive resection and EEA
  - 1/2 circumference be treated by resection and anastomosis
- Appropriate hydration to prevent hypotension and compromised circulation
- Anastomosis in healthy bowel with adequate blood supply; without tension
- Meticulous and precise haemostasis
- Selection of proper needle size, suture
- Omental covering, if possible
- Dead space obliterated with live tissue and properly drained
- Drains kept away from anastomosis site

Abdominal Wall Closure

- Complicated when managed by open abdomen or fistula through center of abdomen
- Nonabsorbable mesh is not indicated if wound is infected

Strategy

- No preoperative fascial defect—primary closure
- Preoperative fascial defect
  - <5 cm—primary closure with or without fascial relaxation
  - >5 cm—component separation technique
  - Very large defect—mesh, vascularised flaps

Phase-5: Postsurgical Phase

- Early postsurgical recovery and late rehabilitation and convalescence
- Recurrence of fistula—strongest predictor of mortality

Factors Predicting Recurrence After Elective Repair of ECF

Patient factors	Surgical factors
Open abdomen	Timing of surgery (<4 weeks, >36 weeks)
Origin of fistula (small bowel > large bowel)	Multiple inadvertent enterotomies at reoperation
Underlying inflammatory bowel disease	Oversewing of enteric defect, rather than resection and anastomosis
"Frozen abdomen" or residual intra-abdominal infection	Use of stapled anastomosis, compared to hand-sewn anastomosis
	Need to perform mesh closure of abdominal wall

14.12 RADIATION ENTERITIS

Etiology

- Ionizing radiation—photon (X-rays or gamma rays) or particle based
- High energy photons—create ionizing electrons which break chemical bonds
- X-ray and gamma rays—create 1000 ionizing tracks per Gray—produce reactive oxygen species from water (hydroxyl radicals, singlet oxygen, superoxide, hydrogen peroxide) and cause indirect damage to cells
- Oxygen presence is very important to generate free radicals and also to help in cell repair

- Ionizing radicals—cause double strand breaks of DNA
- Acute effects—due to depletion of progenitor cells which are radiation sensitive
- Crypt cells deplete within days of radiotherapy
- Non-proliferating differentiated cells will take over function which may get sloughed over time. So symptoms are delayed till 2 weeks
- Progenitor cells depletion occur and their regeneration can occur. This happens more with fractionation of radiation
- Stem cells are more radioresistant—due to presence of antioxidants

	Acute	Chronic
Incidence	70–80%	1.5–15%
Timing	2–4 weeks	6–24 months
Histology	Inflammatory infiltrate crypt mitosis decreased	Endarteritis Fibrosis
	Crypt micro abscesses seen	Lymphatic dilatation
	Ulcerations seen	Tissue necrosis
Causes of symptoms	Malabsorption and bacterial overgrowth	Obstruction Fistula Intestinal failure (malabsorption short bowel syndrome) Neoplasia (recurrent or new)

Clinical Features

- **Acute disease** lasts for 2 weeks, causes pain, and bloating
- Chronic—18 months to 6 years—due to obliterative arteritis of submucosal vessels—submucosal fibrosis—thrombosis and vascular insufficiency.
- TGF—beta plays important role
- Mostly affect ileum and I-C valve due to fixed location and proximity to pelvis
- May perforate or stricture

Factors Affecting Radiation Enteritis

- Dose >5000 cGy
- Previous abdominal surgery
- Chemo agents like 5-FU, Doxorubicin, MTX
- Comorbidities
- RT technique

Prevention

- Use of modern RT techniques—minimize exposure
- Use evening RT schedule—circadian rhythm
- Reduction of field size, conformal RT techniques, IMRT
- Retroperitonealisation of small bowel, omental transposition, absorbable mesh slings

Drugs—to prevent radiation enteritis:
- Sucralfate
- Superoxide dismutase—free radical scavenger
- Antioxidants—vitamin A, E
- Pentoxyphylline
- Probiotics
- ACE inhibitors, statins
- Most effective radioprotective—Amifostine (WR-2721)—binds to free radicals and protect cells
- Glutathione
- Growth hormone, GLP-2, IGF-1

Diagnosis

- ARE—pain, vomiting resolve in 2–6 weeks
  - May have bacterial overgrowth
  - CRP, ESR may be raised
- CRE—ulcerartion, stricture
  - OGD scopy, colonoscopy
  - CT/MRI—enteroclysis
  - Plasma citrulline—a marker for radiation enteritis

Treatment—acute phase

- Antispasmodics
- Opiates—for diarrhea
- Hyperbaric oxygen—increase angiogenesis
- Steroids
- Elemental diet
- Antibiotics
- Cholestyramine—to bind bile salts—reduce diarrhea

Surgery

- In 1–2% cases who received abdominal/pelvic radiation—may require surgery
- A third—(30%) of CRE patients require some surgery
- Most common indication—obstruction—65–80%
- Fistula—10 to 30%, perforation 1–10%, intestinal failure—20%

- If resected—one end of intestine should be from non-irradiated part
- Extensive adhesiolysis should be avoided
- Rigid fixed loops in pelvis—better bypassed
- Perforation areas are resected and anastomosed or exteriorized

14.13 PERITONEUM AND PERITONEAL CAVITY

Peritoneum

- Consists of single sheet of squamous epithelium (flattened polyhedral cells) of mesodermal origin called mesothelium, lying on a thin connective tissue stroma
- Surface area—1 to 1.7 m²—approximately same as total body surface area
- In males—peritoneal cavity is sealed
- Females—open through ostia of fallopian tubes
- Parietal peritoneum covers—abdominal wall surface and inferior surface of diaphragm
- Visceral peritoneum—covers most surfaces of intra peritoneal organs and anterior surface of duodenum, left and right colon, pancreas and kidneys
- Peritoneal cavity is divided into spaces by
  - Eleven ligaments/mesentery
- Coronary, gastrohepatic, hepatoduodenal, falciform, gastrocolic, duodenocolic, gastrosplenic, splenorenal, and phrenicocolic ligaments, transverse mesocolon and SB mesentery

9 Potential Spaces

- Right and left subphrenic, subhepatic, supra and inframesenteric, right and left paracolic gutters, pelvis and lesser space
- These ligaments—direct the flow of fluid inside peritoneum
- Blood supply to visceral peritoneum—from splanchnic blood vessels
- Parietal peritoneum is supplied—by branches of intercostal, subcostal, lumbar, and iliac vessels
- Innervation—parietal peritoneum is richly innervated—can localize pain
  - Visceral—poorly situated around blood vessels—when irritated, pain is poorly localized to the midline

Physiology

- Bidirectional, semipermeable membrane
- Promotes sequestration of bacteria

- Facilitates inflammatory cells from microvasculature into peritoneal cavity
- Normally contains <100 ml of sterile fluid
- Circulation of fluid driven by movement of diaphragm
- Intercellular pores in peritoneum on inferior surface of diaphragm (stomata)—communicate with lymphatic pools in diaphragm and then to subpleural lymphatics and thoracic duct
- Relaxation of diaphragm during exhalation—open stomata (pores) and also negative intrathoracic pressure—draw fluid, particles and bacteria into stomata
- Contraction during inhalation—propels lymph through mediastinal lymph channels into thoracic duct
- Fluid movement is in cephalad direction
- Peritoneum can absorb large volumes of fluid
- Can produce fluid—ascites
- Can produce exudate in peritonitis
- When injured—healing occur not from edges but by development of new mesothelial cells throughout the surface of the defect. So even large defects heal rapidly

Peritoneal Reaction to Infection

- Bacteria are rapidly removed—through diaphragmatic stomata and lymphatics
- Peritoneal macrophages—release proinflammatory mediators—migration of leucocytes into peritoneum from vasculature
- Degranulation of peritoneal mast cells release histamine and cause local vasodilatation and extravasation of protein rich fluid with complement and immunoglobulins into peritoneum
- Protein—opsonize bacteria and cause phagocytosis
- Bacteria are sequestrated in fibrin to form abscess, thus limiting generalized spread

Peritonitis

- Inflammation of peritoneum—usually bacterial
- In DU perforation—fluid run down right paracolic gutter causes pain in RIF—Valentino's syndrome
- Gram negative bacteria produce endotoxin (lipopolysaccharides) and cause release of TNF from host leucocytes—which cause systemic absorption and endotoxic shock

- Clostridial species—produce exotoxins
- Non-GIT cause—From fallopian tube—most common Chlamydia and gonococci cause thinning of cervical mucus and spread of bacteria
- Perihepatitis—from scar tissue on Glisson's capsule-transperitoneal spread of organisms—**Fitz-Hugh-Curtis syndrome**
- Localised peritonitis—body localizes infection by having less peristalsis, adhesions and by omentum
- Guarding—involuntary abdominal wall contraction to protect viscus from examining hand
- Rigidity—involuntary constant contraction of muscles
- Rebound tenderness-on releasing the pressing hand—parietal peritoneal irritation
- Generalized peritonitis—diffuse spread

Chylous Ascites

- Collection of chyle in peritoneum. Seen in
  - Obstruction of cisterna chyli with exudation
  - Injury to retroperitoneal lymphatics
  - Exudation from lymphatics without fistula
- Most common cause in adults—intra-abdominal malignancy obstructing base of mesentery
  - Lymphoma—most common
  - Also in other intra-abdominal malignancies, carcinoid
  - Postop injury in RPLND
- **In children**—congenital
  - Primary lymphatic hypoplasia—lymphedema—chylothorax, ascites

Features

- Ascites, dyspnea
- Low SAAG ascites—<1.1 mg/dl
- Triglycerides 2 to 8 times higher than plasma

For diagnosis—CT, lymphoscintigraphy, lymphangiography

Treatment

- Improve nutrition, treat the cause
- Low fat, high protein diet
- Medium chain TG preferred—directly absorbed by enterocytes into splanchnic blood and in liver converted as FFA and glycerol
  - (Long chain TG metabolites are absorbed through splanchnic vessels as chylomicrons)

- Diuretic
- Paracentesis
- Fibrin glue

Peritonitis

- **Primary**—bacterial, fungal, mycobacterial, chlamydia- in the absence of GI perforation
- **Secondary**—in GI perforation

Spontaneous Bacterial peritonitis (Primary Bacterial Peritonitis)

- Bacterial infection of ascitic fluid in the absence of intra-abdominal source
- Most common in cirrhosis. Also in nephrotic syndrome CCF
- Extremely rare in high protein ascites like malignant
- Most common organisms—*E. coli*, Klebsiella, pneumoniae
  – In children—group A streptococcus, *Staph aureus*
- Seldom produced by anaerobes—because of their incapacity to translocate to intestinal mucosa and the presence of high oxygen in intestinal wall
- Cirrhosis induce impaired GI motility which alter gut flora and translocation of bacteria. Upon impaired clearance produce low protein in ascites which prevent opsonization of bacteria
- **Diagnosis**—paracentesis—peritonitis with low protein ascites
  – >250 neutrophils/cmm
  – Culture—monomicrobial
  – Culture positive in only 40%
  – Most common *E. coli*, Klebsiella, streptococcus
- Broad spectrum antibiotics—third generation cephalosporins—choice
- If responds—no need for repeated paracentesis
- Complications—hepatic failure, hepatorenal syndrome
- SBP—1-year survival—30%, 2-year—20%

Primary Pneumococcal Peritonitis

- In nephrotic syndrome and cirrhosis in children
- Healthy girls affected from vaginal and fallopian infection
- In boys—secondary to respiratory tract infection or middle ear infection
- Pelvic peritonitis—diarrhea and increased frequency of micturition
- Leukocytosis with >90% polymorphs
- After correction of fluid—surgery may be indicated
- Laparotomy—**pus odorless and sticky**—diagnostic

Familial Mediterranean Fever (Periodic Peritonitis)

- Recurrent pain abdomen
- History of previous appendicectomy
- More in Arabs, Jews
- Mutation to MEFV (Mediterranean fever) gene— this gene produces a protein pyrin—expressed in leucocytes
- Children are more affected
- Treatment is mainly conservative
  – Surgery to exclude other causes
- Colchicine used in recurrent attacks

Intraperitoneal Abscess

- Most common site—pelvis—of appendix and fallopian tubes origin and other abdominal causes
- Causes bulging anterior rectal wall
- Pain anorexia, fever with rigors
- May rupture into rectum, which may produce relief.

Treatment

- CT guided aspiration
- Drained into rectum or vagina through posterior fornix
- Rarely suprapubic aspiration—but may contaminate peritoneal cavity
- Laparotomy almost never needed

Left Subphrenic Abscess

- Common cause—stomach operations, tail of pancreas, spleen or splenic flexure infections
- Left subphrenic space is bound on right—falciform
  – Superiorly—diaphragm
  – On left—spleen, gastrosplenic omentum
- Most common cause—pancreatitis
- Perforated gastric ulcer rarely cause in this space— as this space is obliterated by adhesions

Right Subphrenic Space

- Between right lobe of liver and diaphragm
- Posteriorly—right coronary and right triangular ligaments
- Left—falciform ligament
- Common causes—perforated cholecystitis
  – Perforated DU
  – Duodenal cap blow out after gastrectomy

Right Subhepatic Space

- Transversely beneath liver—in Rutherford Morison's pouch
- Bound above by liver, below by transverse colon and hepatic flexure, left by foramen of Winslow, right by right lobe of liver and diaphragm
- Deepest space
- Most common site of subphrenic abscess
- Usually from Appendix, GB, DU
- "Pus somewhere, pus nowhere, pus under the diaphragm"

Treatment

- CT guided aspiration/catheter drainage
- Surgery may be indicated—rarely

Malignancies of Peritoneum

Mesothelioma

- Most common primary malignancy of peritoneum
- Epithelioid type is the most common etiology
- Malignant transformation of squamoid epithelium covering peritoneal cavity
- Exposure to asbestos-causative
- More in males—50s
- Has predilection for pelvic peritoneum
- Causes pain abdomen, intractable ascites and omental mass
- Can involve viscera—obstruction—difficult to differentiate from carcinomatosis from viscera
- Pseudomyxoma peritonei—do not involve other viscera
- Advanced mesothelioma remains confined to abdomen but carcinomatosis can spread
- Can extend locally to pleura more than hematogenous spread

Staging

T1-PCI 1 to 10
T2-PCI 11 to 20
T3-PCI 21 to 30
T4-PCI31 to 39
N1-LNs positive
M1-metastasis

Treatment

- Debulking by CRC advisable in epithelioid type
- Chemo, RT
- HIPEC

Peritoneal Inclusion Cysts

- Caused by accumulation of ovarian fluid—contained by peritoneal adhesions
- For this, need active and functioning ovary and peritoneal adhesions
- Normal peritoneum absorb fluid. This may not happen if the peritoneum is inflamed or in the presence of adhesions
- Only seen in premenopausal ladies with previous history of pelvic/abdominal surgery
- Few mm to cm
- Cysts are non-neoplastic, reactive mesothelial proliferation
- Investigations—USG/MRI

Treatment

- OCP
- Guided drainage
- Surgery to relieve adhesions

Peritoneal Loose Bodies (Peritoneal Mice)

- From appendix epiploica, after axial rotation—necrosis—detachment
- Also in subacute pancreatitis
- Hyaline bodies—contain saponified fat surrounded by fibrin
- Seen in pouch of Douglas or in hernial sac
- Produce no symptoms

Adhesions

- Strands of fibrous tissue formed following surgery-between injured tissues
- After injury-bleeding—increased vascular permeability—extravasation of fibrinogen rich fluid—temporary fibrin matrix—inflammation—cell migration—activation of coagulation cascade—results in thrombin formation—converts fibrinogen to fibrin—in the absence of fibrinolysis—adhesion forms in 5–7 days—matrix gets organized with collagen secretion by fibroblasts
- Fibrinolysis—key whether adhesion persists
- Ischemic tissue loses its ability to breakdown fibrin and inhibits fibrinolysis in adjacent tissues

Adhesions—responsible for 60–70% small bowel obstruction

Adhesion—Prevention

- Reduce ischemic tissue
- Hemostasis
- Preferring laparoscopic surgeries
- Drugs: Aspirin, steroids, vitamin E, anti-clotting agents, antibiotics—not much use
- Barrier method—4% icodextrin solution applied inside abdomen at the time of surgery
- Interseed TC7—mesh-like product—oxidized regenerated cellulose—quickly forms gelatinous mass around healing tissues, and absorbed in 2 weeks

- Hyaluronic acid/carboxymethyl membrane
- All reduce adhesions, but no reduction in small bowel obstruction
- Also increase anastomotic leaks

Mesentery and Omentum

- Omentum—originate from dorsal and ventral midline mesenteries of embryonic gut
- Early stages—alimentary canal a straight tube suspended by dorsal and ventral mesentery-stomach rotates 90 degree on longitudinal axis—lesser curve faces to the right—much of the ventral mesentery resorbs—portion between ligamentum venosum and porta to duodenum and lesser curve persists and forms lesser omentum
- Dorsal mesogastrium forms—greater omentum
- Small bowel mesentery originate from dorsal mesentery—attached form left side of L2 vertebra to RIF anterior to SI joint
- Omental fat is involved in metabolic functions:
  - Increased visceral fat in omentum is an independent risk factor for insulin resistance and high TG levels
  - 'The abdominal policeman'—name by Rutherford Morison
  - Can prevent a hernia—plugs the neck

Omental Cysts

- Uni or multilocular—from congenital or acquired obstruction of lymphatic channels
- Lined by lymphatic endothelium
- Most common in children and young—can undergo torsion, rupture
- Investigations—USG/CT
- Treatment—excision

Omental Torsion/infarction

- Axial twisting of omentum along its long axis
- Causes venous congestion and later arterial occlusion and gangrene
- **Primary**—no cause—involve right side of the omentum
  - Due to anatomic abnormalities—accessory omentum, tongue like projections
  - **Secondary**—due to tumor, adhesion
    - Associated with hernias, cysts, scarring
- More common in men
- Right-sided pain, perotonitis, mass
- DD—appendicitis, cholecystitis, twisted ovarian cyst

- Investigation—CT is the choice
- Surgical resection is the treatment
- **Most common neoplasm of mesentery, peritoneum and omentum—metastasis**
- Most common metastasis to omentum—from ovary
- Most common primary malignant neoplasm of mesentery—lymphoma

Mesenteric Cysts

- Most common non-neoplastic cysts—mesothelial cysts
- Cysts contain chyle or clear fluid
- Occur in SB mesentery—60%
- Colon mesentery—40%
- More in women, age around 45
- One-third occurs in children
- Present with mass, pain
- Cysts caused by disruption of lymphatics in mesentery by trauma, mechanical obstruction or congenital
- Lined by single layer of columnar cells
- 45% found incidentally
- Tillaux's sign—abdominal mass lesion only mobile laterally—whereas in omental cysts they move freely in all directions. Presence of a zone of resonance around the cyst
- CT—cyst with no solid component
- 3% may contain sarcoma which may be solid

Four types

- Chylolymphatic
- Enterogenous
- Urogenital remnant (retroperitoneal)
- Dermoid

Chylolymphatic Cysts

- Most common variety
- From congenitally misplace lymphatic tissue with no efferent communication with lymphatic system
- Most frequently in ileal mesentery
- Lined by thin flat endothelium
- Contain clear lymph or milky chyle
- More often unilocular
- Usually solitary
- Blood supply independent of intestine. So, can be enucleated

Enterogenous Cysts

- From a diverticulum of mesenteric border of intestine—sequestrated from intestinal canal—during embryonic life

- Or from duplication of intestine
- Thicker walled
- Lined by ciliated mucous membrane
- Content mucinous—colorless/yellowish
- Cysts have common blood supply with intestine. So, removal need resection of intestine
- In retroperitoneum
- Attains large size
- DD—hydronephrosis, retroperitoneal STS
- May be unilocular or multilocular
- Many derived from remnants of Wolffian duct-contain clear fluid

Mesenteric Cysts—Management

- Preferred treatment—enucleation
- Sometimes—resection
- Aspiration—very high recurrence
- Internal drainage in large cysts
- Resection in 50–60% of children, one-third of adults
- If cannot be resected—partial excision with marsupialization—in 10%
- If marsupilised—cavity of cyst sclerosed with tincture iodine, 10% glucose or diathermy
- Recurrence—0–13%

Acute Mesenteric Lymphadenitis

- Causes right lower quadrant pain, mesenteric LNE and normal appendix
- Seen in children and young—equal sex
- DD—appendicitis
- In children—due to Yersinia enterocolitica
- Similar to appendicitis—central pain shifts to RIF—tenderness RIF
- Generally WBC count and temperature—normal or slightly high
- Usually discovered on surgery
- Nodes nearest to the attachment of mesentery are largest
- Nodes are not adherent to mesentery

Sclerosing Mesenteritis (Mesenteric Panniculitis)—Mesenteric Lipodystrophy

- Rare inflammatory disease—sclerosing fibrosis, fat necrosis with lipid laden macrophages, calcification
- Early myxomatous later progress to fibrosis
- Marked thickening of mesentery of small intestine—with fat necrosis and discoloration
- Causes, multiple nodules on mesentery—or single mass
- Most common site—root of mesentery—encasing vessels and cause shortening and retraction of

mesentery without causing invasion—can cause venous and lymphatic obstruction
- Rarely affects mesocolon
- Cause—unknown
- Prior surgery, autoimmune, paraneoplastic
  - Mesenteric panniculitis—originally described in Weber-Christian disease, isolated lipodystrophy and mesenteric lipogranuloma

Clinical

- More in men—5th decade
- Most are asymptomatic—incidental
- Pain, obstruction, mass (in >50%)
- DD—carcinomatosis, carcinoid and sarcoma

CT Scan

- Fatty mass from base of mesentery with well-delineated margins which separate from normal mesentery—'tumoral pseudocapsule'
- Normal adipose tissue surrounding mesenteric vessels—'fat ring sign'
- Presence of normal mesenteric vessels coursing through the fatty mass without vascular obstruction or deviation
- Intra-abdominal mass displacing adjacent loops without invading
- Pseudocapsule and fat ring causes 'the misty mesentery'—due to increased mesenteric fat attenuation:
  - Misty mesentery is also seen in pancreatitis, inflammation, cancer infiltration
- Biopsy—to diagnose
- Most resolve spontaneously
- Treated with steroids and anti-inflammatory
- Surgery when in confusion about diagnosis or in obstruction

Internal Hernias

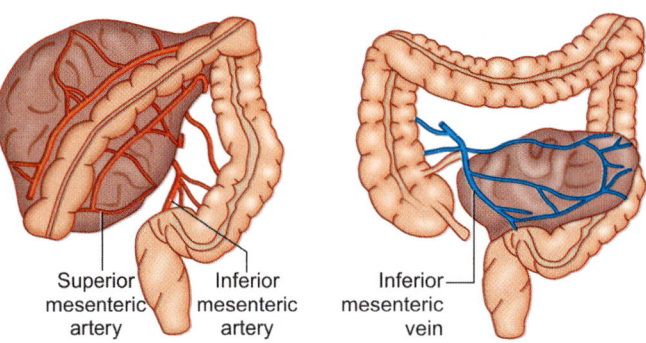

Superior mesenteric artery   Inferior mesenteric artery   Inferior mesenteric vein

Etiology

- Abnormal retroperitoneal fixation of mesentery leads to anomalous positioning of intestine (mesocolic, paraduodenal)
- Abnormally larger internal foramina/fossa—foramen of Winslow, supravesical
- Incomplete mesenteric surfaces with presence of an abnormal opening—mesenteric hernia
- Acquired

Paraduodenal (Congenital Mesocolic)

- Comprise 50% of congenital internal hernias
- Men in 3–4 decades
- Found 75% on left side and 25% rightsided
- Congenital type—SI herniates behind mesocolon—result in abnormal rotation of midgut

Right mesocolic hernia—prearterial limb of midgut loop fails to rotate around SMA

- Most of the SI remains to the right of SMA
- Normal counterclockwise rotation and fixation of cecum and right colon happen to right side and small bowel gets trapped behind mesentery of right colon
- Ileocolic, RCA and MCA—lie within anterior wall of the sac
- SMA—courses along medial border of the neck of hernia
- Hernia happens into a potential space called Waldeyer fossa—this space is normally obliterated as SMA and right colon mesentery fuse with retroperitoneum
  - With the presence of small bowel as hernia—fusion of mesentery does not happen
- In 1%—prearterial segment of small bowel fails to complete >90 degrees of rotation—leaves it on right side and postarterial segment completes 270 degrees rotation.

Left Mesocolic Hernia

- Caused by *in utero* herniation of SI between IMV and posterior parietal attachments of descending colon to retroperitoneum
- IMA and IMV—components of hernial sac
- 75% mesocolic hernia occurs on left side

Herniation into the potential space—*Landzert fossa* which is usually closed at 5–10 weeks of gestation

- In 1–2% space persist
- Splenic flexure, left colon and pancreas are displaced anteriorly
- Afferent limb is formed by D4 and efferent limb can be formed by bowel as distal as ileum

Mesocolic (Paraduodenal) Hernia: Clinical

- Usually present with acute or chronic obstruction
- Barium—small bowel displaced to right or left of abdomen
- CECT—shows the involved vessels

Left Mesocolic Hernia

- CT—clustering of bowel on left upper quadrant, posterior to stomach

Right Mesocolic Hernia: Treatment

- Reduction and obliteration of space
- Incision of lateral peritoneal reflections of right colon—reflection of cecum and right colon to the left—entire gut assumes a position of nonrotation of pre- and post-arterial midgut
- Opening of the neck of hernia by surgical division will injure SMA and SMV and also it will not help to free the herniated bowel

Left Mesocolic Hernia—Treatment

- Incision of peritoneal attachments and adhesions along right side of IMV—reduction of herniated SI from beneath IMV
- Vein is allowed to return to left of base of mesentery
- Neck of hernia is closed by suturing peritoneum adjacent to vein to retroperitoneum
- If dense adhesion—difficulty in reducing contents—IMV and ascending colic artery can be ligated

Mesenteric Hernia

- Intestines herniate through abnormal orifice in mesentery of SI or colon
- Most common location—near ileocolic junction—pericecal
  - Produce intestinal obstruction
- Treatment
- Reduction of hernia and closure of mesenteric defect

Intersigmoid hernia—5% of all congenital internal hernia

Foramen of Winslow Hernia

- Comprise 5–10% congenital IH
- Borders—caudate lobe, IVC, duodenum and hepatoduodenal ligament
- In two-thirds—only small bowel, and in one-third cecum also herniates
- Present with proximal small bowel obstruction and GOO
- Obstruction to CBD causes jaundice
- Bowel may undergo necrosis but may be contained. So may not get peritonitis

- Children draw knees to chest which reduces tension at hepatoduodenal ligament
- **CT**—show bowel loops on right retrogastric space displacing stomach anteriorly
- Surgery—reduction—may injure structures
- If malrotated cecum present—resection—as there may be associated cecal volvulus

Acquired Internal Hernia

- Most common site after liver transplant-through transverse mesocolon
- In Roux en-Y-gastric bypass, the most common indication for reoperation is obstruction at anastomoses
  - Incidence of internal hernia—2 to 8%
  - Weight loss provides more abdominal space and leading to internal hernias

3 Defects in Roux-en-Y Anastomosis

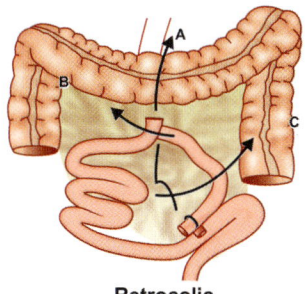 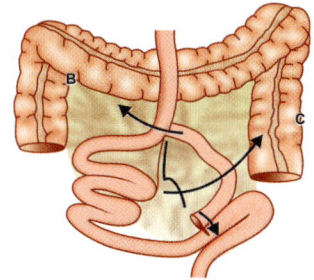

Retrocolic   Antecolic

A—Transverse mesocolic defect
B—Peterson's defect
C—Brolin's defect

- Defect in the mesentery at JJ anastomosis—**Brolin space**
- When Roux limb traverses mesocolon, aperture created by crossing of the two bowel mesenteries—Peterson defect
- Retrocolic passage—space in transverse mesocolon
- Closure of all these defects with nonabsorbable running sutures at index operation indicated
- Retrocolic anastomosis causes more hernias
- Most common hernia in antecolic anastomosis—Peterson hernia

CT Scan

- Localized bowel, swirl sign
- Laparoscopy

Treated by surgical repair

Retroperitoneal Fibrosis

- Chronic inflammation and fibrosis surrounding abdominal aorta and iliac arteries—extend laterally to develop structures like ureters
- First in low lumbar region, then spreads laterally and upwards to encase common iliac vessels, ureter and aorta
- 70%—idiopathic called Ormond disease
- 30%—associated with drugs (ergot, dopaminergic), infections, trauma, bleeding, radiotherapy, metastasis, lymphoma, carcinoid tumor
- Idiopathic—associated with abdominal aorta aneurysms
- Process begins at aortic bifurcation—spreads cephalad
- Usually confined to central and paravertebral space
- In 15%—extends outside retroperitoneum—peri-pancreatic, periduodenal and pelvis
  Other associations
  - Systemic autoimmune disease
  - HLA—DRB1 03
  - Associated with other diseases like Hashimoto, SLE, PSC
  - Also in immunoglobulin related disease
  - Seen in association with Dupuytren's contracture and Peyronie's disease
- More in men, 40–50 years
- Pain abdomen and back, edema limbs
- Varicocele, hydrocele
- Constitutional symptoms precede local symptoms—fever, fatigue
- Lab—azotemia, elevated CRP, ESR
- Ureteral involvement—in 80–100% of cases

CT: Noncontrast

- Homogenous fibrous plaque surrounding lower aorta and iliac vessels
- Isodense with surrounding muscle

MRI of Early Lesion

- High signal intensity in T2 weighted—due to high water content and hypercellularity
- Histology—vary—high cellular content interspersed with bundles of collagen
  - Acellular with more fibrosis

Treatment

- Steroids
- Immunosuppressants—if steroid not responsive mycophenolate, cyclosporine, cyclophosphamide methotrexate, tamoxifen
- Surgery—for ureteral obstruction—urterolysis, intraperitonel transposition and omental wrapping—in refractory cases
- Early—ureteric stenting—steroids
- AAA—repaired if >4.5 to 5 cm

Retroperitoneal Abscess (Psoas)

- Causes—most common these days in rich countries—hematogenous spread from occult source—especially in immunocompromised, IV drug abuse
  - Direct spread from GI/urinary source
  - Earlier—Pott's spine
- Pain, fever
- Hip held in fixed flexion
- Pain on passive extension
- Treatment is CT-guided aspiration

14.14 ABDOMINAL COMPARTMENT SYNDROME AND TEMPORARY ABDOMINAL CLOSURE
Other Names of Open Abdomen

- Laparostomy
- Etappenlavage

Definition

- Abdomen is not closed primarily or partially closed in order to prepare for a later definitive closure
- First by ogilvie—used a piece of canvas—1940s
- A concept that emerged out of previous failures to manage abdomens that either could not be closed or should not be closed
- In infected abdomen
- Trauma
- Surgeon related/suboptimal circumstances

Goal

- Save the life by first surgery
- Closure planned when patient is stabilized
- To close the fascia as soon as possible
- Ideally within 8 days
- Risk of abdominal compartment syndrome, Inflammation and edema—may delay closure

Primary Aim

- Maximize tissue perfusion
- Minimize intra-abdominal complications
- Meticulous care of bowel
- Cover of the bowel from environment
- Reduce mortality

Indications for Temporary Abdominal Closure

- Damage control
  - Severe hemorrhage
  - Lethal triad—acidosis, hypothermia, coagulopathy
- Intra-abdominal hypertension (IAH) and abdominal compartment syndrome (ACS)
- Questionable visceral viability
- Severe intra-abdominal sepsis

Damage Control Surgery (DCS)

- In severe trauma, sepsis and infarction
- To limit the surgery to the minimum
- Control hemorrhage and contamination
- Minimum procedure done and patient is shifted to ICU
- Treat and stabilize lethal triad
- After optimization—reoperation—definitive procedure
- Usually within 24–72 hours

IAH and ACS

- Intra-abdominal pressure is a function of
  - Intra-abdomen contents
  - Abdominal wall dispensability (wall musculature and diaphragm)
- Normal IAP 0–5 mm Hg

IAH

- Sustained or repeated elevation of IAP >12 mm Hg
  - 3 measurements 4–6 hours apart
  - Measured in a relaxed patient at the end of expiration
- Directly related to the inflammatory/trauma response
- Leads to significant decrease in organ perfusion
- Decrease in splanchnic circulation and ACS with organ dysfunction

ACS (Abdominal Compartment Syndrome)

- Sustained IAP >20 mm Hg
- With or without abdominal perfusion pressure <50 mm Hg

- At least 3 values are taken 1–3 hours apart
- Associated with one or more organ failures not present previously
- Primary, secondary and tertiary

Primary ACS Causes

- Caused by intra-abdominal pathology
- Closure of abdomen in adverse conditions
- In trauma, after DCS
- Ileus, edema, bleeding
- Coagulopathy, capillary leak, and due to abdominal packing
- Massive fluid resuscitation
- Transfusion
- Reduction of large hernia
- Pregnancy, large tumors

Secondary ACS

- ACS in the absence of intra-abdominal pathology or intervention

Causes

- Iatrogenic
- Shock—large volume of fluid
- Burns after fluid management
- Critically ill, hypothermic
- Sepsis
- Shock and ischemia—increased capillary permeability—edema, ascites

Tertiary ACS

- Following prophylactic attempts like medical and surgical interventions to prevent primary or secondary AC

ACS—Pathophysiology

System	Effect	Manifestations
Renal	Renal vein compression Cortical arteriolar compression	Oliguria Rising creatinine
Pulmonary	Upward pressure on diaphragm Decreased compliance and functional residual capacity Increased airway resistance	Hypoxia Hypercarbia Elevated airway pressure Decreased tidal volume
Cardio-vascular	Decreased venous return Increased afterload	Decreased cardiac output
Cerebral	Increased intrathoracic pressure with decreased cerebral venous outflow	Elevated intracranial pressure
Splanchnic	Decreased perfusion of liver and intestine	Metabolic acidosis Bowel ischemia

Diagnosis

- Similar features in primary and secondary
- Diagnosis of secondary is often missed
- Features of hypoxia, difficulty in ventilation
- Oliguria, CO reduced
- CVP, PCWP elevated
- Pulmonary failure, cardiac failure—death
- Urinary bladder pressure measurement
  - Using Foley's—instill 50 ml saline, clamp, insert needle and measure
  - Using 3 way Foley—inject saline into one—measure through the other
  - Serially connect a Foley's into a stopcock and transducer
- IVC pressure
- Gastric/rectal pressure

- **Grade 1:** IAP 10–15 cm water
- **Grade 2:** IAP 16–25 cm water
- **Grade 3:** IAP 26–35 cm water
- **Grade 4:** IAP >36 cm water

- 1 mm Hg = 1.36 cm of H_2O

Treatment

- High index of suspicion
- Careful fluid resuscitation
- Grade 1 and 2—careful observation
  - Muscle relaxants, sedation
  - Aspiration/drainage of fluid
- Grade 3 and 4—may need decompression
- In raised intracranial pressure with ACS—decompression is indicated
- Following decompression—sudden reduction in preload—toxins release, which can result in cardiac arrest

Temporary Abdominal Closure
Ideal TAC Technique

- Easy to use and apply
- Tension free
- Protect abdominal contents
- Prevent evisceration
- Preserve skin/fascia
- Quantify third space fluid loss
- Minimize loss of abdominal domain
- Lower infection
- Keep patient dry
- Cost effective

Dynamic Abdominal Visceral Coverage
- Artificial burr

Tension Free, Atraumatic Abdominal Visceral Coverage
- VAC
- Vacuum pack

Management of Open Abdomen
- General management
- Wound management
- Definitive wound closure

General
- IV Fluids
- Prevent hypothermia
- Analgesia/sedation
- Nutrition—enteral/parentetral
- Enteroclysis/fistuloclysis
- Intraperitoneal lavage and fluid therapy

Hypothermia—Management
- Passive methods to keep temperature >37 degree C
  - Limbs into plastic bags
  - Air warmers on ventillators
  - Air warming blankets
  - Proper wound managing systems
- Active methods
  - Infusion of warm fluids
  - Warm saline bladder irrigation
  - Warm gastric lavage

Wound Management
- Nonadherent dressings
- Secondary dressings for absorption of fluids
- Optimizing for definitive closure
- Dressings are done in OT
- Simple approximation of skin
- Bogota bag
  - Sterile plastic bag
  - Can visualize bowel
  - Can lose abdominal domain
  - Abdominal space obliterated
- SSG done after granulation tissue is formed
- Negative Pressure Wound Therapy
  - Locally prepared—suction
  - Commercial (–125 mm) Hg
- Allow to granulate later SSG and to develop incisional hernia which is managed later

Complications
- Infection—treated by
  - Dressings done in OT
  - Wound debridement
  - Antibiotics
- Bleeding
- Fistula formation

Definitive Closure
Delayed Primary
- Should be by day 10

Secondary Closure
- Staged repair using flaps
- Meticulous surgical job
- Sharp dissection
- Preserve vascularity
- Done by senior surgeon
- CT scan for evaluation
- Consider
  - Bowel edema,
  - Contamination
  - Poor tissue strength/necrosis

Closure
- Skin cover
  - Allow granulation tissue to form over bowel—SSG
  - Ventral hernia formed is managed later
- Absorbable mesh/biological
  - Bridge repair
  - SSG
  - Biological mesh is prepared from dermal matrix which provides the scaffold. May not provide adequate wound strength
- Component separation technique
- Cavity abdominal reapproximation anchor closure system (ABRA)

14.15 PERITONEAL CARCINOMATOSIS AND PMP
- Shedding, implantation and dissemination of a tumor, localized or widespread to peritoneum
- Due to intracavitary dissemination of tumor

Historical background: First reported by a gynecologist, R. Werth, in 1884

- Unusual reaction of the peritoneum to a jelly-like substance in relation to an ovarian neoplasm.
- In the first quarter of the 20th century, Naeslund suggested
  - Simultaneous occurrence of an appendiceal mucocele and cystadenoma of the ovary with PMP

- At the end of the century, new treatment strategy emerged, pioneered by **Sugarbaker**
- Combination of extensive surgery with intra-peritoneal chemotherapy

Definition—PMP (Pseudomyxoma Peritonei)

- A condition in which tumour perforation has seeded the peritoneum with mucinous tumour cells.
- Mucinous ascites arising from a ruptured ovarian or appendiceal adenocarcinoma

Epidemiology

- 40–50 years of age
- Incidence—1–2/million/year
- Predominance of women—2 to 3 times
- Approximately 10% epithelial appendiceal neoplasm develop PMP
- 20% in mucinous appendiceal neoplasms

Pathology

Origin

- Appendix, generally mucinous adenoma—most common
- Colon, stomach, pancreas, ovary, and urachus
- The primary tumor consists
  - Mucinous cystadenoma
  - Cystadenocarcinoma with low malignant potential
- PMP—does not give rise to extra-abdominal metastasis—cause symptoms due to tumor bulk

Histology

Ronnett, et al. Proposed Three Subtypes

- Disseminated peritoneal adenomucinosis (DPAM)
- Peritoneal mucinous adenocarcinoma (PMCA)
- Intermediate type PMP (PMCA-I)

Clinical

Disseminated Peritoneal Adenomucinosis (DPAM)

Low-grade lesion

- Abundant extracellular mucin
- Lack of cytological atypia or mitotic activity
- Usually from mucinous neoplasms of the appendix
- Good prognosis

Peritoneal Mucinous Adenocarcinoma (PMCA)

- High-grade metastatic adenocarcinoma
- Abundant mucinous epithelium with architectural and cytologic features of carcinoma
- Derived from the appendix and colon

Intermediate Type PMP (PMCA-I)

- Predominant features of DPAM
- Focal areas of PMCA
- Prognosis between that of DPAM and PCMA

Classification of pseudomyxoma peritonei

Acellular mucin

Low-grade mucinous carcinoma peritonei

High-grade mucinous carcinoma peritonei

High-grade mucinous carcinoma peritonei with signet ring cells

---

Clinical Presentation

- 30 to 50% patients have "Jelly belly" (abdominal distension), global deterioration
- Intestinal obstruction associated with compressing tumor and ascites which produce nonshifting dullness
- 50 to 80% patients—local symptoms, reflecting the location of the primary or metastatic tumor
  - Appendicitis-like symptoms
- Development of new hernia

Laboratory Tests and Immunohistochemical Markers

- CA-125
  - Gynecological marker to exclude an ovarian neoplasm
  - Not widely used as a tumor marker
  - Elevated in benign or inflammatory diseases
  - Sensitivity—60%
- Cytokeratin (CK) 20, CEA, and CDX-2—+ve in primary tumors of colorectal or appendiceal origin
- CK 7—negative in appendiceal tumors in 70%
- CK7, WT-1, PAX 8,—+ve in primary tumors of ovarian origin
- IL-9 +ve in 95% pts
- CEA elevation—55 to 75% of pts
- CA 19–9 elevation—60% to 68% of pts

Tumor Assessment

- USG abdomen:
  - Useful in appendiceal mucocele or PMP
  - Usually in combination with CT

- Sparse cellular density of both low and high grade lesions limits the benefits of FNAC
- CT scan with oral, rectal, and IV contrast
  - Gold standard and diagnostic
  - Mucinous ascites
  - Higher density (5 to 20 HU) compared to normal ascites
  - Low attenuation of soft tissue masses
  - Rim-like calcifications
  - Septae
- PET CT—to assess tumor burden—in carcinomatosis

Sugarbaker Peritoneal Cancer Index (PCI)

- Used in decision-making process as abdomen is explored
- Size of intra-peritoneal nodules must be assessed
- Lesion size score (LS) is used
  - LS 0—No visualization of malignant deposits in particular abdomino-pelvic region
  - LS 1—Nodules <0.5 cm
  - LS 2—Nodules 0.5–5 cm
  - LS 3—Nodules >5 cm
- Regions—13
  - Abdomino-pelvic regions—9

  Small bowel regions—4
- Maximum score—39 (13 × 3)

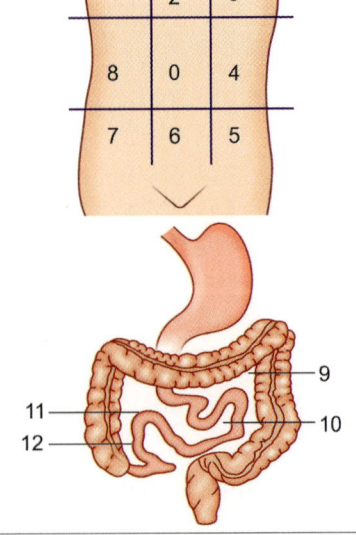

Peritoneal Cancer Index

Regions
0. Central
1. Right upper
2. Epigastrium
3. Left upper
4. Left flank
5. Left lower
6. Pelvis
7. Right lower
8. Right flank
9. Upper jejunum
10. Lower jejunum
11. Upper ileum
12. Lower ileum

Regions
0. No tumor
1. Tumor up to 0.5 cm
2. Tumor up to 5
3. Tumor >5 cm

Gilly's Classification in PC

- Stage 0—No lesion (positive cytology)
- Stage 1—Malignant granulations <5 mm, localized to one part in abdomen
- Stage 2—<5 mm, diffuse to whole abdomen
- Stage 3—Localized/diffuse 5 mm to 2 cm
- Stage 4—Localized or diffuse >2 cm
- Findings recorded before and after surgery

Simplified Preoperative Assessment For Appendix Tumor (SPAAT)

- Based on preoperative CT scan, five regions in abdomen are considered
- Score range: 0–7
- Score more than 3 indicate poor prognosis
- Shortening of small bowel injury is called 'cauliflowering' of bowel

Treatment

- Traditional surgical treatment
  - Consists of
  - Cytoreductive surgery
    - □ Removal of all mucinous ascites
- Long-term survival could be achieved by surgery alone
- Combined modality treatment
  - Introduced in the 1990s by Sugarbaker
  - Aims at achieving cure or at least long-term remission

Aggressive Cytoreductive Surgery (CRS)

- Removal of peritoneum from all five regions
  - Right and left hemidiaphragm
  - Right and left paracolic gutters
  - Pelvis
- Omentectomy
- Removal of involved mesentery—resections Gastrectomy, splenectomy, anterior resection, sigmoidectomy, colectomy, cholecystectomy
- Resection of internal gynaecological organs
- Glissonial capsule removal
- CC 0—complete cyto reduction—the goal
- CC 1—residual tumor <2.5 mm
- CC 2—residual nodule 2.5 mm to 2.5 cm
- CC 3—residual nodules >2.5 cm

Hyperthermic Intraperitoneal Chemotherapy (HIPEC)

- Direct delivery into the peritoneal cavity
- Permits high concentrations of drugs directly toward the tumor deposits
- Without important systemic side effects
- Hyperthermia enhance the penetration of cytostatic drugs and synergism with various cytostatic drugs
- Effective only in minimal residual macroscopic disease because of the limited penetration depth of drugs
- For HIPEC to be effective—CRS residual tumor size should be <2 mm

3 Techniques

- Open (coliseum technique)
- Semiclosed—plastic sheet cover
- Closed—temperature maintenance is good, but drug distribution is not achievable
- If the chemotherapeutic agent is oxaliplatin—drug perfusion is for 30 minutes
- If Mitomycin C, needs—90 minutes
- Also give IV chemotherapy called bidirectional chemotherapy
- After HIPEC, drains are introduced to all 5 peritonectomy regions—for early postop chemotherapy
- HIPEC should be performed intra-operatively before anastomoses, to maximize uniform drug distribution and tumor exposure
- In h/o prior surgery, adhesiolysis should be performed to prevent nonuniform drug distribution
- Mitomycin—C given as an intraperitoneal drug, either as single drug or in combination—12 mg/m^2
- Doxorubicin—15 mg/m^2
- Cisplatin—50 mg/m^2
- Duration for perfusion
  - 41C × 90 min
  - 43C × 30–40 min
  - 42C × 60 min

Rationale for Hyperthermia

- Ideally 42–43 degree C
- Synergesic effect of heat and chemo
- Heat induces DNA damage, protein denaturation, inhibition of oxidative metabolism
- Causes vasodilation and oxygen delivery to the tumor, thereby increasing delivery and effect of chemotherapy
- Heat—reduce interstitial pressure—increase cytotoxicity

Neoadjuvant IP and IV Chemo

- Surgery is done after 3–4 cycles

Early Postop IP Chemo (EPIC)

- Chemotherapy is given through drain tubes—post-op days 1 to 5
- Drugs given for 1 hour and all drains closed for next 23 hours changing the position of patient to mix—after this drugs are allowed to flow out over 1 hour—repeated over next 4 days

Indications for CRS and HIPEC

- Pseudomyxoma
- Mesothelioma
- CRC with peritoneal seeding
- Perforated CRC
- Recurrent CRC with ovary metastasis
- Recurrent ovary cancer
- Malignant ascites

Contraindications

- Poor general condition
- Extraperitoneal metastasis
- Diffuse PC
- Extensive liver metastasis (relative)
- Ureteric and biliary obstruction
- Extensive SI and mesentery involvement
- Extensive hepatoduodenal ligament involvement

Complications

- Incidence—35–45%
- Chemotherapy toxicity to kidneys, bone marrow, liver, lungs—3–5%
- Organ damage secondary to hyperthermia
- Surgical complications—26–30%
- Small bowel fistula
- Mortality—0–6%

14.16 ABDOMINAL TUBERCULOSIS

- Chronic granulomatous disease
- *M. tuberculosis*—microaerophilic bacteria
- Yakshma = weakness, in vedas
- Tubercula, latin = small lump
- 24, March, 1882: Robert Koch discovered *M. tuberculosis*
- India—the largest share in TB—25%—then—China—South Africa

- Extrapulmonary TB—16–20% in immunocompetent
  - 45–50% in HIV patients

Extrapulmonary TB (EPTB)

- Abdominal TB—6th among EPTB
- Lymphatic—gut—skeletal—miliary—meningeal—abdominal in that order
- Abdominal TB comprises 10% of EPTB **pathophysiology**
- **Hematogenous** from active PTB or miliary TB—bacilli spread through portal circulation or abdominal arteries
  - Mainly affects solid organs—spleen, liver, pancreas, kidney, peritoneum
- **Ingestion** of infected sputum from PTB—mucosal layer of GIT infected in areas of stasis—lodge in submucosal lymphoid tissue—form epithelioid tubercles—granulomatous inflammation—coagulative and liquefactive necrosis—cheesy material (caseous necrosis)—bursts out—ulcerate mucosa and into deeper layers—bacilli later affects LN and peritoneum
- **Direct spread**
  - From adjacent organs like fallopian tubes, vertebrae
  - Mainly affects peritoneum and LN
- **Lymphatic route** to LN
- Most common site involved in ATB: Peritoneum (60%)
  - GIT (40%), mesenteric LN: 25%

GIT TB

Esophageal TB

- 0.3 to 1%
- From lymphatic spread, from LNs or hematogenous from endobronchial TB
- Most common site—midesophagus, due to proximity to LNs
- Presentation similar to malignancy
- Can develop traction diverticulum

Gastroduodenal TB

- Constitute 2–3 %
- Acidic juice, thick mucosa, less number of lymphatic tissue and rapid transit—prevent gastroduodenal TB
- Most common sites—distal stomach and D3
- Intrinsic form present as gastric ulcer
- Extrinsic form present with perigastric LNs and GOO—more common

Ileocecal TB

- Most common site of GIT TB—40–90%, due to
  - Stasis near IC valve, narrow lumen
  - Abundant lymphatic tissue
  - Favourable pH
  - High absorption and close contact of infective agent

GIT TB: 3 Types

- Ulcerative—ulcer develops early due to rupture of submucosal LN
  - Ulcer may be linear, transverse or circumferential
  - Pain, diarrhea, bleeding
- Hypertrophic/ulcerohypertrophic
  - Due to good immune response of the host
  - Enlarged LNs and hypertrophic mucosa
  - Presents as lump
- Fibrous stricture (sclerotic)
  - Healing stage
  - Pain, obstruction—'napkin ring' stricture

Clinical Features

- Most common pain abdomen—70–90%
  - Fever 40–70%
- One-third presents acutely—obstruction, perforation

Colorectal TB

- Second most common site of GIT TB—
- Cecum—most common—then sigmoid
- Linear or transverse ulcers cause narrowing

Peritoneal TB

- Most common ATB
- 1–6% of all EPTB
- Affected age 3–4 decades, women—spread from fallopian tubes
  - Also hematogenous and lymphatic

3 Types

Gross ascitic or wet type

- Free fluid or loculated or encysted
- Fluid with high protein and lymphocytes

Fixed fibrotic or plastic type

- Involves mesentery or omentum—bands and matted bowel loops
- Obstruction

- Sclerosing encapsulating peritonitis (abdominal cocoon)
  - Partial type—membranous sac covering small bowel
    □ Complete type—covers small bowel, colon and solid organs causing obstruction and mass

Purulent form—more common in females

Solid organ TB

- Spread—hematogenous
- In liver causes hepatitis—diagnosed by biopsy
- Pancreas TB is rare

LN TB

- Mesenteric—tabes mesenterica
- Omental and retroperitoneal
- Most common type of ATB in children and young
- Produce pain weight loss, mass abdomen

Clinical Features

- General—fever, weight loss, malaise
- Abdominal—pain distension
  - Gola formation—moving ball of wind
  - Mass

Diagnosis

- Definitive diagnosis by demonstration of *M. tuberculosis* by microbiologic, histologic or molecular methods

Mantoux Test

- Tuberculin test by Koch in 1890
- In 1912 Charles Mantoux—intradermal injection of antigen
- Purified protein derivative extracted from cultures of *M. tuberculosis*
- 5 tuberculin unit injected intradermally on volar aspect of forearm—interpreted after 48–72 hours
- In immunosuppressed >5 mm—significant
- In immunocompetent >10 mm is significant
- Low specificity
- Low or no value in diagnosis

Diagnosis

Interferon-gamma Release Assay (IGRA)—Quanti FERON-TB Gold

- Detects interferon gamma response by T lymphocytes, when stimulated by specific proteins like ESAT-6 (Early Secreted antigenic target of 6 kDa) and CFP-10 (culture filtrate protein 10)
- No cross reactivity to other mycobacteria—more specific

- No role in endemic areas—does not differentiate between latent and active disease

Mycobacterial Culture

- Gold standard in peritoneal and solid organ TB
- Takes a long time

Molecular Methods

Nucleic Acid Amplification Tests (NAAT) Like PCR

- Shock treatment (acute temperature changes)—breaks the cell wall
- Chemical lysis
- DNA purification
- Then the pathogen's DNA specific region is amplified and detected by agarose gel electrophoresis
- Effective in paucibacillary (10 bacilli/ml)

Reverse Transcriptase PCR (RT-PCR)

- Detects m-RNA
- Can differentiate viable from non-viable *M. tuberculosis*, as m-RNA decompose very fast in dead cell
- Used for both diagnosis and monitoring drug resistance

FISH

- Uses oligonucleotide probe labelled with fluorophore
- More sensitive than PCR

Xpert *M. tuberculosis* (detection of rifampicin resistance—MTB/RIF)
- Targets rpoB gene, critical in identifying *M. tuberculosis* mutations related to rifampicin resistance

Immuno PCR

- Ultra sensitive assay—detects antigens
- Combines ELISA with NAA of PCR
- Very accurate—but costly

Radiology

X-ray may show

- Obstruction
- Perforation

Barium Follow Through

- **Chicken intestine**—hypersegmentation of barium due to increased peristalsis in the intestine with ulceration and inflammations
- **Hour-glass stenosis**—multiple strictures and dilated loops
- **Fleischners or inverted umbrella sign**—with wide open ileocecal valve with thickened loops and narrow terminal ileum

- **Goose neck deformity**—retracted, fibrosed cecum and dilated terminal ileum and loss of i-c angle
- **Purse string stenosis**—localized stenosis near i-c valve with smooth cecum and distended terminal ileum
- **Stierlin sign**—due to acute on chronic inflammation. Affected segment does not retain barium, with normal appearance of columns on either side—also in CD
- **String sign**—stricture, also seen in CD
- **Pulled-up cecum**

Intestinal TB Barium Studies

Group 1: Highly suggestive of TB if one or more is seen

- Ileocecal valve deformed with dilated ileum
- Contracted caecum with abnormal ileocecal valve or terminal ileum
- Ascending colon stricture with shortening or involvement of ileocecal region

Group 2: Suggestive of intestinal TB if one or more is seen

- Contracted caecum
- Ulceration or narrowing of terminal ileum
- Multiple narrowing of small bowel
- Stricture of ascending colon

Group 3: Non-specific changes

Group 4: Normal study

CT Scan

- Can detect both intra and extraluminal pathology
- Wall thickening
- CECT—peripheral enhancement of LN
  - LN involvement of mesenteric, upper paraaortic and omental region—common
  - Lower paraaortic LNE—seen more in lymphoma
- CT enteroclysis
- CECT in—peritoneal TB—smooth, mildly thickened
  - In carcinomatosis—nodular, irregular thickening of peritoneum

USG

- Ascites/loculated
- LNE—matted—caseation with calcification—distinguishes from lymphoma and malignancy
- Bowel wall thickening
- Pseudokidney sign—I-C complex with pulled-up cecum

Endoscopy/Biopsy

- Ulcerative/ulceroproliferative—dd malignancy
- Histology—granuloma seen only in LN not on walls—vs CD seen on walls
- Double balloon endoscopy and capsule endoscopy TB—multiple 1–2 cm transverse/oblique ulcers with necrotic base

Others

- FNAC/EUS-FNAC
- Ascites—low SAAG (<1.1 g/L)
- AFB in ascites smear positive in <3%
- AFB culture of ascites—positive in one-fifth (20%)
- ADA (adenosinedeaminase)—raised in TB ascites >36 IU/L
- Ascitic gamma interferon with ADA
- Multiplex PCR with antigens IS6110 and MPB64

Laparoscopy

- Tubercles with caseation
- Fibrous bands extending from parietal to visceral peritoneum—**stalactic** bands

Histopathology

- Central caseous necrosis
- Granulomatous inflammation >400 micrometer with macrophages, Langhans giant cells (50–80%)
- AFB staining in 5–10%
- Granulomas in CD—noncaseating, non-confluent and <200 micrometer

Paustian's Criteria for Diagnosis of Abdominal TB

- Any of the 4 criteria—establishes diagnosis
  1. Histology of specimen shows tubercle with granuloma
  2. Operative findings suggestive of TB. Mesenteric LN with caseation
  3. AFB staining positive
  4. Tissue culture for Mycobacteria
- Logan modified—added response to ATT

Diagnostic method	Time taken for final outcome
Interferon-gamma release assay	24 hrs
Ziehl-Neelsen staining	30 mins
Lowenstein-Jensen culture	6–8 weeks
BACTEC	6–12 days
Nitrate reductase assay	15–18 days
Thin layer agar culture	15–18 days

TREATMENT

- Mainly medical
- Surgery for complications
- ATT-2 months of Rif, INH, Pyrazinamide, Ethambutol followed by 4 months of Rif and INH
- Some advice 9–12 months
- In HIV added ART irrespective of CD4 count—Efavirenz added
- Liver failure occurs in 2nd week—in INH and Rif combination if so stop them and start second line drugs—Fluoroquinolones, Amikacin with Ethambutol and Streptomicin

Role of Surgery

- GOO-GJ preferred—not pyloroplasty
  - Vagotomy if bleeding

Ileocecal and SI TB

3 Types

- **Bypass**—when cannot be resected—but forms blind loop
- **Stricturoplasty**
  - Possible in up to 50% luminal narrowing
  - In multiple strictures and single short stricture
  - In long stricture >10 cm or multiple short strictures over a short segment—resection is preferred
- **Radical or curative**—resection right hemicolectomy

New Modalities

- New drugs
- Delamanid, Bedaquiline in MDR, PA-824
- Oxazolidinones (cycloserine, linezolid)

New Delivery Systems

- **Nanotechnology**—'nanoparticle' = colloidal particles size <1 micrometer
- **Nano dispersion/nano emulsions**—thermodynamically stable oil in water dispersions
- **Nanosuspension**—submicron colloidal dispersions of pure drugs stabilized with surfactants. Reduction in size—increases solubility and bioavailability
- **Niosomes**—thermodynamically stable liposome like vesicles. Increase bioavailability

Anorectal and Perianal TB

- Anal TB—0.8% of cases
  - Pathogenesis

- Ingestion
- Hematogenous
- Direct spread
- Through lymphatics
- Rectal TB—most common manifestation—Hematochezia (85%), constitutional, constipation
- Anal TB—most common—multiple fistula
- Massive bleeding is rare in ATB—due to obliterative endarteritis

Anorectal and Perianal TB: Classification

Type of lesion	TB type	Manifestations
Ulcerative	Pulmonary/GI	Superficial ulceration, haemorrhagic base, well-defined boundaries
Verrucous	M. bovis	Wart, haemorrhoidal nodule, abscess, fistula
Lupoid TB	TB anywhere in body	Nodule which turns into clean cut ulcer, mucopurulent discharge
Miliary	Disseminated TB	Involves any organ

Acid Fast Smear

- Detects only when 10^5 bacilli per ml present
- Efficacy increased by concentration techniques like Petroff's method and staining with Auramine Ofluorescent dye using LED
- **Diagnosis**
- CT/MRI
  - Multiple fistula
  - Extra sphincteric tracts
  - LNE
  - Osteomyelitis

14.17 MESENTERIC ISCHEMIA
Definition

Interruption to the normal circulation to the bowel resulting in dysfunction and sometimes infarction

- Not a common etiology for abdominal pain
- Often unrecognized or misdiagnosed
- Delay could be critical

History

- One of the earliest descriptions—Elliott in 1895
- Association between SMA and ischemia—Councilman, 1894

- 1951-Klass—first report of surgical embolectomy for AMI
- 1958-Derrick—first use of surgical bypass in CMI
- Later decades focus shifted to revascularization
- Catheter directed techniques
- Development of angiography—USG/Doppler—CTA
- Focus on early diagnosis

Three main arteries: CA, SMA, IMA
- CA-origin at T12-L1 level at an acute angle from aorta
  - Largest branch—splenic artery
- SMA at L1 level
- IMA at L3 level

Variants of Celiac Axis

- Common celio-mesenteric artery variant seen in 1%
- Replaced RHA—from SMA in 20% from GDA in 2%, celiac axis in 1%
- Replaced LHA—from LGA in 18%, GDA in 1%, celiac trunk in 2%

SMA

- Supplies entire small bowel except D1
- First branch—inferior pancreaticoduodenal artery
- Second branch—middle colic artery
- 4–6 jejunal branches and 10–14 ileal branches
- Final branch—ileocolic artery—appendicular artery arises from inferior branch

IMA

- Critical point of Griffith at splenic flexure between LCA and SMA branches
- Sudek's point at rectosigmoid
- Splanchnic organs receive 25% (10–35%) of cardiac output and have 25% of total blood volume at rest

SMV

- Formed by confluence of—ileocolic vein (receives appendiceal vein, distal ileal, and right colic veins), segmental ileal and jejunal veins and gastrocolic trunk—anterior to head of pancreas
- Gastrocolic trunk drains—right gastroepiploic, middle colic, anterior superior pancreaticoduodenal veins
- Splenic veins are joined by IMV, left gastric vein, short gastric veins, pancreatic veins, and left gastroepiploic vein—joins SMV under the neck of pancreas to form portal vein

Micro Circulation

- Mucosal flow is 3 times as that of muscle layer
- Shunting blood away from mucosa occurs with
  - Sympathetic tone
  - Angiotensin II
  - High pH
  - High oxygen tension

'Metabolic' theory and *'Muscular'* theory of mesenteric ischemia

Metabolic Theory

- High metabolic demand generates anaerobic metabolites which relax arteriolar smooth muscle lead to delivery of high volumes
- Low pH due to anaerobic environment lead to better oxygen delivery

Muscular Theory

- Transmural arteriolar pressure modulates arteriolar spasm
- Low wall tension (low flow) lead to low arteriolar muscular tone and less spasm and more blood delivery
- High arteriolar wall tension (high flow states) leads to more muscular tone and less delivery of blood
- Digoxin and alfa agonists instigate spasm

Increases intestinal blood flow:
- Food intake
- Digested food
- Osmolality >1500 mOsm/L
- Gut pH <2.5
- Bile acids—in ileum
- Proteins
- Glucose
- Long chain fatty acid—most potent

Mesenteric Ischemia
Classification

- Acute mesenteric ischemia (AMI)
  - Arterial
    - Embolus (EAMI)
    - Thrombosis (TAMI)
  - Venous thrombosis (VAMI)
- Nonocclusive mesenteric ischemia (NOMI)
- Chronic mesenteric ischemia (CMI)
- Rare causes

  Fibromuscular dysplasia

Median Arcuate Ligament Syndrome
 – Takayasu's arteritis

EAMI and TAMI (Embolic and Thrombotic AMI)

- Emboli and acute on chronic thrombi—most common pathologies
  - EAMI—most common cause
- Elderly
- More common in males
- Cardiac embolization—most common cause
  - AF
  - PostMI
  - Ventricular/valvular thrombus
  - Rarely arterial—arterial emboli
- Mostly lodge at SMA—due to its acute origin and high flow states
- Females have more acute angle of origin of SMA from aorta
- 50% emboli lodge distal to origin of middle colic artery so that ischemia isolated to jejunum, ileum and ascending colon—spares duodenum and proximal jejunum

TAMI

- Account for 50%
- Typically seen in elderly women
- With known POVD
- H/o claudication, carotid disease
- Can occur during hypotension and following catheter manipulation

Clinical Features

- Sudden onset periumbilical pain
- Preceded by palpitations, arrhythmias, MI, catheterization
- Urge to defecate
- Loose stools
- Agitated/anxious
- May have history of AF
- Flat, scaphoid abdomen
- Usually nontender
- Pain out of proportion to signs
- Peritoneal signs appear once gangrene/perforation
- Can have multiple emboli—
  - Look for other pulses

Diagnosis

- Triad
  - New onset AF
  - Severe pain abdomen
  - Pain out of proportion to signs

- Lab
  - Acidosis
  - Elevated lactate—in late stages
  - Elevated amylase
  - intestinal fatty acid binding protein (IFABP)
  - Alfa-glutathione S-transferase
- X-ray
  - Thumb printing, free air, in perforation
- Duplex ultrasound
  - Needs experience
  - Obesity, bowel gas—obscure the view
- Conventional angiography
  - Gold standard—but used only if intervention is needed
  - Not routinely used
  - Has specific therapeutic uses

CT Features of AMI

CTA—is the choice—the features
- Bowel wall edema
- Thinning of the wall
- Low attenuation of the wall
- Dilatation of the wall
- Artery/vein obstruction
- Fat stranding of mesentery
- Ascites
- Pneumatosis intestinalis
- Air in veins—pneumatosis portalis

Management

- Early diagnosis and treatment
- Delay causes morbidity and mortality
- Younger the age the better
- AMI usually single vessel—SMA
- Patients may have multisystem problems and there is no time to correct those

Aim

- Open surgery—standard of care
- Adequate revascularization/bowel viability
- Remove all frankly ischemic bowel
- Second look laparotomy/laparoscopy

Embolus—Therapy

- Usually lodge at take-off of right colic artery
- Duodenum and proximal jejunum—well perfused
- SMA pulse disappears 5–8 cm from origin
- Embolectomy is the choice
  - Expose the SMA
  - Heparin
  - Transverse arteriotomy

– Fogarty catheter is used

– Repair the arteriotomy

– Hemostasis

• Doppler to assess vascularity

Embolus-Therapy

Catheter Directed

• If no indication for laparotomy

• Lytic therapy and papaverine

• Takes time to clear the artery

Acute Thrombosis: Treatment

• *SMA obstruction—flush with aorta*

• Ischemia to duodenum and proximal jejunum occur

• Pulseless SMA from origin

• Revascularization—treat the orifical disease by

– Stenting

– Bypass

• Simple embolectomy is not enough

Bypass Procedures

• Aortomesenteric bypass

• Iliomesenteric bypass

• Endarterectomy

• *Treatment is similar to CMI*

• Need to consider

– Comorbidities

– Bowel viability

– Inflow sites

Stenting

• Better in sick patients with comorbidities

• Intraoperative retrograde stenting and patch closure of artery

– No need to cross-clamp aorta

• Can be done in gangrene and perforation

• Minimal graft contamination

• Viability checked after procedure

NOMI

• Flow impeded by spasm—no luminal obstruction

• Occur in ICU/critically ill patients

• Due to

– Drugs

– Sympathetic reaction to shock, sepsis

Clinical Features

• Pain insidious and progressive

• Critically ill patients

• Assessment difficult

• Loose bloody stools

• Abdomen soft scaphoid

• Usually thought about other commoner diagnosis

Diagnosis

• Mainly clinical

• ICU patients on alfa agonists/vasopressin/digoxin

• Lab

– Hemoconcentration

– Leucocytosis

– Elevated lactate

• X-ray and CECT—may be normal

• Duplex, grey scale imaging—small artery with resistive flow

• *Arteriography—highest sensitivity*

– Only way to demonstrate small vessel spasm

• Classic features

– Narrowing of multiple SMA branches

– Impaired filling intramural vessels

– 'String of lakes' appearance of run off vessels

– 'Defoliated tree' appearance

• CTA—also useful

Therapy

• Directed at

– Adequately perfusing bowel

– Overcoming spasm

• Direct catheter delivery of papaverine 30–60 mg/hour

• Prostaglandin E1 (Alprostadil) 20 mcg bolus followed by 60–80 mcg/24-hour infusion

• Systemic anticoagulation recommended

• Follow-up angiography in 12–24 hours

• Laparotomy simultaneously—if indicated

• Use pressors with minimal effect on splanchnic circulation like Dopamine, Dobutamine

• Antibiotics can be given

VAMI

• Mesenteric venous thrombosis account for <10% of all AMI

• Most common in SMV

• Different from other causes of AMI

• Seen in 50–60 years of age

• Equal gender distribution

• No cardiac disorders/POVD

• Have procoagulant states

- Mortality less than arterial origin
- MVT—Mesenteric venous HTN—reduction in arterial delivery—edema—ascites
- Stomach, duodenum, colon—less affected due to rich collaterals
- Small bowel most affected—less collaterals

Clinical Features

- Less rapidly progressive—over days
- Vague insidious pain
- Present with many days of pain ,distension and loose stools
- Melena—not common occult blood is seen
- H/o coagulopathy, trauma, pancreatitis, or malignancies
- Abdominal distension
- Periumbilical tenderness
- Ascites
- Peritoneal signs seen in infarction
- Leucocytosis—most common lab abnormality
- Elevated lactate, LDH

Diagnosis

CECT with venous phase is the choice

- Dilated SMV with ring enhancement
- Nonopacifying SMV
  - Specific venous protocols
  - Bowel wall thickness >3 mm
- Ill-defined bowel wall, thick mesentery
- Ascites
- Duplex not useful

Therapy

- Fluid resuscitation
- Anticoagulation—mainstay
  - Heparin/fractionated heparin
  - Warfarin and prolonged anticoagulation
  - Life long anticoagulation in patients with hypercoagulable states
  - In others for 3–6 months
- Laparotomy is decided on clinical and CT evidence
- Removal of gangrenous bowel—may need wider margins of resection
- Routine surgical thrombectomy and lytic therapy—not recommended
- Endovascular treatment—not routine
  - TIPS with mechanical aspiration thrombectomy/lysis
  - Percutaneous transhepatic thrombolysis
  - Indirect thrombolysis via SMA catheter
  - Thrombolysis via catheter in SMV

- Mortality—25–30%
  - In those who require bowel resection—(45–50%)
- Sepsis and multiorgan failure—major cause
- Need 3–6 months of anticoagulation
- For hypercoagulable states—lifelong anticoagulation

AMI: To Consider

- Role of damage control surgery
- Issue of short bowel syndrome
- Time for anastomosis
- Role of planned second look surgery—in case of extensive bowel ischemia, resect only the frankly gangrenous parts and do a second look laparotomy 48–72 hours later

	SMA Thrombosis	SMA Embolus	NOMI	SMVT
Appearance	Pale and contracted bowel		Patchy ischemia	Congested and dilated
Distribution	Small bowel complete	Spares proximal bowel	Patchy throughout	Diffuse or segmental
SMA pulse	Absent proximal pulse	Strong proximal, absent distal	Weak pulse along length	Good pulse

Assessment for Viability
On Table Evaluation of Viability
Clinical

- Color
- Sheen
- Peristalsis
- Mesenteric pulsations
- Bleeding from cut ends
- **Pulse oximetry**
  - Measures O_2 saturation—not blood flow
- **Polarographic measurement of O_2 tension**
  - Measures tissue O_2 tension
  - Using probes
- **Near Infrared and Visible Light Spectrophotometry**
  - Uses principles of light transmission and absorption—measures concentration of Hb O_2 saturation
  - Handheld device
- **Intravital microscopy**
  - Directly visualize and quantify changes at capillary level—using fluorescent labelled plasma of blood cells

- **Doppler USG scan**
- **Hydrogen gas clearance**
- **Radioisotope studies**
  - IV, intra—arterial or submucosal injection—studies blood flow
- **Fluorescence studies**
  - Perfusion fluorometry
  - Sodium fluorescein IV—bowel illuminated with UV light
  - Laser fluorescence angiography LFA
    - *Injection indocyanine green—illumination* by Laser/IR
- **Infrared imaging**
  - Thermal difference studied
- **Laser Doppler Flowmetry (LDF)**
  - Doppler shift
  - Studies the amount of blood cells
- **Bowel wall contractility measurement**
  - Electronic Contractility Meter (ECM)
  - EMG
- **pH measurement**
  - Tonometry
  - Ischemia causes acidosis which can be detected
- **Microdialysis**
  - Microprobes in seromuscular layer
  - Measures lactate/glucose ratio
  - Can assess anastomosis-postop

On Table Evaluation: Most Useful

- Doppler Ultrasound
- Fluorescein and perfusion fluorometer

New Methods
Radiological
- CE—MRA
- 7 Telsa—MRI-noncontrast

Biochemical
- Intestinal Fatty Acid Binding Protein (I-FABP)
- Alfa Glutathione Transferase (GST)
- D-Lactate

Chronic Mesenteric Ischemia (CMI)
- Constant hypoperfusion of small bowel with two or more mesenteric vessels occluded or stenosed

- Severe atherosclerosis of multiple mesenteric arteries
- Rich collaterals make it—uncommon entity
- Most are asymptomatic

Causes
- Osteal atherosclerosis—most common cause
- Fibromuscular disease
- Median arcuate ligament syndrome
- Arteritis

Clinical Features
- Female, 7th decade
- Smoker
- Long standing pain abdomen
- Hypertension, POVD, CAD, DM
- Post prandial pain abdomen—within 30 minutes
- 'Gastric steal' phenomenon—after food intake, due to the extensive collateral supply, blood is diverted from SMA region to CA region into the stomach—aggravating the chronic ischemic SMA supply—patient experiences early pain
- 'Intestinal angina' is like Claudication
- Food fear (sitophobia)
- Weight loss
- No characteristic findings
- Flat, scaphoid abdomen

Triad-pathognomonic: Postprandial Pain, Foodfear, Weight Loss
- Differential diagnosis—cholecystitis, ulcer disease, malignancy

Diagnosis
- Duplex US
  - Due to cachexia, there will be less of abdominal fat. So these patients are ideal candidates
- Oregon/Wisconsin, Dartmouth criteria

Duplex velocity criteria

Oregon/Wisconsin criteria—suggestive of >70% stenosis if the measured

Celiac artery peak systolic velocity >200 cm/s

SMA >275 cm/s

Dartmouth criteria—suggestive of >50% stenosis, if the measured

Celiac artery end diastolic velocity >55 cm/s

SMA >45 cm/s

- **CTA**
  - Modality of choice
- **MRA**—Gadolinium contrast
  - Efficacy similar to CTA
- **Angiography**
  - Invasive
  - Resources necessary
  - More to deliver specific therapy
- Trauma to vessels

Therapy
- Indicated in symptomatic

Goals
- Relieve symptoms
- Restore normal digestion
- Prevent bowel infarction
- Prophylactic intervention—not indicated

Endovascular or Open Method
- Trade off between
  - Invasiveness vs durability
- Depend on patient factors

CMI: Stenting
- Preferred in
  - Debilitated not fit for anesthesia
  - Diagnosis is less clear but extensive mesenteric atherosclerosis exist
- Mostly through femoral approach or left brachial artery
- Primary stenting in
  - Osteal or 'spillover' plaques
  - Heavy calcification
  - Luminal obstruction
- Angioplasty alone in
  - Nonatherosclerotic lesions in mesenteric circulation

CMI: Bypass
Inflow options
- Based on CTA and intraop findings
- Antegrade bypass
  - From supraceliac aorta to SMA
- Retrograde bypass—preferred in emergency
  - From infrarenal aorta or

- Iliac artery—right iliac artery is preferred
- Aortoceliac and aorto SMA bypass
- Saphenous vein is used if single vessel bypass is done
- Prosthetic graft-Dacron, PTFE—if two vessels are bypassed
- Postop Duplex to confirm

Retrograde Bypass
- Advantages
- Clamp placement below renal artery—less stressful
- Exposure more familiar to surgeons

Endarterectomy
- Not a common procedure
- Indications
  - Gross contamination preventing a conduit
  - Exuberant or 'coral reef' type plaque
  - In disease of both supraceliac and infrarenal aorta
- Trap door aortotomy—endarterectomy

Results and follow-up
- Long-term patency better in bypass
- Bypass operative mortality nearly 5%
- Follow-up with duplex, CTA
- Antiplatelet therapy for life
- Cessation of smoking
- Control hypertension
- Statins

Endovascular Therapy
- Primary stenting preferred over angioplasty which causes restenosis—covered stents are used
- Femoral approach or left brachial approach

Less Common causes
Fibromuscular Dysplasia
- Extremely rare cause
- Nonatherosclerotic fibrodysplastic stenosis
- Involve media and intima-fibrosis
- Web-like obstruction
- Renal, carotid and iliac artery involvement—more common
- Can develop CMI
- Treated by angioplasty

Median Arcuate Ligament Syndrome

- Compression of celiac artery by median arcuate ligament
- Can cause CMI
- Due to diaphragmatic movement on celiac artery
- At end of expiration, abdominal contents and vasculature move superiorly causing obstruction
- During inspiration, they move downwards relieving obstruction

Median Arcuate Ligament Syndrome

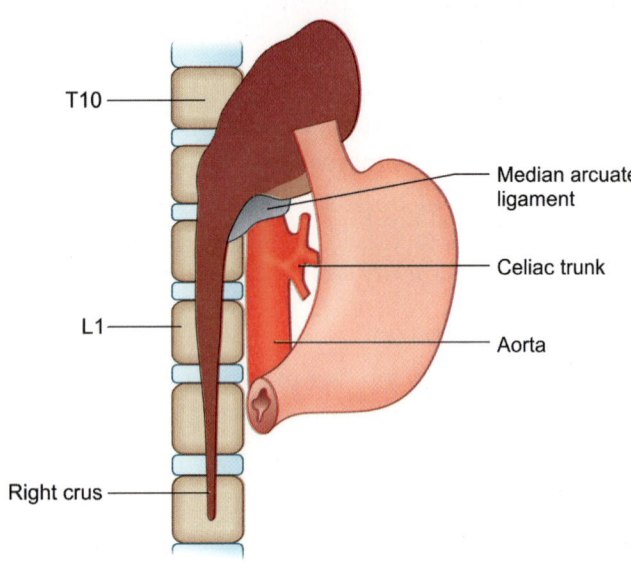

- Can be demonstrated with Doppler
- Crampy pain, nausea, vomiting
- Diagnosis by exclusion
- Patients commonly—psychiatric, substance abuser
- Treatment—surgical decompression
  - Reserved for symptomatic
  - Objective evidence of obstruction should be there on imaging

Takayasu's Arteritis

- Rare cause of CMI
- Women in 40s
- Weight loss, pain, food fear
- Angiography—diagnostic
- SMA and IMA are involved
- Steroids, methotrexate
- Surgical—similar to CMI

14.18 ABDOMINAL TRAUMA
Areas of Abdomen

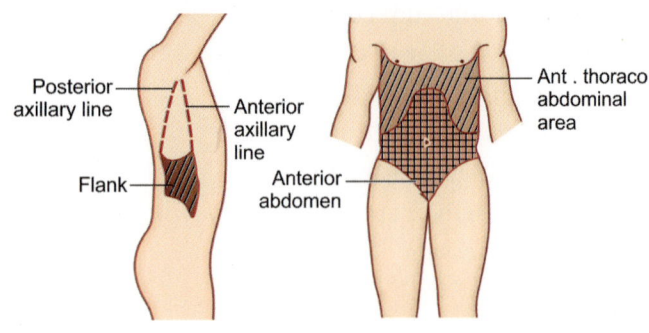

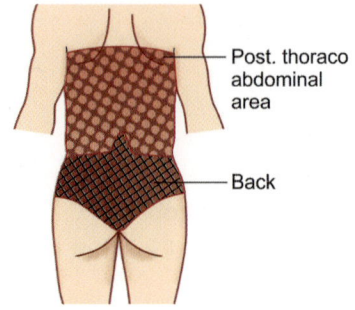

Mechanism of Injury

- Blunt
- Penetrating
- Blast

Blunt Trauma

- Direct blow
  - Steering wheel, handle
  - Cause compression and crushing
- Shearing injuries
  - Inappropriate restraint devices
- Deceleration
  - Differential movement of body parts
  - Spleen, liver injuries
  - Bucket handle injuries of mesentery

Blunt Injury of Organs

- Spleen (nearly 50%)—most common
- Liver (nearly 40%)
- Small bowel (5–10%)
- Retroperitoneum—15%

Penetrating Injury
Stab Injury

- Liver—most common—40%
- Others—small bowel, diaphragm, colon

Gunshot Wounds

- Transfer more kinetic energy
- Trajectory is important and produce cavitation, and bullet fragmentation
- Most common—small bowel 50%

Blast Injuries due to

- Penetrating fragments
- Patient being thrown away
- Combination of blunt and penetrating trauma

A B C D E of Resuscitation

Assessment and Management

- History
- Physical examination
- Investigations

History

Blunt Injury

- Vehicle speed
- Type of collision
- Condition of other passengers
- Height of fall
- History from on lookers
- Penetrating injury
  - Time of injury
  - Type of weapon
  - Distance from assailant
  - Magnitude and location of pain

Physical Examination

- Proper exposure
- Examine lowerchest, abdomen, perineum
- Flanks, scrotum, vagina, rectum, buttocks
- Back is examined by log rolling
- Look for tenderness and guarding
- Bowel sounds
- Assess the pelvis
- Perineal hematoma
- Urethral bleeding
- Pelvic tenderness
- Per rectal examination
- Per vaginal examination
- Gluteal examination

Further Evaluation is Indicated in

- Altered sensorium
- Injuries to ribs, pelvis, spine
- Prior equivocal examination
- Prolonged loss of contact
- Seat belt sign

Gastric Tubes

- Reduce gastric dilatation
- Reduce aspiration
- Before diagnostic peritoneal lavage
- Exclude upper GI injury

Urinary Catheter

- Relieve retention
- Output monitoring
- Detect GU trauma
- Avoid if suspecting urethral trauma

Investigations

- Blood investigations
- Hemogram
- Blood grouping
- Amylase
- RFT

X-rays

- Only in stable patients
- In thoraco-abdominal trauma

FAST

- False negative can occur in
  - Obese
  - Hollow viscus injury
  - Repeat if needed
  - Detects if >100 cc blood

e-FAST

- Evaluation of thorax for hemopneumothorax
- Better than X-ray chest

Paracentesis

- Four quadrant aspiration
- Positive study, if—aspirate blood, bile, fecal matter
- Negative tap—nonspecific
- False negative in 20–30%

DPL

- Subumbilical canula
- Aspirate first
- 1 Liter NS of RL instilled and 20% of the fluid should be aspirated (200 ml)

Positive DPL

- GI contents, bile
- Vegetable fibers
- >10 cc blood in unstable
- >100000 RBC/ml in abdominal trauma and > 10,000/ml in thoracoabdominal stab wounds
- WBC >500/ml
- Amylase >19 IU/L
- Alkaline phosphatase >2 IU/L
- Bilirubin >0.01 mg/dl

DPL done in

- In hemodynamically abnormal
- Blunt or penetration
- Rarely used these days

Relative Contraindications for DPL

- Previous laparotomy
- Obesity
- Advanced cirrhosis
- Coagulopathy

Types

- Open
- Semiopen
- Closed infraumbilical (Seldinger)

CECT

- Not indicated in unstable
- Or if delays the procedures
- Can assess retroperitoneum
- Solid organs
- Bowel injury

Laparoscopy

- Penetrating wounds-to assess peritoneum
- Diaphragmatic injury
- No role in blunt injury with hemoperitoneum

Other Studies

- Urethrography
- Cystography/CT cystography
- IVU
- GI contrast studies

Evaluation of Specific Penetrating Wounds

- History
- Serial physical examination
- FAST
- DPL
- Triple contrast CT

Immediate Management

- Initiation of resuscitation
- Rapid assessment of source of bleeding
- IV Fluids/blood
- Massive Transfusion Protocol = PRBC, Plasma, Platelets in 1:1:1 ratio

Laparotomy in Penetrating Wounds Indications

- Hemodynamic instability
- Gunshot wounds with transperitoneal trajectory
- Signs of peritoneal irritation
- Peritoneal penetration
- Evisceration
- GI/GU bleeding

Nonoperative Management—in

- Hemodynamically stable
- Serial examinations normal
- Serial FAST satisfactory
- Normal DPL
- CT confirmation
- Diagnostic laparoscopy done and found normal

Indications for Laparotomy

Blunt Injury

- Hypotension
- Positive FAST
- Bleeding
- Positive DPL
- CECT evidence

Penetrating Abdominal Trauma Index-PATI

- 14 organs are considered in this assessment, and are allotted risk factor score which varies with different organs
- Duodenum, Pancreas—score is 5
- Liver, colon, major vessels—score is 4
- Spleen, kidney—score is 2
- Biliary, stomach, SI, ureter—score is 2
- Bone, minor vascular, bladder—score is 1
- Each organ is graded 1–5 on injury estimate
- Organ score = Risk factor X injury estimate
- PATI = sum of all organ scores
- Maximum score possible-200
- If > 25 there is chance of complications

Laparotomy General Steps

- Liberal incision
- Blood evacuated
- Falciform ligament divided
- Sponges in four quadrants
- Entire GI tract, lesser sac inspected
- Retroperitoneum, solid organs
- Consider damage control

Damage Control Surgery Considered in

- Difficult hemostasis
- Coagulopathy
- Acidosis
- Hypothermia
- No expertise
- Multiple injuries
- And followed by elective relaparotomy in 24–72 hours

Damage Control Surgery—Stages

1. Patient selection
2. Control of bleeding and contamination

3. ICU management

4. Definitive surgery

5. Abdominal closure

Splenic Injury

- Most common organ injured in blunt trauma
- Mortality 9–10%
- Mechanism
  - Direct compression—parenchymal fracture
  - Deceleration—tear of parenchyma—subcapsular hematoma
- Bleeding may have stopped before operation but there is more chance of rebleeding

Role of Investigations

- If hemodynamically unstable
  - May be FAST or DPL
- No CT if unstable

AAST Splenic Injury Scale

Injury grade	Injury type	Description of injury
I	Hematoma Laceration	Subcapsular, <10 surface area Capsular tear, <1 cm parenchymal depth
II	Hematoma Laceration	Subcapsular, 10% to 50% surface area; Intraparenchymal, <5 cm in diameter Capsular tear, 1 to 3 cm parenchymal depth that does not involve a trabecular vessel
III	Hematoma Laceration	Subcapsular, >50% surface area or expanding; ruptured subcapsular or parenchymal hematoma; intraparenchymal hematoma > =5 cm or expanding >3 cm parenchymal depth or involving trabecular vessels
IV	Laceration	Laceration involving segmental or hilar vessels producing major devascularisation (>25% of spleen)
V	Hematoma Laceration	Completely shattered spleen Hilar vascular injury devascularizes spleen

Non-operative Management

- Grades I, II, III
  - Hemodynamically stable (normal BP, no tachycardia, no shock, no metabolic acidosis)
- Or stabilized after IV fluids

- No ongoing bleeding
- No other indications for laparotomy

Immediate Laparotomy

- Hemodynamic instability
- Ongoing bleeding
- Grade 4 or 5 with hemodynamically instablility. If stable can attempt nonoperative management
- Other injuries
- Bowel injuries
- Most common cause for splenectomy—trauma
- Minimal invasive surgery—contraindicated in major trauma
- Splenectomy is the definitive management
- Splenorrhaphy—by laser, cautery, thrombin gelatin sponges, fibrin glue, absorbable mesh
- Spleen autotransplantation into a pouch made by omentum—in young and with no bowel injury
- Postsplenectomy vaccines for
  - *H. influenzae, spneuminiae, N. menigitidis*

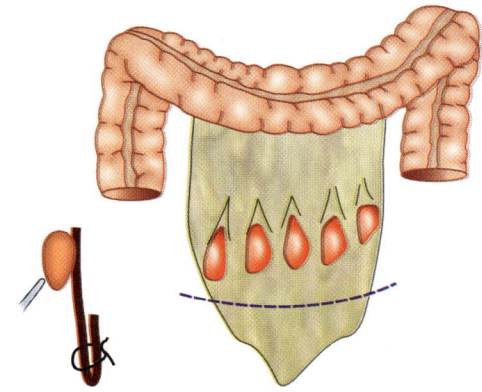

Splenic Injury

Stable Patients

- FAST
- CECT
- Angiography—embolization—only in stable patients
- Continuous monitoring
- Angio embolisation at the main splenic artery just distal to dorsal pancreatic artery is called proximal embolization. This can cause global ischemia-affects immunocompetence
  - Or selectively at the bleeding vessel
- Radiologic feature predictive of future surgery—presence of AV fistula

Liver Trauma

- Most common organ injured in penetrating abdominal injury
- Second most common in blunt injury—after spleen

AAST liver trauma scale

Liver Injury Grade

Grade I	<10% of surface area	<1 cm in depth
Grade II	10–50% of surface area	1–3 cm
Grade III	>50% of surface area or >10 cm in depth	>3 cm
Grade IV	25–75% of a hepatic lobe	
Grade V	>75% of a hepatic lobe	
Grade VI	Hepatic avulsion	

Nonoperative Management

- Lesser grades (I, II, III)
- Stable
- No ongoing bleeding
- Controlled with angioembolisation
- If patient is stable and no bowel injury—standard of care is nonoperative—regardless of the grade or extent of injury
- Success rate is more than 90%

Adjuncts for Nonoperative Management

- Angiography embolization—if a blush seen on contrast
- CT guided percutaneous drainage
- ERCP—in high output bile drainage
- Delayed laparoscopic lavage

Surgery

Operative techniques for control of liver injury

Cautery
Argon beam coagulation
Individual vessel ligation
Parenchymal reapproximation with large mattress sutures
Selective hepatic artery ligation
Resectional debridement
Hepatic lobectomy
Omental packing
Packing and planned reoperation

Surgery

- Liberal laparotomy
- Mobilise liver—triangulars, falciform
- Compress liver
- Debride devitalized parts
- Omentum pack

Pringle Maneuver

- Time kept to minimum
- Inflow occlusion of 15 minutes at a time is advised
- Cumulative 120 minutes is safe
- Rumel tourniquet can be used for Pringle's maneuver

- If Pringle fails to control bleeding—may be from aberrant LHA in the lesser omentum as the source or from HV

If Bleeding is Not Stopped—it Could be Venous Bleeding

- Damage control
- Atriocaval shunt
- Ligation of veins

4 Ps
- Push (bimanual compression)
- Pringle (portal vein/hepatic artery/bile duct)
- Plug (holes due to penetrating injury—silicone tubing, sengstaken Blakemore tube)
- Pack

- In bleeding—angioembolisation can be done
- No need to suture the liver unless we need haemostasis.
- Hepatic artery injury tied; portal vein injury repaired
- Closed suction drain must be left *in situ*
- Liver parenchyma necrosis most common complication of severe liver injury following surgery
- Rebleeding is most common complication of non-operative management

Hepatic Packing: Tenets

- Control arterial bleeding (angiography)
- Ideal for venous bleeding and coagulopathy
- Use before excessive bleeding develops
- Compress in superior to inferior direction
- Use nonadherent material
- Count sponge
- Avoid tension—ACS
- Packs removed—24–72 hours later
- Subcapsular hematoma—not intervened—if no arterial blush
- In hepatic avulsion—veno-venous bypass or liver autotransplantation

Bleeding from HV

- Posterior—inferior traction on falciform ligament—Pringle—packing—if still bleeding—try outflow occlusion
- Outflow occlusion
  - Infra and suprahepatic IVC clamping leads to hypotension
  - Atriocaval shunt (Shrock)—by median sternotomy
  - Complete hepatic vascular isolation and repair

Renal Trauma

- Mostly in blunt trauma
- CECT

- One shot IVU
- USG
- MRI

Renal injury classification	
Grade 1	Contusion or non-expanding subcapsular heamatoma, no laceration
Grade 2	Non-expanding peri-renal haematoma, cortical laceration <1 cm deep without extravasation
Grade 3	Cortical laceration >1 cm without urinary extravasation
Grade 4	Laceration through corticomedullary junction into collecting system or segmental renal artery or vein injury with contained haematoma or partial vessel laceration, or vessel thrombosis
Grade 5	Shattered kidney or renal pedicle or avulsion

- Nonoperative in Grade I, II, III, Stable
- CECT/angiography should be done and angio-embolization
  - Operative management in unstable
- Anterior exploration
- Control of pedicle
- Explore if expanding/pulsatile hematoma
- Renal preservation is the rule

Duodenal Injuries

- Most are due to penetrating injuries—4%
- Blunt—0.1%
- Vague clinical features—due to retroperitoneal nature
- CECT—choice

Duodenum injury scale		
Grade	*Type of injury*	*Description of injury*
I	Hematoma	Involving single portion of duodenum
	Laceration	Partial thickness, no perforation
II	Hematoma	Involving more than one portion
	Laceration	Disruption of <50% of circumference
III	Laceration	Disruption of 50–75% of circumference of D2
		Disruption of 50–100% of circumference of D1, D3, D4
IV	Laceration	Disruption of 75% of circumference of D2
		Involving ampulla or distal common bile duct
V	Laceration	Massive disruption of duodenopancreatic complex
	Vascular	Devascularization of duodenum

Treatment

- Obstructing hematomas
  - Gastric decompression, TPN—contrast study after 5–7 days—if obstruction persists after 2 weeks—surgery
- Hematomas found incidentally—not explored—unless concern for full thickness injury
- Perforation:
  - Simple closure
  - D1—extensive—debridement and EEA as it has good blood supply and mobility
  - D2 is more tethered and repair results in lumen narrowing, so patched with Roux-Y-DJ
  - Injury distal to papilla and proximal to SMV/SMA with tissue loss treated with Roux-Y-DJ with distal duodenum oversewn
  - Injury to D3, D4—resected and DJ

Pancreatic Trauma

- Penetrating injury—more common-accounts for 70%
- Delayed diagnosis—more complications
- Common in crush injury—steering wheel/seat belt
- Need high index of suspicion
- Mortality—10–25%
- Early mortality due to bleeding, late mortality is due to SIRS, MODS
- In blunt injury—neck in the prevertebral segment—most common site
- Seatbelt sign will be positive

American Association for the Surgery of Trauma Organ Injury Scaling: Pancreas	
Types of injury	
Grade I	
Hematoma	Minor contusion without duct injury
Laceration	Superficial laceration without duct injury
Grade II	
Hematoma	Major contusion without duct injury or tissue loss
Laceration	Major laceration without duct injury or tissue loss
Grade III	
Hematoma	Distal transection or parenchymal injury with duct injury
Grade IV	
Laceration	Proximal transection or parenchymal involcing ampulla
Grade V	
Laceration	Massive disruption of pancreatic head

Vascular Structures Around Pancreatico Duodenal Complex, Arranged in 3 Layers

- Deepest—IVC and right renal pedicle
- Middle PV, SMA/V

- Uppermost—GDA and pancreatic duodenal arcades
- Penetrating injuries can be formidable in this location

CECT—if needed may be repeated—in 8–12 hours edema sets in due to pancreatic juice leakage—makes it more evident

- Amylase—elevated in 80% with blunt injury to pancreas—more sensitive if done 3–6 hours after injury than immediately
- MRI/ERCP
- **'Hard signs' on CT of pancreatic injury**
  - Active bleeding
  - Hematoma/laceration
  - Diffuse enlargement/edema
  - Low pancreatic attenuation
- If CT equivocal—ERCP/MRCP may be done

Nonoperative management
- In stable
- Grade I and II

Surgery

- Kocherisation

Aird's maneuver—after dividing splenorenal, splenocolic and splenophrenic ligaments, spleen and tail of pancreas are lifted

Cattel-Braasch Maneuver

To expose D3 and D4
- Carrying the peritoneal incision around cecum and along the line of fusion of small bowel mesentery to the posterior peritoneum—up to ligament of Treitz
- Complete reflection of midgut on to chest wall
- Entire midgut remains suspended by SM pedicle
- Hematomas on pancreas unroofed—to see duct disruption

Mattox Maneuver

- Left-sided medial visceral rotation
  - Spleen, pancreas and left colon are reflected anteriorly towards midline, exposing aorta and origins of left renal artery, SMA and celiac artery.
- Helpful in zone 1 and 2 abdominal injury

Treatment

- Conservative-in minor contusions
- Simple drainage, when limited tissue destruction in the head—with ERCP stenting
- Debridement
- Distal pancreatectomy

- Whipple (trauma Whipple)—when massive destruction of head
- Pyloric exclusion
- Intra-operative pancreatogram may help to see duct injury—by direct canulation of papilla, if duodenum is open or via cystic duct
- Grade II injury distally to left of SMV—distal pancreatectomy—splenectomy if bleeding and in unstable

Major Injury to Right of SMV

- Extended distal pancreatectomy
- Central pancreatectomy
- If unstable—simple drainage only—damage control—ERCP stenting is done
- **Pyloric exclusion**—gastrotomy—pylorus sutured using prolene/staplers—GJ done—GD continuity is established in 4–6 weeks time
  - This is to divert gastric content—to prevent stimulation of pancreas in high grade pancreatic duodenal injuries

In Very Severe—Whipple—Trauma Whipple

- Staged Whipple—resection is done in first stage and anastomosis in second stage 24–48 hours later
- Gall bladder is preserved and CCJ is done instead of HJ—after excluding low entry of CD and making sure that it is not transected
- Minor laceration not involving pd—managed with external drainage
- In unstable patient—as damage control—SMV and PV may be ligated

Retroperitoneal Zones

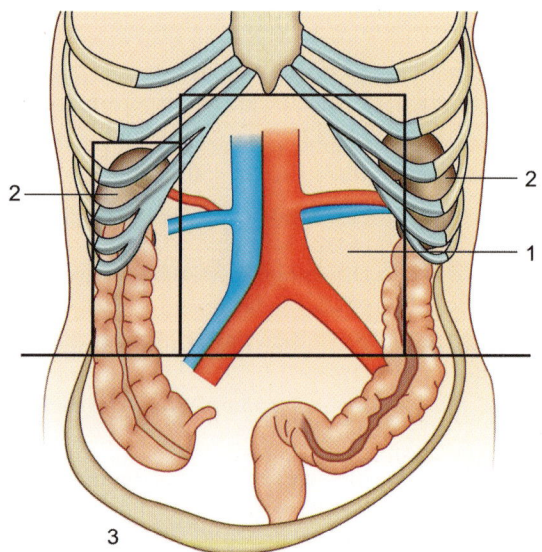

- **Zone 1 hematoma**—requires exploration as they usually involve aorta, IVC, visceral vessels except in dark hematoma behind liver, suggestive of vena cava injury which is managed by gentle packing.
- **Zone 2 hematoma**—usually renal injury, explore only if hematoma is expanding and in continuous bleeding.
- **Zone 3 hematoma**—hematoma from pelvic fracture, should not be explored unless in severe bleeding.

14.19 SMALL BOWEL TRANSPLANT (SBTX)

Significance
- Final curative option in patients with intestinal failure
- After futile medical and surgical attempts
- Offers relief from complications associated with TPN
- Better quality of life

Statistics
- Survival rates greater for isolated small bowel transplant than multivisceral transplant

Indications
Short Bowel Syndrome (SBS) Patients with
- IFALD—intestinal failure associated liver disease
- Parenteral nutrition failure
- Recurrent catheter related infections (CRIs) > 2/year
- Thrombosis of 2 of the six major central access veins
- Severe dehydration and electrolyte imbalance
- Established liver disease or impending liver failure.

Donor Evaluation
- Hemodynamically stable
- Geographically close
- Blood type
- Cold ischaemia time—must not be prolonged
- Child recipient—EBV/CMV screening of cadaveric donor

Diagnostic Evaluation of Intestinal Transplant Candidate
- Biochemistry—LFT, platelet count
- Serology—CMV, EBV, Hepatitis
- Endoscopy—upper and lower GI
- Pathology—liver biopsy

- Radiology—barium follow through and enema, CT abdomen and pelvis, Doppler study of jugular and subclavian veins.
- Cardiac evaluation

Procedure
- Entire jejunum and ileum ± colon and associated vasculature, effort to maintain as much functional bowel as possible
- Vascular anastomosis as applicable—usually SMA and SMV
- **8–10 cm distal to ligament of Treitz:** Side-to-side graft to native jejunojejunal anastomosis
- End allograft ileostomy—for graft surveillance for rejection (repeated biopsies)
- Later, side-to-side graft ileum to native colon anastomosis, approximately 15 cm from the ileostomy

Variations
- Isolated small bowel transplant (SBTx)—irreversible intestinal failure in absence of concomitant liver failure
- Combined liver—intestinal transplant (SB-LTx)—when patients with liver failure have a coexisting irreversible intestinal disease
- MVTx (multivisceral transplant)—for abdominal catastrophise like extensive intestinal resection, severe trauma, multiple enterocutaneous fistulas, chronic diffuse mesenteric arterial thrombosis—foregut and midgut transplantation ± liver, kidneys, and large intestine
- Multivisceral allograft—donor stomach present
- Modified multivisceral allograft—donor liver excluded, donor stomach present
- Cluster allograft—emphasizes anatomic structure of various organs with vascular supply from a common pedicle (donor aorta)
- SI being more immunogenic, need more potent immunosuppression
- Induction is with monoclonal antibodies (alemtuzumab, or basilixizumab)

Complications
- Postop haemorrhage
- Biliary leak—in SB-LTx, choledochojejunostomy may be considered in early postop period
- Arterial thrombosis—results in necrosis
- Venous thrombosis—causes outflow obstruction
- GI leaks usually occur in 1st postop week
- GI bleeding may occur which may be due to rejection or infection, can be diagnosed by end ileostomy scopy

Infection

- EBV/CMV infection—bleeding ulcers visualised via endoscopy
- EBV associated post-transplant lymphoproliferative disorder (PTLD)
- PTLD—ranges from self-limiting mononucleosis to lymphoma
- CMV—most common viral infection post-transplant- 34% incidence

Rejection

- Acute cellular rejection (ACR) rates—SBTx—nearly 80%, SB-LTx—nearly 70%, MVTx—nearly 60%
- High rejection rate is due to highly immunogenic small bowel allograft with lymphoid tissue and dendritic cells
- In MVTx and SB-LTx the protective effects are from the liver tissue
- Surveillance endoscopy—twice weekly—1st 6 weeks, decreasing frequency thereafter
- Presents with diarrhoea—damage to gut mucosal barrier—bacterial sepsis, fever
- Rejection is confirmed by endoscopy and biopsy, treated with steroids and refractory cases treated with antilymphocyte antibody, anti-CD 3 antibody

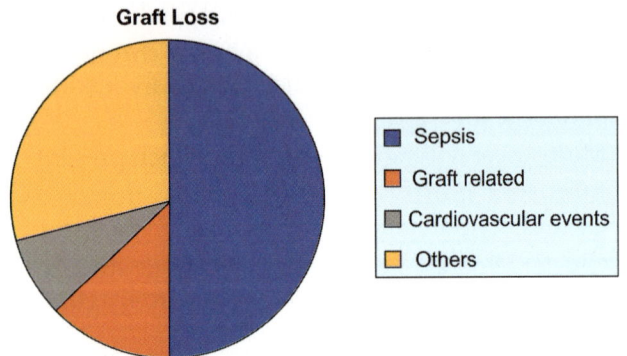

Graft Loss

- Sepsis
- Graft related
- Cardiovascular events
- Others

14.20 LIVER TRANSPLANTATION

- First liver transplantation: Thomas Starzl

Indications of Liver Transplantation

Cirrhosis (most common)

- Alcoholic
- Hepatitis (hep B and C)
- Primary biliary cirrhosis
- Sclerosing cholangitis
- Biliary atresia
  - Acute fulminant liver failure
- Fulminant hepatic failure

- Drug induced
  - Metabolic liver diseases
  - Wilson
  - Alpha 1 antitrypsin deficiency
  - Primary hepatic malignancy

Most Common Indication in Children—Biliary Atresia

> **King's College criteria is used for orthotopic liver transplantation in acute liver failure**

- **Types of liver transplantation**
  - Heterotopic—donor liver implanted in alternative site rather than normal anatomic site
  - Auxiliary—native liver remains *in situ* and whole or partial liver transplant added
  - Orthotopic—donor liver implanted in normal anatomic position after recipient hepatectomy
  - Piggyback—orthotopic liver transplant that preserves recipient IVC
  - Split—cadaveric donor liver divided with portion transplanted to each of two recipients
  - Reduced size LT—liver can be reduced to functional units of appropriate size for the recipient
  - Auxiliary partial orthotopic (APOLT)—left lobe of recipient liver excised and donor liver occupies vacated space.
  - Auxillary heterotopic—whole liver or lobe placed in subhepatic space

Living donor transplants—donation by an adult to another adult can be right lobe or left lobe. Adult to a child donation is usually the left lateral lobe (segments 2 and 3). T tube or stent is used in biliary anastomosis. Mortality in donor is 0.4%

Contraindications to Liver Transplantation

Absolute

- Active, untreated sepsis
- Uncorrectable, life-limiting congenital anomalies
- Active substance or alcohol abuse
- Advanced cardiopulmonary disease
- Extrahepatobiliary malignancy
- Metastatic liver secondaries
- Cholangiocarcinoma
- AIDS
- Life-threatening systemic diseases

Relative

- Age >65
- Prior extensive hepatobiliary surgery
- Portal vein thrombosis
- Renal failure not attributed to liver disease
- Previous extrahepatic malignancy
- Severe obesity
- Severe malnutrition/wasting
- Intrahepatic sepsis
- Uncontrolled psychiatric disorder
- Severe hypoxemia secondary to right to left intrapulmonary shunt
- Severe pulmonary hypertension
- Preoperative assessment of transplant candidates
- Child-Pugh-Turcote system
- MELD score—minimum score for transplant is 15

Bile Duct Anastomosis in Orthotropic Liver Transplantation

Choledochocholedochostomy

- This is end to end anastomosis between donor common bile duct and recipient common bile duct
- This is the preferred bile duct anastomosis, used when the recipient bile duct not diseased
- **Choledochojejunostomy**
  - Roux-en-Y configuration anastomosis between the end of the common bile duct and the side of a loop of jejunum
  - This is an alternative bile duct anastomosis and is performed when CBD-CBD anastomosis is not possible

The Technique

- Removal of recipient liver-mobilise liver, bile duct is divided. Vascular clamps placed in suprahepatic IVC, infrahepatic IVC, PV and HA and divided

- Transplantation-suprahepatic IVC, infrahepatic IVC, PV, HA—in that order
- Finally bile duct is anastomosed
- Piggyback technique—leaves host IVC intact and anastomosis is done between donor suprahepatic IVC to the confluence of hepatic veins, the donor infrahepatic IVC is ligated

Complication of Liver Transplantation

- Early—primary nonfunction, acute rejection, ischemic reperfusion injury
- Late—chronic rejection, disease recurrence
- Bile leak, anastomotic stricture, ascending cholangitis—the Achilles heel
- Vascular complications—HA thrombosis—may present as raising levels of transaminases, fever and bile leak. May require urgent retransplantation
- PV thrombosis—present with features of portal hypertension
- HV occlusion—present with ascites
- Stenosis
- Infection
- Most common disease which recurs after transplant is HCV infection
- Recurrence of malignancy—high in cancers of breast, bladder, sarcomas
- Low recurrence in uterine, testicular, papillary carcinoma thyroid
- Increase in cancers seen in post-transplant—most common skin cancers

Immunosuppression in Liver Transplantation

- Corticosteroids—primary immunosuppressant (PI)—used for 6 months
- Cyclosporine and tacrolimus also PI used life long
- OKT3 and IL-2 receptor antibodies are used in induction used for 5 days and 2 weeks respectively
- Mycophenolate, an adjunct primary agent, is used when necessary.

Tables

Carcinoma Esophagus

Tx	Primary tumor cannot be assessed
To	No evidence of primary tumor
Tis	High grade dysplasia, defined as malignant cells confined to epithelium by basement membrane
T1	Tumor invades lamina propria or muscularis mucosae or submucosa
T1a	Tumor invades lamina propria or muscularis mucosa
T1b	Tumor invades submucosa
T2	Tumor invades muscularis propria
T3	Tumor invades adventitia
T4	Tumor invades the adjacent structure
T4a	Resectable tumor invading pleura, pericardium, azygos vein, peritoneum or diaphragm
T4b	Unresectable tumor invading other adjacent structures, such as aorta, vertebral body, or airway

NX	Regional nodal status cannot be assessed
N0	No regional lymph node involvement
N1	Regional lymph node metastases involving 1 or 2 nodes
N2	Regional lymph node metastases involving 3 to 6 nodes
N3	Regional lymph node metastases involving 7 or more nodes

*Regional nodes include periesophageal nodes from cervical to celiac axis.

M0	No distant metastasis
M1	Distant metastases

Stage (SCC)	T	N	M
0	Tis	N0	M0
I	T1	N0-1	M0
II	T2	N0-1	M0
	T3	N0	M0
III	T3	N1	M0
	T1-3	N2	M0
IVA	T4	N0-2	M0
	Any T	N3	M0
IVB	Any T	Any N	M1

Stage (adenocarcinoma)	T	N	M
0	Tis	N0	M0
I	T1	N0	M0
IIA	T1	N1	M0
IIB	T2	N0	M0
III	T2	N1	M0
	T3-4a	N0-1	M0
IVA	T1-4a	N2	M0
	T4b	N0-2	M0
	Any T	N3	M0
IVB	Any T	Any N	M1

Carcinoma Stomach

Tx	Primary tumor cannot be assessed
To	No evidence of primary tumour
Tis	Carcinoma *in situ*: Intraepithelial tumour without invasion of the lamina propria, High grade dysplasia
T1	Tumor invades lamina propria or muscularis mucosae or submucosa
T1a	Tumor invades lamina propria or muscular mucosae
T1b	Tumor invades submucosa
T2	Tumor invades muscularis propria
T3	Tumor penetrates the subserosal connective tissue without invasion of the visceral peritoneum or adjacent structures
T4	Tumor invades the serosa (visceral peritoneum) or adjacent structures
T4a	Invades serosa
T4b	Invading other adjacent structures/organs

A tumour may penetrate muscularis propria with extension into the gastrocolic or gastrohepatic ligaments or into greater or lesser omentum without perforation of visceral peritoneum classified as T3. If there is perforation of the visceral peritoneum covering the gastric ligaments or the omentum, should be classified as T4

NX	Regional lymph node(s) cannot be assessed
N0	No regional lymph node metastasis
N1	Metastasis in one or two regional lymph nodes
N2	Metastasis in three to six regional lymph nodes
N3	Metastasis in seven or more regional lymph nodes
N3a	Metastasis in seven to 15 regional lymph nodes
N3b	Metastasis in 16 or more regional lymph nodes

M0	No distant metastasis
M1	Distant metastases

Stage	T	N	M
0	Tis	N0	M0
I	T1	N0	M0
	T2	N0	M0
IIA	T1	N1-3	M0
	T2	N1-3	M0
IIB	T3	N0	M0
	T4a	N0	M0
III	T3	N1-3	M0
	T4a	N1-3	M0
IVA	T4b	Any N	M0
IVB	Any T	Any N	M1

Carcinoma Pancreas

T Category	T Criteria
T0	No evidence of primary tumor
Tis	Carcinoma *in situ*
TX	Tumor cannot be assessed
T1	Tumor limited to the pancreas, size <2 cm
T1a	< = 0.5 cm in greatest dimension
T1b	>0.5 cm but <1 cm in greatest dimension
T1c	1–2 cm in greatest dimension
T2	Tumor limited to the pancreas, size >2 cm and < = 4 cm in greatest dimension
T3	Tumor limited to the pancreas, size >4 cm in greatest dimension
T4	Tumor invading celiac axis, the superior mesenteric artery, and or common hepatic artery regardless of size

NX	Regional lymph nodes cannot be assessed
N0	No regional lymph node involvement
N1	One to three regional lymph node involvement
N2	Four or more regional lymph nodes

M0—no metastasis, M1—metastasis

Stage	T	N	M
Stage 0	Tis	N0	M0
1A	T1	N0	M0
IB	T2	N0	M0
IIA	T3	N0	M0
IIB	T1-3	N1	M0
III	T1-3	N2	M0
	T4	Any N	M0
IV	Any T	Any N	M1

Carcinoma Gall Bladder

TX	Primary tumor cannot be assessed
T0	No evidence of primary tumor
Tis	Carcinoma *in situ*
T1	Tumor invades the lamina propria or muscular layer
T1a	Tumor invades the lamina propria
T1b	Tumor invades the muscular layer
T2	Tumor invades the perimuscular connective tissue on the peritoneal side, without involvement of the serosa (visceral peritoneum) Or tumor invades the perimuscular connective tissue on the hepatic side, with no extension into the liver
T2a	Tumor invades the perimuscular connective tissue on the peritoneal side, without involvement of the serosa (visceral peritoneum)
T2b	Tumor invades the perimuscular connective tissue on the hepatic side, with no extension into the liver
T3	Tumor perforates the serosa (visceral peritoneum) and/or directly invades the liver and/or one other adjacent organ or structure, such as the stomach, duodenum, colon, pancreas, omentum, or extrahepatic bile ducts
T4	Tumor invades the main portal vein or hepatic artery or invades two or more extrahepatic organs or structures

Nx	Regional lymph nodes cannot be assessed
N0	No regional lymph node metastasis
N1	Metastases to one to three regional lymph nodes
N2	Metastases to four or more regional lymph nodes

M0	No distant metastasis
M1	Distant metastasis

0	Tis	N0	M0
I	T1	N0	M0
IIA	T2a	N0	M0
IIB	T2b	N0	M0
IIIA	T3	N0	M0
IIIB	T1-3	N1	M0
IVA	T4	N0-1	M0
IVB	Any T	N2	M0
IVB	Any T	Any N	M1

Hepatocellular Carcinoma

TX	Primary tumour cannot be assessed
T0	No evidence of primary tumor
T1	Solitary tumor $< = 2$ cm, or >2 cm without vascular invasion
T1a	Solitary tumor $< = 2$ cm
T1b	Solitary tumor >2 cm without vascular invasion
T2	Solitary tumor >2 cm with vascular invasion, or multiple tumors, none >5 cm
T3	Multiple tumors, at least one of which is >5 cm
T4	Single tumor or multiple tumors of any size involving a major branch of portal vein or hepatic vein, or tumors with direct invasion of adjacent organs other than the gallbladder or with perforation of visceral peritoneum

NX	Regional lymph nodes cannot be assessed
N0	No regional lymph node metastasis
N1	Regional lymph node metastasis

M0	No distant metastasis
M1	Distant metastasis

T	N	M	STAGE
T1a	N0	M0	IA
T1b	N0	M0	IB
T2	N0	M0	II
T3	N0	M0	IIIA
T4	N0	M0	IIIB
Any T	N1	M0	IVA
Any T	Any N	M1	IVB

Carcinoma of Distal Bile Duct

Tx	Primary tumor cannot be assessed
Tis	Carcinoma *in situ*/high-grade dysplasia
T1	Tumor invades the bile duct wall with a depth less than 5 mm
T2	Tumor invades the bile duct wall with a depth of 5–12 mm
T3	Tumor invades the bile duct wall with a depth greater than 12 mm
T4	Tumor involves the celiac axis, superior mesenteric artery, and/or common hepatic artery

Nx	Regional lymph nodes cannot be assessed
N0	No regional lymph node metastasis
N1	Metastasis in one to three regional lymph nodes
N2	Metastasis in four or more regional lymph nodes
M0	No distant metastasis
M1	Distant metastasis

Stage	T	N	M
0	Tis	N0	M0
I	T1	N0	M0
IIA	T1	N1	M0
	T2	N0	M0
IIB	T2	N1	M0
	T3	N0-1	M0
IIIA	T1-3	N2	M0
IIIB	T4	N0-2	M0
IV	Any T	Any N	M1

Carcinoma of Intrahepatic Bile Duct

Tx	Primary tumor cannot be assessed
T0	No evidence of primary tumor
Tis	Carcinoma *in situ* (intraductal tumor)
T1	Solitary tumor without vascular invasion, ≤5 cm or >5 cm
T1a	Solitary tumor ≤5 cm without vascular invasion
T1b	Solitary tumor >5 cm without vascular invasion
T2	Solitary tumor with intrahepatic vascular invasion or multiple tumors, with or without vascular invasion
T3	Tumor perforating the visceral peritoneum
T4	Tumor involving local extrahepatic structures by direct invasion

Nx	Regional lymph nodes cannot be assessed
N0	No regional lymph node metastasis
N1	Regional lymph node metastasis present

M0	No distant metastasis
M1	Distant metastasis

Stage	T	N	M
0	Tis	N0	M0
IA	T1a	N0	M0
IB	T1b	N0	M0
II	T2	N0	M0
IIIA	T3	N0	M0
IIIB	T4	N0	M0
	Any T	N1	M0
IV	Any T	Any N	M1

Colorectal Carcinoma

TX	Primary tumor cannot be assessed
T0	No evidence of primary tumor
Tis	Carcinoma *in situ*
T1	Invades submucosa
T2	Invades muscularis propria
T3	Invades through muscularis propria into pericolorectal tissues
T4	Invades visceral peritoneum or invades/adheres to adjacent organs or structures
T4a	Invades through visceral peritoneum
T4b	Directly invades or adheres to adjacent organs/structures

NX	RLNs (regional lymph nodes) cannot be assessed
N0	No RLN metastasis
N1	1–3 RLNs are positive or any number of tumor deposits are present and all identifiable LNs are negative
N1a	1 RLN + (positive)
N1b	2 or 3 RLNs +
N1c	No RLN +, but there are tumor deposits in • Subserosa • Mesentery • Non-peritonealised pericolic, or perirectal/mesorectal tissues
N2	4 or more RLN +
N2a	4–6 RLN +
N2b	7 or more RLN +

M0	No distant metastasis by imaging or clinically
M1	Metastasis to one or more distant sites or organs or peritoneal metastasis
M1a	One site or organ without peritoneal metastasis
M1b	2 or more sites or organs without peritoneal metastasis
M1c	Metastasis to the peritoneal surface with or without other organ metastasis.

Appendicular Neuroendocrine Tumor

TX	Primary tumour cannot be assessed
T0	No evidence of primary tumor

T1	Tumor 2 cm or less in greatest dimension
T2	Tumor more than 2 cm but less than or equal to 4 cm
T3	Tumor more than 4 cm or with subserosal invasion or involvement of mesoappendix
T4	Tumor perforates the peritoneum or directly invades other adjacent organs or structure (excluding direct mural extension to adjacent subserosa of adjacent bowel)
Nx	Regional lymph nodes cannot be assessed
N0	No regional lymph node metastasis
N1	Regional lymph node metastasis present

M0	No distant metastasis
M1	Distant metastasis
M1a	Confined to liver
M1b	Metastasis in atleast one extrahepatic site
M1c	Both hepatic and extrahepatic metastasis

Stage	T	N	M
0	Tis	N0	M0
I	T1-2	N0	M0
IIA	T3	N0	M0
IIB	T4a	N0	M0

IIC	T4b	N0	M0
IIIA	T1-T2	N1/N1c	M0
	T1	N2a	M0
IIIB	T3-T4a	N1/N1c	M0
	T2-T3	N2a	M0
	T1-T2	N2b	M0
IIIC	T4a	N2a	M0
	T3-T4a	N2b	M0
	T4b	N1-N2	M0
IVA	Any T	Any N	M1a
IVB	Any T	Any N	M1b
IVC	Any T	Any N	M1c

Adenocarcinoma Small Bowel

T0	No evidence of primary tumor
TX	Primary tumor cannot be assessed
Tis	High grade dysplasia/carcinoma *in-situ*
T1	Invades lamina propria or submucosa
T1a	Invades lamina propria
T1b	Invades submucosa
T2	Invades muscularis propria
T3	Invades through muscularis propria into the subserosa, or extends into nonperitonealised perimuscular tissue without serosal penetration
T4	Perforates the visceral peritoneum or directly invades other organs or structures

NX	Cannot be assessed
N0	No regional lymph nodes metastasis
N1	Metastasis in one or two regional lymph nodes
N2	Metastasis in 3 or more regional lymph nodes

M0	No distant metastasis
M1	Distant metastasis present

Stage	T	N	M
0	Tis	N0	M0
I	T1-2	N0	M0
IIA	T3	N0	M0
IIB	T4	N0	M0
IIIA	Any T	N1	M0
IIIB	Any T	N2	M0
IV	Any T	Any N	M1

Bibliography

1. *Shackelford's Surgery of the Alimentary Tract*, 8th edition.

2. *Blumgart's Surgery of the Liver, Biliary Tract and Pancreas*, 6th edition.

3. *Schwartz's Principles of Surgery*, 11th edition.

4. *Bailey and Love's Short Practice of Surgery*, 27th edition.

5. *Sabiston Textbook of Surgery*.

6. *AJCC Cancer Staging Manual*, 8th edition.

7. *DeVita, Hellman, and Rosenberg's Cancer: Principles and Practice of Oncology*, 11th edition.

8. *Maingot's Abdominal Operations*, 13th edition.

9. *Greenfield's Surgery: Scientific Principles and Practice*, 6th edition.

Index